AROMATHERAPY
FOR VIBRANT HEALTH & BEAUTY

ROBERTA WILSON

Avery Publishing Group
Garden City Park, New York

The information and procedures contained in this book are based upon the research and the personal and professional experiences of the author. They are not intended as a substitute for consulting with your physician or other health care provider. The publisher and author are not responsible for any adverse effects or consequences resulting from the use of any of the suggestions, preparations, or procedures discussed in this book. All matters regarding your physical health should be supervised by a health care professional.

Cover designer: William Gonzalez and Rudy Shur
In-house editor: Amy C. Tecklenburg
Typesetter: Bonnie Freid
Printer: Paragon Press, Honesdale, PA

Cover photograph by Roberta Wilson. The photograph includes the following fresh or dried botanicals: lavender flowers, chamomile flowers, pine needles, cedar leaf, juniper berries, cypress needles, rose petals, eucalyptus leaves, helichrysum flowers, jasmine flowers, geranium leaves, coriander seeds, orange peel, rosemary leaves, sage leaves, frankincense tears, and myrrh tears.

Library of Congress Cataloging-in-Publication Data

Wilson, Roberta, 1951–
    Aromatherapy for vibrant health and beauty : a practical A-to-Z
  reference to aromatherapy treatments for health, skin, and hair
  problems / Roberta Wilson
     p. cm.
  Includes bibliographical references and index.
  ISBN 0-89529-627-6
  1. Aromatherapy.   I. Title
RM666.A68W57   1994
615'.321—dc20   94-5343
                                    CIP

10 9 8 7 6 5 4 3

Contents

Part Four   Ways of Using Aromatherapy

Appendix

Acknowledgments

While I was researching this book, almost everyone associated with aromatherapy graciously gave me information and help whenever I asked for it. I wish to thank all of you for your kindness and cooperation.

I am especially grateful to several people without whom my job would have been much more difficult, if not impossible. My special thanks to Marcel Lavabre at Aroma Vera, Michael Scholes of Aromatherapy Seminars, and Kurt Schnaubelt at Pacific Institute of Aromatherapy for sharing their immense knowledge in their certification courses and for patiently answering my endless lists of questions; to Christine Malcolm of Santa Fe Fragrance for supporting me during my research, for willingly sharing her knowledge, for reading and critiquing my manuscript, and for helping me to verify information about essential oils; to Rob McCaleb at the Herb Research Foundation, for his valued opinion on my manuscript and for checking the accuracy of the botanical information; and to Annette Davis, Eric Davis, and Annemarie Buhler of Time Labs for their generosity and their willingness to share valuable information.

I wish to thank Jan Kuśmirek of The Kuśmirek Group in Somerset, England, for drawing upon his vast knowledge of aromatherapy, botanicals, and essential oils, and graciously giving me easy-to-understand answers to all my many questions. I am grateful also to Francis Alliot, M.D. of Paris, France, for his explanations of how he uses essential oils in his medical practice and for answering all my questions; to Jean-Claude LaPraz, M.D., also of Paris, for sharing his vast knowledge and for helping me gain a greater understanding of medical aromatherapy; to Corey Resnick, N.D., Prevail Corporation, Gresham, Oregon, for his thorough explanations of various bodily functions; to Bruce A. Mann, M.D., of Albuquerque, New Mexico, for checking the accuracy of my medical information; to Patty Ross, Lori Malone, and Susan Dvorsky at Aroma Vera, who promptly supplied me with information whenever I needed it; to Marianne Griffeth of Prima Fleur Botanicals, for supplying me with books, information, and feedback; to Frank Wilson, Helen Browning, and Susan Weeks, for editing my manuscript and giving valuable support

v

and feedback; and to all the suppliers who provided me with essential oils and raw materials for experimenting with the blends contained in this book. I extend my appreciation to my publisher, Rudy Shur, for his patience and persistence in convincing me that his suggestions could make my book so much better; and to Amy Tecklenburg, my editor at Avery Publishing, for enhancing the quality of this book with her input, helping me to clarify my ideas, and making the whole publishing process a fun experience. My thanks also to Catherine Hannigan for graciously assisting me with the styling of the botanicals for the cover photograph, and to Gloria Giannini for providing many of the beautiful flowers and herbs pictured. And most of all, I thank my skin care clients, students, friends, and members of my family, who showed such excitement about and interest in aromatherapy, and who, by asking me to make them aromatherapy blends, convinced me that there was a need for this book.

Foreword

I first met Roberta Wilson in 1988, when I gave a lecture in Los Angeles on essential oils. She asked to interview me for an article on skin care. Little did I suspect that this would be the beginning of a friendship based on our shared passion for aromatics. It therefore gives me great pleasure to see *Aromatherapy for Vibrant Health & Beauty,* the fruit of Roberta's intensive research and the expression of her deep faith in the virtues of aromatherapy.

As a professional perfumer committed to the use of natural aromatics, I am impressed with the clarity and breadth of this book. As I read through the formulas, I could smell each one, tempting and enticing me to read further—and to try them all myself.

Roberta offers valuable insights into the underlying connections between a healthy mind, a healthy body, and a healthy planet. Achieving mind-body-planet harmony depends upon the conscious, considerate, and sustainable use of renewable resources. The benefits of using essential oils in our daily lives go far beyond the pleasures of scent; essential oils bring us possibilities for alleviating ailments of both physical and psychical origin. While all fragrances, both natural and synthetic, can alter *moods,* only natural essences support our overall well-being, as well as that of the earth.

Personal perfumes, baths, compresses, environmental scents, skin care products, inhalations, and more—you will find all aspects of how to benefit from aromatherapy covered in this book. It provides an up-to-date, accurate, and remarkably complete resource guide that will make it easy for you to experience for yourself the wonderful formulas Roberta has developed.

Before 1940, perfumes were derived almost entirely from botanicals and were regarded as precious commodities. Each perfume creation was a treasury of aromatics gathered from all over the globe. From the 1940s on, however, inexpensive synthetic aromatics, which are primarily coal- and petroleum-based, replaced the more costly botanicals. Today, environmental awareness, especially among those who make social responsibility and ecological consciousness a priority, is finally swinging the pendulum of fashion back in favor of natural essences.

At the same time, the discovery and distillation of new natural aromatics are opening up exciting horizons, adding interesting nuances to existing types of fragrances and expanding the potential for aromatherapy applications. In my travels around the world, I have met with scientists and other researchers involved in different aspects of the cultivation of aromatic and medicinal plants, and have seen many exciting developments. There are researchers in Australia, France, and Tasmania who are working to discover potential aromatics for flavor and fragrance applications. They are researching some plants that have not been used in the last century and others that have never before been considered. There are preservation foundations that provide funding to South American tribal peoples in order to prevent further cutting and clearing of rainforests, so that scientists may learn about long-term therapeutic properties of the plants that grow there. There are scientists and research institutes that specialize in medicinal, aromatic, and fragrance plants and that are developing ways to enhance the production of such crops. There are also organizations involved in the cultivation, study, and preservation of plants that are in danger of becoming extinct.

With improved methods being developed for isolating essences from their plant sources, there are very few limits to the number of new aromatics and medicines possible. In countries throughout the world, many companies are very interested in expanding their crops and distillations to meet higher demand. Abandoned or underutilized production facilities are being put back into service, and new ones that employ highly improved extraction methods are being built. Roberta discusses these new technologies in her section on essential oils. The production capacity is unlimited and growers throughout the world are clamoring for

jobs and cash crops. Growers, distillers, and extractors, however, cannot produce increasing quantities of botanical crops or botanical oils simply on speculation. They can do so only if there is a market for their products. As more people become familiar with aromatherapy and its many benefits, there will be a greater demand for pure essential oils and these industries will continue to grow, to the benefit of our health and well-being and to that of our planet.

There is a naive belief among many perfume and cosmetic professionals that the growing interest in natural products can be satisfied by making changes in packaging, labelling, and marketing, without ever changing the ingredients. For example, most fragrances that are advertised as "rose" and "jasmine" do not contain the naturally derived botanical essences of these plants. Unfortunately, many consumers and manufacturers assume that they do, because they have been told by their fragrance suppliers that the products are "natural."

Despite this, a growing segment of the population is questioning the legitimacy of label and advertising claims and is searching for genuinely natural products. In this book, Roberta not only presents valuable guidelines to assist you in the selection and evaluation of genuine, pure essential oils; she also offers dozens of formulas for treating a wide variety of conditions. You will know that they are as fresh and pure as possible—just as nature intended them—because you choose the ingredients and make the blends yourself.

One thing that differentiates this book from dozens of others on the subject is the author's insistence upon the use of authentic essential oils and the importance of reliable sources for obtaining them. Today, ecological consciousness is growing, and it is being shaped by an awareness of the problems of ecological imbalance. Many people in the commercial fragrance industry say that they are forced to use synthetics rather than natural essences because essential oils are too expensive. But coal and petroleum, and their derivatives—including synthetic fragrances—will escalate in price as supplies decline. Furthermore, the prices of these products will also surely rise as society requires that more of the costs of environmental cleanup be factored into the price equation. This domino effect will carry price increases along to *all* products derived from coal and petrochemicals. If we calculate the full and real costs of producing and using synthetic fragrances—the long-term consequences for the earth—we can see that in comparison, whole botanical essences are not nearly as costly as they seem. And they offer us so many wonderful benefits because they contain the vitality and energy of once-living plants and flowers.

One of the best features of this book is its discussion of common conditions that can be helped with aromatherapy, either as treatment or prevention. As Roberta makes very clear, good results derive from a combination of common-sense, easy-to-make lifestyle changes (such as changes in diet, exercise, and attitude) with the responsible use of essential oils as a complement to other treatments. As we become better acquainted with the causes of *dis*-ease and take more responsibility for our own health, we are learning to look into all possible treatment options, as well as learning the right questions to ask our health care professionals. Frequently, for example, we are advised to decrease stress, but seldom are natural prescriptions written for this. With the guidance of this book, we can enhance the quality of our lives. Roberta conveys the information required to use essential oils skillfully. She also objectively discusses situations in which essential oils should *not* be used, as well as any potential problems that might arise.

With this book, Roberta Wilson has made a valuable contribution to the literature on aromatherapy by making her knowledge readily available in a down-to-earth format that will be easily understood by everyone.

Christine Malcolm
Executive Director,
Aroma Research Institute of America
President, Santa Fe Fragrance Inc.

Preface

Since the day in the early 1980s when I first discovered lavender oil, I have been fascinated by aromatherapy. I felt as if I had found a long-lost friend. Aromatherapy filled a gap in my life—both a personal and a professional one. I immediately incorporated essential oils into my skin care practice, into my private life, and into my study of herbs, nutrition, and holistic healing. Using these concentrated plant extracts to improve physical and emotional health seemed like the perfect addition to my natural beauty treatments and lifestyle.

Curious by nature, I became a sponge for knowledge about aromatherapy, soaking up every drop of information I could find on the subject, particularly on ways to use aromatherapy. Unfortunately, at the time, only a few books were available, and their highly technical approach was somewhat discouraging and confusing. As a beginner, I was more interested in how essential oils could help me than I was in their chemical composition.

Through the years I've combed library and bookstore shelves, searching for books on the practical applications of aromatherapy. Today, although over two dozen aromatherapy books are in print, simple and easy-to-understand books with explicit instructions for using essential oils are still scarce.

I have spent much of the past ten years researching aromatherapy and attending numerous aromatherapy classes. I have taken two certification programs, interviewed French physicians who use medical aromatherapy, and written over two dozen articles on aromatherapy. I have become familiar with at least 110 different essential oils, and have mixed hundreds of blends for myself, my friends, and my clients. Everyone has responded with encouragement and enthusiasm.

Through the years I have also educated people—friends, neighbors, strangers, children, senior citizens, clients, skin care professionals, cosmetic manufacturers, health food store retailers, and the general public—about aromatherapy. I have come to realize that many people are simultaneously interested in and intimidated by aromatherapy. My primary objective in writing this book is to provide a complete, useful reference to help people learn how they can use aromatherapy to improve the quality of their lives. In the pages that follow, I will provide the important information you need so that you can use aromatherapy safely and effectively, without overwhelming you or inundating you with more information than you can use. At the same time, I have eliminated most of the guesswork by providing precise instructions for making aromatherapy blends to treat over fifty common conditions. To keep it simple, I have omitted the chemistry and botany of essential oils. First of all, there are already many good books that address these subjects in detail (some of them are listed in the reference section at the end of this book). Second, I believe that unless aromatherapy is presented in an easy, enjoyable manner, you probably won't use it. And only by using aromatherapy will you discover its many pleasures and benefits.

Though this book is simple and easy to follow, it is not intended only for beginners. Veteran aromatherapists, skin care specialists, massage therapists, cosmetic manufacturers, and health care professionals will all find plenty of practical information and useful formulas here that can complement the treatments they already use.

Aromatherapy plays a vital part in my life. From saving me from the stresses of hectic days to keeping my skin youthful and attractive; from soothing my sore throats to making my breathing easier; from freshening my home to fragrancing my bath water; from providing me with delightful, emotionally soothing perfumes to furnishing me with great gifts for loved ones, essential oils have been my faithful friends and constant companions for the last decade.

My study of aromatherapy has awakened more than my sense of smell. I have become acutely aware of my other senses and my many abilities. Aromatherapy has also inspired in me a deep, abiding reverence for plants. These sometimes sturdy, sometimes fragile—but always amazing—chlorophyll factories give us the gift of life. Without them we would surely starve and suffocate.

Beyond providing the basics of life, plants beautify our planet. In doing so, they sustain another aspect of human survival—the satisfaction of our senses. Their delightful perfumes seduce our sense of smell. Their rainbows of colors decorate our homes, offices, gardens, parks—the entire earth—and delight our sense of sight. They spice up our lives and our foods and satisfy our sense of taste. Their feathery leaves and silky petals tantalize our sense of touch. Without plants we could not live. And even if we could, would we want to? How dull life would be if we were deprived of the rich splashes of pastels and vibrant shades of flowers and greenery that color the earth!

I have written this book for several reasons. Writing is a true love of mine; it is something I must do. I especially love writing about essential oils and aromatherapy. I enjoy educating people about anything I've found valuable in my life, and essential oils head the list of tools that have helped me. Beyond my personal reasons, I saw the need for a book that would encourage people to incorporate aromatherapy into their daily lives by showing them exactly how to use it. I hope this book will spark your curiosity about aromatherapy, inspire you to experiment with essential oils, and make you want to continue seeking knowledge about aromatherapy.

I am excited about sharing my discoveries with you. In writing this book, I have expanded my own knowledge about aromatherapy, and what I have learned has validated my work over the previous few years. As we embark on this adventurous journey of the senses, I hope aromatherapy will enhance your health and well-being and improve the quality of your life.

Thank you and bon voyage!
Roberta Wilson

PART ONE

The
Basic Principles
of
Aromatherapy

What Is Aromatherapy?

Aromatherapy is the practice of using naturally distilled essences of plants to promote the health and well-being of your body, mind, and emotions. These essences, called essential oils, can restore balance and harmony to your body and to your life.

Essential oils can be used in a variety of ways. You can inhale them directly from the bottle. You can use them for skin care, hair care, and body care, as well as for numerous other beauty purposes. You can use them for personal hygiene and oral hygiene. You can take aromatherapy baths. You can soak your tired, aching feet in a foot bath fragranced with essential oils. You can give and receive aromatherapy massages. You can breathe in aromatherapy blends to relieve congestion, clear your head, and make your breathing easier. You can make delightful fragrances with essential oils.

Aromatherapy can help prevent or ease an assortment of ailments. Essential oils can boost your immune system and help you stay well. You can treat aches, pains, and injuries with essential oils. Essential oil compresses can relieve the pain or discomfort of a wide variety of problems. Aromatherapy can also help you reduce stress, lift depression, and restore or enhance emotional well-being. You can even disperse essential oils in the air throughout your home or office to help improve your productivity or to alter your moods.

In this book you will discover hundreds of aromatherapy blends, each designed for a specific purpose, as well as many different ways you can incorporate aromatherapy into your life. You will also learn how to choose and experiment with essential oils on your own. Aromatherapy offers a natural approach to health and beauty care that you can use to make your life healthier and more enjoyable.

The History of Aromatherapy

Aromatherapy is nothing new. Virtually all ancient cultures recognized the value of botanicals and aromatic plants and practiced primitive forms of aromatherapy. Ancient people used botanicals to adorn their bodies, to maintain physical health, and for religious purposes. The ancient Egyptians were among the first practitioners of aromatherapy. Fragrance was a dominant aspect of their lives, particularly for pharaohs and priests. Priests often doubled as physicians and perfumers, and they guarded the secrets of their craft closely. Royalty and the rich lavished on themselves such botanicals as cedarwood, coriander, cypress, elemi, frankincense, juniper, myrrh, and rose, often anointing each part of the body with a different essence.

THE ANCIENT WORLD

The first perfumes were incense. The word "perfume," in fact, is derived from the Latin *per,* meaning "through," and *fume,* meaning "smoke." Incense burned day and night in early Egyptian temples. The Egyptians also used botanical gums, ointments, perfumed powders, and scented oils, waters, and wines. During elaborate religious rituals, Egyptians anointed their bodies with aromatic oils and burned elemi, frankincense, myrrh, and sandalwood incense to glorify their gods. Incense helped them to heighten their spiritual experiences by deepening meditation, inspiring inner transformation, and purifying the spirit. They used benzoin, cedarwood, juniper, and thyme incense to freshen the air and to expel evil spirits. What ancient Egyptians considered evil spirits, we would probably equate with psychological or emotional problems.

The Egyptians were famous for embalming their dead. Embalmers would hollow out the body cavities of the dead and fill them with aromatic plants and ointments. If the deceased was from a wealthy family, myrrh and cedarwood would be used. Less costly plants, such as cinnamon, elemi, sandalwood, and thyme, were used to preserve the bodies of the common people. Beauty and cosmetics were of prime importance to Egyptians, both in daily life and in preparing for the afterlife. In fact, the world's first cosmetic chemists may have been Egyptian embalmers who transferred their knowledge of preserving the flesh of the dead to treating the skin of the living.

Aromatic oils were the key ingredients of the earliest cosmetics. The ancient Egyptians believed in bathing frequently and anointing their bodies with botanicals to keep their skin healthy and youthful, as well as to protect against the harshness of the climate and the sun. Perfuming their bodies, the ancient Egyptians believed, made them more attractive and alluring. Indeed, Cleopatra supposedly seduced Mark Antony with her extravagant use of roses and other aromatics. Many of the perfumed oils and ointments used in ancient Egypt also had healing properties, and served as medicines as well.

At around the same time, Ayurvedic medicine—the oldest known form of medicine—was developing in India. The Vedic texts mentioned the healing properties of such aromatic plants as coriander, ginger, myrrh, sandalwood, and rose. The *Kamasutra* suggested using sandalwood for lovemaking and for beauty purposes. Sandalwood was also an important part of early Indian religious and spiritual rites. The practice of perfumery was described in early Sanskrit literature, and ancient Indians took full advantage of the abundant aromatic plants of their country. Perfumery lore was intertwined with Indian legends and spiritual beliefs. Indians especially enjoyed the sweet scents of sandalwood, rose, and jasmine.

Hindu worshippers anointed themselves with perfumed oils to purge themselves of spiritual impurities and wash away their sins. In the temples, priests burned incense made of benzoin, sandalwood, and patchouli to banish evil spirits. At weddings, fires burning sandalwood and other scented woods, aromatic oils, and incense emitted lovely aromas into the air. A Hindu bride's feet would be anointed with a sacred scented oil, and at the end of the wedding ceremony, the guests would toss scented rice at the newlyweds to validate their marriage vows.

Following their exodus from Egypt, the ancient Hebrew people travelled to what is now Israel, bringing with them a knowledge of incense and perfumery. Frankincense soon burned in their temples. Moses made a special holy oil from olive oil, myrrh, calamus, cassia, and cinnamon, and anointed priests with it. During their captivity in Egypt, the Hebrews had adopted the Egyptian custom of scenting their bodies with aromatic oils and their homes with incense. However, Hebrew law forbade the private use of certain aromatics that were designated as sacred. These were reserved for use only in the temple by consecrated priests.

Hebrew law did require that maidens, before being presented at the royal court, undergo a year-long purification process with myrrh and many other fragrant oils. When a heavily perfumed Jewish bride arrived at her wedding, all the guests joined in the celebration and were also anointed with sweet-scented oils.

The Bible mentions the use of numerous aromatic essences, including cedarwood, cinnamon, coriander, cypress, frankincense, juniper, mint, myrrh, myrtle, pine, rose, and spikenard. Well known is the tale of the Magi presenting gifts of gold, frankincense, and myrrh—three of the most valuable commodities of that time—to the baby Jesus.

The Babylonian empire was the main source of fragrant botanicals during ancient times. Babylonians themselves consumed vast quantities of such scents as cedarwood, cypress, fir, juniper, myrtle, pine, and rose. While in Egypt only the wealthy enjoyed perfumes, Babylonian law compelled all citizens to douse themselves with fragrance—probably to subdue offensive body odors. On festive occasions, Babylonians burned immense amounts of aromatic woods and incense and saturated their entire bodies with scented oils.

Other ancient cultures made use of aromatic botanicals as well. The Assyrians burned tons of frankincense in religious rituals and drenched their bodies with botanical perfumes made from frankincense. They used cedar, cypress, and myrrh in cosmetics and for medicinal purposes. During the regal gatherings of King Antiochus Epiphanes of Syria, thousands of people were anointed with precious perfumes while aromatic incense burned all around. Every guest left these feasts with a garland of frankincense and myrrh.

The ancient Chinese and Japanese used perfumes in religious rituals. In both cultures, aromatic woods and herbs were burned at funerals. The Chinese used jasmine to venerate their ancestors; mourners would carry burning jasmine incense along with a funeral procession. Both the Chinese and Japanese used botanicals for personal hygiene and beauty purposes, which they considered very important. Chinese women massaged fragrant jasmine oil into their bodies after bathing. The Chinese used some botanicals, such as cinnamon, ginger, and jasmine, to help restore health and balance to the ill.

Some ancient Africans also anointed their bodies with botanicals, primarily to soften their skin and protect it from the searing effects of the sun. In preparation for an African wedding ceremony, a bride and groom would coat their bodies with scented oils and unguents, both to beautify their bodies and to deter evil on their wedding day. Many ancient Africans bathed their bodies with oils that were sweetly scented with aromatic roots and woods. The regular application of these oils helped their skin maintain its suppleness and elasticity and also prevented skin disorders.

THE GREEKS AND ROMANS

The ancient Greeks learned about aromatics and botanicals from the Egyptians. They respected the healing power of fragrant botanicals and perfumes, which they considered medicines. Perfumes played a major role in Greek mythology. Aphrodite, the Greek goddess of love, supposedly delivered perfume to earth from the heavens. The Greeks believed that plants were of divine origin, and that plant extracts therefore possessed spiritual and godlike qualities. They honored their gods and goddesses at elaborate feasts and squandered vast quantities of aromatics during these celebrations. Wishing to partake of the good fortune of their deities and to be equally blessed, the Greeks enthusiastically adorned their bodies with an abundance of personal fragrances in hopes of gratifying the gods.

The ancient Greeks believed that the therapeutic and medicinal perfumes they used on their bodies would also have favorable effects on their minds, especially in treating ailments of an emotional or nervous nature. Healing the mind, they felt, would restore physical health. During their daily routines, they anointed each part of their bodies with a different aromatic oil. Wealthy Greeks built altars in their homes at which they held daily rituals involving the burning of incense. Perfumes were also an essential part of funerals, and the dead were buried with bottles of their favorite fragrances.

The ancient Romans gained their knowledge of both medicine and perfumery from the Greeks. They enjoyed using aromatics for cosmetics, hygiene, massage, and medical treatments. Bathing was an important ritual for the Romans, and the public baths were centers for cultural activities. The ancient Romans added aromatic oils to steam baths and hot tubs, and followed their baths by massages with scented oils. In addition to scenting their bodies and hair, the Romans fragranced their clothing and homes with botanicals. Aromatics and perfumes also played a part in all government ceremonies. Following each conquest of the Roman empire, the Romans introduced botanicals to their new subjects.

THE MEDIEVAL PERIOD

With the collapse of the Roman Empire in the fifth century A.D., the influence of Roman civilization in Europe all but disappeared, and the use of expensive and rare botanicals for beauty, bathing, and perfumery declined dramatically. Much ancient knowledge of perfumery was lost to the continent forever.

While Europeans allowed aromatic fragrances and medicines to vanish into obscurity for some centuries, the Arabs continued to explore perfumes' myriad applications. Avicenna, a tenth-century Arab physician, discovered a means of extracting the aromatic essences of flowers by distillation. His first creation was rose oil. Soon many other essential oils were equally easy to obtain. The popularity of perfume spread rapidly among the Arabs, Moors, and Spaniards. By the thirteenth century, as trade resumed between Europe and the East, the use of essential oils for beauty, health, hygiene, and medicinal purposes became common throughout Europe.

THE RENAISSANCE AND BEYOND

By the middle of the sixteenth century, perfumers had become prominent and prevalent throughout Europe. They created essential oil blends, some with claims bordering on the miraculous or magical. Many Europeans believed that bathing was unhealthy and preferred perfuming their bodies to conceal offensive body odors. Essential oils became crucial for this. The use of essential oils was so widespread that even public fountains were fragranced for festivals. During the reign of Henry III of France (1551–1559), perfume use became so extravagant that it was actually wasteful. The French fragranced everything—public fountains,

stationery, wines, and drinking water, as well as their homes, their bodies, their hair, and all of their clothing. Throughout the medieval period in Europe, oils such as juniper, pine, and thyme were used in great quantities to combat and prevent the spread of illness, particularly epidemics and plagues.

In the sixteenth and seventeenth centuries, the religious and philosophical climate of Europe emphasized strictness in religious discipline and lifestyle. This era saw the rise of Puritanism in England. The Roman Catholic church too adopted stricter and more demanding attitudes. This religious atmosphere exerted a mighty influence on people's actions. Many members of the clergy frowned on any personal use of aromatics, partially because pagans and witches had used them in their rites, and partially because religious leaders of the time felt that any display of vanity or adornment detracted from spirituality.

As late as the eighteenth century, puritanically minded people discouraged women from using perfumes and fragranced cosmetics. Some British lawmakers felt that perfume possessed special powers that gave women an unfair advantage over men, and proposed a law to prohibit women from wearing scents. Perfumes and cosmetics, according to these men, were forms of witchcraft that allowed women to seduce men and lure them into marriage while the men were not in full command of their senses. The law failed to pass, however, and the sale of perfumes, cosmetics, and medicines continued. Essential oils remained the most powerful antiseptics available until modern chemicals appeared.

As modern science evolved in the late nineteenth century, essential oils fell from favor. Synthetic chemicals soon replaced botanical ingredients in medicines and beauty products. By the early twentieth century, modern perfumers were using more synthetic fragrances than natural oils in their scents.

The natural beauty and health benefits of essential oils and aromatics were all but forgotten as scientists and perfumers switched to cheaper, more readily available man-made chemicals. Today, only the most costly commercially available fragrances contain even the tiniest amounts of pure essential oils.

AROMATHERAPY TODAY

The modern revival of essential oils began during the 1920s, with the work of René-Maurice Gattefossé, a French chemist and perfumer who coined the term *aromatherapy*. While experimenting in his laboratory, Gattefossé severely burned his hand. He immediately plunged it into the nearest liquid, which happened to be a bowl of lavender oil. He later noticed that his hand healed very rapidly and without scarring. After his speedy recovery, Gattefossé dedicated the rest of his life to researching the therapeutic aspects of essential oils, and his studies helped to revive an ancient, almost forgotten art.

During the past two decades, with the emerging trends toward holistic health and natural skin care, there has been another resurgence of interest in aromatherapy. Concern about the environment and the desire of many people to be closer to nature are probably partially responsible for this. In addition, the escalating costs of conventional medicine and concern about the numerous adverse side effects of many modern drugs and the harsh synthetic chemicals in cosmetics, plus the growing awareness of the advantages of preventive health care, are contributing to aromatherapy's popularity. As people take increasing responsibility for their own physical and emotional health, aromatherapy is becoming a welcome addition in more and more people's lives. Today, aromatherapy is experiencing its greatest popularity in centuries, as people are becoming aware of its potential for enhancing the quality of their lives.

What Aromatherapy Can Do for You

Through essential oils, nature has provided us with a network of therapeutic plant essences that have valuable healing properties. These highly concentrated essential oils are ideal for treating an array of physical, mental, and emotional problems. People around the world are searching for safe, effective, and environmentally responsible alternatives to conventional medicines and cosmetics. Those who have discovered aromatherapy have found exactly what they need to help maintain and improve their health and take care of their skin, hair, and bodies. Women, men, and children are all benefitting from the use of aromatherapy.

Aromatherapy works with your body in a very natural, holistic way. By gently activating your body's own healing energies, aromatherapy helps to restore balance to your body, mind, and spirit. Aromatherapy complements almost any other type of therapy or healing practice, whether conventional or alternative.

Aromatherapy offers you an easy way to enhance the quality of your life and improve your health. Aromatherapy can prompt your body and mind to function more efficiently. It can help boost your immune system. Often, you can prevent common ailments or illnesses with aromatherapy. If you do get sick, you can use aromatherapy to minimize the discomforts and speed up your recovery. Aromatherapy can help you get back on your feet after an illness. It also makes a safe and effective first aid treatment.

Aromatherapy can help you reduce and manage stress. Since none of us seems to be spared from modern-day stress, any reduction in stress will certainly improve or enhance the quality of our lives and restore balance to our lives. Stress plays a major role in almost all illnesses, both physical and mental. The regular use of essential oils can help you control stress, alleviate anxiety and tension, and minimize the physical aches and pains they cause. You can use aromatherapy to relax and unwind after a stressful day at work, at home, or on the road. Or you can use it to refresh and recharge yourself so that you can keep up the pace of your busy life.

Aromatherapy has a positive influence on the emotions. Many essential oils can help you regulate your moods. Some are uplifting and energizing; others are calming and sedating. Some work to restore balance. In Part Two of this book, you will learn about essential oils that can elevate your mood, soothe your emotions, clear your mind, quiet your anger, and even inspire your creativity.

Aromatherapy treatments for the skin, hair, and body can add a new dimension to your beauty or personal hygiene routine. They are among the most natural and effective types of beauty treatments. Aromatherapy can give a healthier appearance to any skin, especially troubled or problem skin. Essential oils can revitalize dry or prematurely aging skin, regulate oily skin, clear problem skin, and add a healthy glow to all complexions. Men as well as women will enjoy using essential oils—in after-shaves, in skin care products, and for hair care.

In addition to offering a natural, holistic approach to enhancing health and well-being, the practice of aromatherapy supports the environment. Growing plants—lots of them—for the production of essential oils helps the planet and helps us. Too many people, in their race to turn the world into a concrete jungle, forget that without plants, humans could not exist. Plants provide us with a most vital element for life—oxygen. They manufacture and circulate this life-sustaining gas so that we may breathe. In doing this they utilize the carbon dioxide we exhale—a waste that otherwise contributes to the greenhouse effect. Besides beautifying its surroundings, every plant that flourishes makes the air a little cleaner, reduces some of the effect of greenhouse gases, and diminishes global warming.

Cultivating crops for the production of essential oils has other environmental advantages. By avoiding chemical fertilizers and pesticides, farmers who grow botanicals using organic methods help to counter soil erosion and reduce the toxic wastes that contaminate waterways and ground water. In developing countries, growing botanical crops can provide farmers with a greater economic return than other, more harmful industries, such as logging, cattle grazing, and growing crops for illegal drugs. People thus have an opportunity to make a better living in ways that are not as destructive to the land or to society.

Growing botanicals can help protect the world's diminishing forests instead of demolishing them. By reducing greenhouse gases, plants may also help preserve the fragile ozone layer. Each time you purchase pure essential oils, you cast a vote for natural botanicals that can have immediate and long-term effects on your health and well-being as well as on the health and well-being of the planet. You send the message to manufacturers that you want to buy products that are good for the planet, that help sustain agriculture around the world, that preserve plant species, and that support life on earth.

You can use your purchasing power to make a significant statement and have a positive influence on the environment. Plants can help us solve some of the problems we face, if we will only let them do what they instinctively want to do—grow. By using botanicals in your everyday life, you can help guarantee plants' survival. And their survival has an important influence on people. We need plants. We cannot live on earth without them.

Using pure essential oils has another far-reaching effect: It can provide a perfect opportunity to connect with nature. In these stress-filled times, we often forget about nature and fail to appreciate the many advantages that the earth offers. In fact, the neglect of nature is, in part, responsible for the current global environmental crisis. Opening a bottle of an essential oil, which was once part of a living plant, and breathing in its fragrant and therapeutic aroma can subtly yet powerfully serve to remind you that you too are an integral part of nature—whether you live on a farm in the rural Midwest or in a penthouse 100 floors above a modern metropolis.

Aromatherapy can make a big difference in your life. In this book, you will learn exactly how you can use aromatherapy for body, hair, and skin care; for creating personal perfumes and fragrancing your environment; for first aid treatments; for relaxation; for maintaining or improving health; for boosting immunity; for reducing stress; and for enhancing or restoring emotional equilibrium. You will learn how to make many different cosmetics, skin oils, massage oils, fragrances, diffuser blends, and therapeutic blends for treating a variety of conditions. You will find out about essential oils—what they are, what they do, and how to select them. You will discover how you can easily use aromatics in your everyday life. In short, you will come to appreciate essential oils for the value they can add to your daily life. In fact, once you begin using them and realize what a difference they can make, you will probably wonder how you ever managed without aromatherapy.

Essential Oils

Essential oils are essences that are extracted from the bark, leaves, petals, resins, rinds, roots, seeds, stalks, and stems of certain aromatic plants. Essential oils are what give plants their characteristic smells. Pure essential oils are extremely concentrated. Many pounds, even tons, of plant material may be required to produce a relatively small amount of essential oil. For example, over 150 pounds of lavender flowers will yield one pound of lavender oil; 5,000 pounds of rose petals produce but one pound of rose oil.

Essential oils are not oils in the same sense that oils like almond, canola, olive, or sunflower oil are. Essential oils are usually very liquid and do not feel greasy at all. They will not leave an oily stain on clothing or paper. Essential oils are sometimes called *volatile oils* because they evaporate readily when exposed to air. They are soluble in vegetable oil and partially soluble in alcohol. However, they do not dissolve in water.

Plants that produce essential oils store them in tiny pockets between their cell walls. As the plant releases the essential oils, they circulate throughout the plant and send messages that help it function efficiently, much as hormones do in humans. Many botanists believe that essential oils activate and regulate such activities as cellular metabolism, photosynthesis, and cellular respiration. Some scientists speculate that essential oils may trigger immune responses that assist plants in coping with stressful changes in climate and environment. Some plants release essential oils that protect them by repelling harmful insects and diseases, while others emit essential oils to attract insects or animals that aid in the plants' pollination and propagation. Essential oils thus play an important part in the survival of plants.

Of the thousands of plants that populate the plant kingdom, relatively few produce essential oils. Even among those that do produce essential oils, many yield such a minute amount that it is not financially feasible to extract them. Other plants produce essential oils, yet the oils smell nothing like the plants; often, this is due to chemical reactions that occur during the extraction process.

Ironically, some of nature's most fragrant flowers—gardenia, lilac, lily of the valley, magnolia, violet, wisteria—yield no essential oils. Some flowers, such as carnation, honeysuckle, and narcissus, yield absolutes through solvent extraction (see page 18), but they are quite costly and smell nothing like the original flowers. Most fruits, with the exception of some citrus fruits, do not produce essential oils. Scents such as apple, banana, cherry, coconut, mango, papaya, peach, pear, pineapple, raspberry, strawberry, and watermelon are not essential oils. These fragrances are artificially synthesized by scientists in chemistry labs.

HOW ESSENTIAL OILS WORK

Essential oils work on several different levels. The first way they affect most people is through the sense of smell. The sense of smell is the most complex and the least understood—and at the same time the most sensitive—of the five senses. Whenever you open a bottle of an essential oil, its volatile aromatic molecules permeate the air. As you inhale the aroma, odor molecules enter your nostrils and drift upward into the olfactory receptors, structures in the nose where smell originates. The olfactory nerves are the only sensory pathways that open directly into the brain.

It takes only eight odor molecules to activate your sense of smell. When the odor molecules reach the mucous membranes in your olfactory apparatus, they are greeted by about 10 million olfactory receptors at the end of each nostril. Atop these receptors are cilia, tiny hairlike projections that wave rhythmically back and forth, waiting to detect scents. Scientists theorize that each of these receptors acts like a "key" that fits a certain odor, allowing it to "unlock," or identify, an aroma. The human olfactory system needs as few as forty odor molecules before it can recognize a specific smell.

Once receptors identify an odor, nerve cells relay this information directly to the limbic system of the brain, or the "smell brain," even before the odor molecules themselves actually arrive. The limbic system is a group of deep brain structures that are involved in the sense of smell and the experience of emotions, among other things. Here odors can trigger memories and influence behavior. In addition, the limbic system works in coordination with the pituitary gland and the hypothalamus area of the brain to regulate the hormonal activities of the endocrine system. Odors can thus trigger the production of hormones that govern appetite, body temperature, insulin production, overall metabolism, stress levels, sex drive, and conscious thoughts and reactions. The limbic system also influences immunity. Through their action on the limbic system, essential oils can have a positive impact on all of these functions. In addition, the limbic system interacts with the neocortex area of the brain, and odors can affect conscious thoughts and reactions.

The limbic system affects the nervous system as well. Desires, motivation, moods, intuition, and creativity all originate within the limbic system. Because they act on the limbic system, smells can make you feel better psychologically in addition to enhancing your physical health. Research shows that people who surround themselves with pleasant scents enjoy higher self-esteem. Smells initiate both physical and psychological reactions by stimulating the release of neurotransmitters and endorphins in your brain. These hormonelike chemicals produce gratifying sensations, even feelings of euphoria, and generate an overall sense of well-being. Neurotransmitters can arouse sexual feelings, reduce stress, relieve pain, and restore emotional equilibrium.

Smells can gain direct access to your emotions and work on a subconscious level to modify emotional imbalances or change behavior. Odors also can trigger long-forgotten memories and alter your attitude. Inhaling certain essential oils can enhance your emotional equilibrium, either calming and relaxing you or stimulating and energizing you. Calming floral fragrances such as neroli, rose, or ylang ylang oil will relax you, while the stimulating scents of black pepper, ginger, or peppermint oil will energize you. Some essential oils work to restore balance, depending on what your body needs. Lavender and geranium are two oils that can establish or enhance a sense of equilibrium.

When you inhale essential oils, they enter into your respiratory system as well as your brain. In your lungs, minute molecules of essential oils attach themselves to oxygen molecules. These oxygen molecules then carry the essential oil molecules into your bloodstream and circulate them, in much the same way that blood delivers nutrients, to each cell in your body. Within the cells, essential oils can activate the body's ability to heal itself and improve health.

Essential oils work through the skin, too. They can stimulate circulation to surface skin cells and encourage cell regeneration, the formation of new skin cells. They can calm inflamed or irritated skin. Some oils can release muscle spasms, soothe sore muscles, and relieve muscular tension.

Because the skin is porous, essential oils are easily absorbed through it. Molecules of essential oils are very tiny and can easily penetrate the skin. Once beneath the skin, they go into the intercellular fluid surrounding the skin cells and can enter your bloodstream. There they can travel to your internal organs and your lymphatic system, and can affect your immune system. Scientists suspect that essential oils stimulate the body's own natural defense systems. For example, certain oils, such as basil, tea tree, and thyme oils, can encourage the production of white blood cells, thereby boosting your body's immune response. In addition, many essential oils fight harmful bacteria, fungi, viruses, and other microbes in the body.

When taken internally, essential oils are ab-sorbed directly into the bloodstream through the digestive system. However, the internal use of essential oils is beyond the scope of this book. A health care professional trained in medical aromatherapy should supervise any internal use of essential oils. Essential oils are the most highly concentrated form of botanical, and it is important to respect their power.

Essential oils can improve your health and well-being in many different ways. Open a bottle of an essential oil and inhale it. Apply aromatherapy cosmetics to your face. Massage aromatherapy skin oils over your body. Take aromatherapy baths. Blend your own perfumes with essential oils. Disperse essential oils throughout your room with a diffuser. No matter how you choose to use aromatherapy, it can work on at least one of the levels mentioned above.

THE EXTRACTION OF ESSENTIAL OILS

During certain hours of the day in certain months of the year, farm workers harvest crops that have been cultivated especially for essential oil production. By gathering the plants at these specific times, they can produce greater quantities of higher quality essential oils. To further ensure the freshness and quality of essential oils, extraction often takes place in or near the fields in portable stills.

Steam Distillation

Steam distillation is the most common method of extracting essential oils. Many old-time distillers favor this method for most oils, and say that none of the newer methods produces better quality oils.

Steam distillation is done in a still. Fresh, or sometimes dried, botanical material is placed in the plant chamber of the still, and pressurized steam is generated in a separate chamber and circulated through the plant material. The heat of the steam forces the tiny intercellular pockets that hold the essential oils to open and release them. The temperature of the steam must be high enough to open the pouches, yet not so high that it destroys the plants or fractures or burns the essential oils.

As they are released, the tiny droplets of essential oil evaporate and, together with the steam molecules, travel through a tube into the still's condensation chamber. As the steam cools, it condenses into water. The essential oil forms a film on the surface of the water. To separate the essential oil from the water, the film is then decanted or skimmed off the top.

The remaining water, a byproduct of distillation, is called *floral water, distillate,* or *hydrosol.* It retains many of the therapeutic properties of the plant, making it valuable in skin care for facial mists or toners. In certain situations, floral water may be preferable to pure essential oil, such as when treating a sensitive individual or a child, or when a more diluted treatment is required.

Cold Pressing

Another method of extracting essential oils is cold-pressed expression, or scarification. It is used to obtain citrus fruit oils such as bergamot, grapefruit, lemon, lime, mandarin, orange, and tangerine oils. In this process, fruit rolls over a trough with sharp projections that penetrate the peel. This pierces the tiny pouches containing the essential oil. Then the whole fruit is pressed to squeeze the juice from the pulp and to release the essential oil from the pouches. The essential oil rises to the surface of the juice and is separated from the juice by centrifugation.

Enfleurage

Some flowers, such as jasmine or tuberose, have such low contents of essential oil or are so delicate

that heating them would destroy the blossoms before releasing the essential oils. In such cases, an expensive and lengthy process called enfleurage is sometimes used to remove the essential oils. Flower petals are placed on trays of odorless vegetable oil or animal fat, which will absorb the flowers' essential oils. Every day or every few hours, after the vegetable oil or fat has absorbed as much of the essential oil as possible, the depleted petals are removed and replaced with fresh ones. This procedure continues until the fat or oil becomes saturated with the essential oil. Adding alcohol to this enfleurage mixture separates the essential oil from the fatty substance. Afterwards, the alcohol evaporates and only the essential oil remains.

Solvent Extraction

Another method of extraction used on delicate plants is solvent extraction, which yields a higher amount of essential oil at a lower cost. In this process, a chemical solvent such as hexane is used to saturate the plant material and pull out the aromatic compounds. This renders a substance called a *concrete.* The concrete can then be dissolved in alcohol to remove the solvent. When the alcohol evaporates, an *absolute* remains.

Although more cost-efficient than enfleurage, solvent extraction has disadvantages. Residues of the solvent may remain in the absolute and can cause side effects. While absolutes or concretes may be fine for fragrances or perfumes, they are not especially desirable for skin care applications.

Some trees, such as benzoin, frankincense, and myrrh, exude aromatic "tears," or sap that is too thick to use easily in aromatherapy. In these cases, a resin or essential oil can be extracted from the tears with alcohol or a solvent such as hexane. This renders a resin or an essential oil that is easier to use. However, only those oils or resins extracted with alcohol should be used for aromatherapy purposes.

Turbodistillation, Hydrodiffusion, and Carbon Dioxide Extraction

Several modern methods of extraction are becoming popular alternatives to traditional steam distillation. Turbodistillation is suitable for hard-to-extract or coarse plant material, such as bark, roots, and seeds. In this process, the plants soak in water and steam is circulated through this plant and water mixture. Throughout the entire process, the same water is continually recycled through the plant material. This method allows faster extraction of essential oils from hard-to-extract plant materials.

In the hydrodiffusion process, steam at atmospheric pressure is dispersed through the plant material from the top of the plant chamber. In this way the steam can saturate the plants more evenly and in less time than with steam distillation. This method is also less harsh than steam distillation and the resulting essential oils smell much more like the original plant.

Supercritical carbon dioxide extraction uses carbon dioxide under extremely high pressure to extract essential oils. Plants are placed in a stainless steel tank and, as carbon dioxide is injected into the tank, pressure inside the tank builds. Under high pressure, the carbon dioxide turns into a liquid and acts as a solvent to extract the essential oils from the plants. When the pressure is decreased, the carbon dioxide returns to a gaseous state, leaving no residues behind.

Many carbon dioxide extractions have fresher, cleaner, and crisper aromas than steam-distilled essential oils, and they smell more similar to the living plants. Scientific studies show that carbon dioxide extraction produces essential oils that are very potent and have great therapeutic benefits. This extraction method uses lower temperatures than steam distillation, making it more gentle on the plants. It produces higher yields and makes some materials, especially gums and resins, easier to handle. Many essential oils that cannot be extracted by steam distillation are obtainable with carbon dioxide extraction. In the future, many botanicals that are not now available may possibly be obtained through carbon dioxide extraction.

THE PURITY AND QUALITY OF ESSENTIAL OILS

Selecting high-quality essential oils is always a challenge. When you first begin buying essential oils, you must rely almost entirely on the reputation of the supplier to guarantee the purity and quality of the oil you purchase (some recommended suppliers are listed in the Aromatherapy Resource Guide in the Appendix). Over time, as you smell different grades of essential oils and compare pure oils to synthetic ones, you will gain experience in recognizing the difference between high-quality essential oils and lower quality oils or synthetics. You'll learn to trust your nose as time goes by.

Pure Essential Oils Versus Synthetic Substitutes

The most important thing to understand when selecting essential oils is the difference between pure essential oils and synthetic products. The practice of aromatherapy requires essences extracted from plants, not synthetic scents made from petroleum byproducts in laboratories. As with any other type of treatment, results are the goal. Synthetic oils can never produce the same desirable results that pure essential oils can. Aromatherapy is a holistic healing method that works by treating individuals as whole beings, not as machines made up of so many isolated parts to be fixed when broken. The body and the mind are integrated. The body affects the mind, and the mind affects the body.

Whole essential oils work best for aromatherapy; they contain all the elements of the plants' essential oils, just as nature created them. They therefore have greater therapeutic benefits than do the isolated components, which lack many of the important properties of the plants. All of the components of essential oils work in a synergistic manner and all are necessary to achieve the best results.

Quality and Price

The highest quality essential oils are extracted from plants that have been cultivated under optimum conditions—they were planted at the right time, in balanced soil, and grown using organic farming methods; they flourished in an ideal climate with the right amount of water and sun; and they were harvested at the most opportune time of day during the most suitable season.

Distillation also affects the quality of essential oils. The type of equipment used, its age, the size of the still, the capacity of the plant chamber, the size and length of the coil in the condenser, and the pressure and temperature of the water in the condenser all affect the finished product. Another consideration is the distillation time. The time required to produce the highest quality oil varies from plant to plant. Some distillers hurry distillation to minimize labor costs and increase profits, but rushing distillation will produce a weak or poor-quality oil. Other producers may add solvents to the water, increase the water pressure, or raise the temperature to produce more oil. Any of these measures will cause the quality of the oil to suffer.

Quality affects the price of essential oils. Growing plants and distilling essential oils are labor-intensive activities, and they can be costly. This is why high-quality pure essential oils are not inexpensive. Some plants are easier to grow and more readily available than others; some oils are easier to extract than others. The price of essential oils depends on the availability of the botanicals, the amount of essential

oils contained within the plants, the ease of obtaining the essential oils, the location of the fields, harvest conditions, cultivation methods, local labor costs, seasonal and regional growing conditions, soil conditions, transportation and shipping costs, types of fertilizers used and their costs, weather, and world economics. In addition, the color, smell, and consistency of essential oils can differ from season to season and year to year. This also affects price. As a rule, the higher the quality of the essential oil, the higher the price.

Adulterated and "Nature-Identical" Oils

When purchasing essential oils, you should be aware of a number of warning signs that indicate you may not be getting the purest product available. Adulteration is the addition of other substances (synthetic or natural) to extend or to alter the appearance, the chemical composition, or the smell of an essential oil. Some suppliers "magically" transform one pound of pure essential oil into ten pounds of adulterated oil. Many manufacturers engage in this practice to expand their profit margins. For example, it's common knowledge that the demand for French lavender oil is so high that each year France sells far more "lavender oil" than it produces. Sometimes companies, knowingly or unknowingly, sell products labeled as pure essential oils that are in fact synthetic or adulterated oils.

Adulterating essential oils with vegetable or carrier oils can be perfectly acceptable—if the label reflects that addition. For example, a facial oil that contains essential oils diluted in jojoba oil is fine, as long as the label doesn't imply that the product is pure essential oil. Unfortunately, some companies fail to disclose all the ingredients in their products. If a company fails to disclose that one of its products contains some other oil in addition to the essential oil, it is deceiving consumers. Likewise, if synthetic scents have been added to essential oils to extend them and the customer isn't notified, the customer is being misled. One way to tell if a product contains anything other than pure essential oil is to place a drop of it on a piece of paper. Pure essential oils will evaporate, leaving no trace, whereas those in carrier oils will leave an oily spot.

There are other signs that may alert you to an adulterated or synthetic oil. If a company sells all of its essential oils for the same price, chances are they aren't pure. Essential oil prices vary dramatically. While one-half ounce of orange oil may sell for several dollars, the same amount of rose oil costs over two hundred dollars. Any rose oil selling for several dollars an ounce is surely synthetic.

If the label on a product doesn't specify "essential oil" or "pure essential oil," the product probably isn't an essential oil. Unfortunately, however, even the words "essential oil" or "pure essential oil" on the label are not a guarantee of purity. Some companies sell synthetic oils mislabelled as essential oils. Companies also often sell products called perfume oils. These are rarely made with pure essential oils. While the label may read Oil of Neroli, Oil of Rose, Rose Oil Perfume, or Jasmine Perfume Oil, the product is likely to be a blend of synthetic oils that attempt to simulate the smell of real flowers. Price may be an indication. If a very expensive essential oil is selling for several dollars as a perfume oil, it's not a pure essential oil. The few companies that make natural perfumes with pure essential oils and other botanicals usually specify on the label that their ingredients are essential oils in a base of alcohol or jojoba oil. These are excellent alternatives to commercial colognes and perfumes.

Sometimes people confuse infused oils with essential oils. Infused oils are prepared by soaking or simmering plants in heated almond, safflower, soy, or other vegetable oils to infuse the oil with some of the properties of the plant. These infused oils are greasy and are not pure essential oils. Common infused oils are aloe vera, arnica, calendula, chamomile, comfrey, mullein, and St. Johnswort. Calendula, chamomile, and St. Johnswort are occasionally available as essential oils.

"Nature-identical" is a very misleading term that you should understand. So-called nature-identical oils are man-made petrochemical-based products that have been scientifically reconstructed to closely mimic the smell and chemical composition of pure essential oils. There's really nothing "nature-identical" about them; they are not from nature, and they certainly are not identical to pure essential oils. The scientists who make these synthetics strive primarily to duplicate the smell. While only a dozen or so chemical components may be responsible for the smell of an essential oil, essential oils contain literally hundreds of components that bestow upon it its unique therapeutic properties. Many of these components are present in such minute amounts that it is impossible to isolate and identify them, yet in many instances it may be these unidentified parts that make the essential oil so effective. In addition, so-called nature-identicals lack the vital energy that essential oils have as a result of coming from plants that once grew in the earth.

The action of an essential oil depends upon the delicate balance and synergy of all its components. With all the marvels of modern science, chemists still cannot duplicate essential oils in their laboratories. Some synthetic oils may smell very much like the real thing, but because they lack all of the genuine oil's many components, they cannot produce the desired therapeutic results. Synthetic substitutes also lack the balance and synergy that pure essential oils have.

Finally, when selecting your essential oils, question the products of any company that sells animal extracts, such as musk or civet oil, as essential oils. All true essential oils come from plants, not from animals. Moreover, almost all of the so-called musk and civet oils sold are synthetic; the smell of real musk or civet oil is so offensive that most people would never even consider wearing it. Be suspicious if a company offers essential oils that don't exist, or sells animal extracts as essential oils. All or most of their other oils may also be synthetic.

STORING AND HANDLING ESSENTIAL OILS

Storing your essential oils properly is important for protecting their freshness and effectiveness, and for extending their shelf life. The properties of essential oils are easily altered by exposure to sunlight and heat. Always keep your essential oils in dark amber bottles in a cool, dry place, away from sunlight or heat. Avoid leaving them in a moist or damp place, such as the bathroom.

Essential oils are very volatile and will evaporate rapidly when exposed to air. In addition, oxygen can compromise their quality or change their chemical compositions. Always keep the bottles tightly capped when not in use. When using essential oils, never leave the bottles uncapped for more than a few seconds. To prevent contamination of your oil, avoid touching the dropper or the opening of the container to your skin or to anything else. Instead, allow the oils to drop from the bottle into the palm of your hand or into the bottle you are using for blending. Most essential oils will remain fresh for one year or longer with proper care and storage. The quality and aroma of some essential oils, such as vetiver and patchouli, actually improve with age.

Pure essential oils are the tools of aromatherapy. Using the highest quality pure essential oils available will ensure that your aromatherapy experiences are as therapeutic and pleasurable as possible. As you become more and more familiar with essential oils, your appreciation of essential oils, their purity, and their potency will grow.

As you read on, you will learn about the specific applications of individual essential oils. You will also learn how to make the blends in this book and how to create some of your own. You are embarking on an aromatherapy adventure that can improve the quality of your life and your health.

Carrier Oils

A carrier oil is any oil that is used to dilute pure essential oils. Carrier oils are extracted from nuts, kernels, seeds, and other parts of plants. Any vegetable oil will work, although some are preferable to others because of their specific properties and the nutrients they contain. It is always wise to mix essential oils with a carrier oil before applying them to your skin. Pure essential oils are so concentrated and so potent that they may irritate or burn your skin, or you might develop a sensitivity to them. In addition, essential oils spread more evenly when diluted in carrier oils. Using carrier oils makes aromatherapy more economical; you use less essential oil and can cover a greater area of skin. Most suppliers of essential oils also offer carrier oils.

CHOOSING CARRIER OILS

The carrier oils most often used in aromatherapy are almond, apricot kernel, canola, grapeseed, hazelnut, jojoba, sunflower, and sesame oils. In addition, avocado, borage, evening primrose, rose hip seed, and wheat germ oils are often added in small percentages to enhance aromatherapy blends. Less commonly used carrier oils include camellia, kukui, macadamia, meadowfoam, olive, peanut, pecan, pistachio, rice bran, soy, and walnut oils.

For aromatherapy purposes, you should choose carrier oils that are unscented, cold-pressed vegetable oils that contain no additives. Many oils—even some of the ones sold in health food stores—are extracted using chemical solvents. Harmful solvent residues can remain in the oil and your skin can absorb them. Cold-pressed, organically grown vegetable oils contain no solvent, herbicide, or pesticide residues.

In addition to using organically grown oils, many people prefer to use only unrefined vegetable oils, because they retain more nutritional value and therefore offer greater therapeutic benefits. The more an oil is refined, the more nutrients it loses. Refining can also change the chemical composition of an oil. If an oil is unrefined, the label should state this.

One common oil that should never be used for aromatherapy is mineral oil. This is a byproduct of the petroleum industry, and it is made up of very large molecules that sit on the surface of the skin and prevent the penetration of essential oils. Coconut oil cannot be recommended, either. Although it is a natural oil, it too has large molecules that interfere with the skin's absorption of essential oils.

A major concern when choosing a carrier oil is how long it remains fresh. When an oil smells "off" or old, it is usually rancid. All triglyceride oils go rancid eventually, but some go rancid more quickly than others. Of all the carrier oils mentioned in this book, only jojoba oil is not a triglyceride oil. Instead, it is a wax ester, and for all practical purposes does not go rancid. For this reason jojoba oil is preferred for fragrance blends or for blends containing precious or expensive oils such as jasmine, neroli, and rose. You can also add a portion of jojoba oil to any aromatherapy blend to lengthen its life.

USE AND STORAGE

To keep your carrier oils as fresh as possible, always refrigerate them until you are ready to use them. This is especially important for oils that go rancid quickly, such as almond, avocado, borage, evening primrose, flaxseed, and rose hip seed oils. Also, you should mix only small amounts of aromatherapy products at any one time, and use them quickly. Essential oils act as mild antioxidants and can extend the shelf life of some carrier oils, but it is best to blend fresh aromatherapy products frequently.

AN INTRODUCTION TO THE CARRIER OILS

All carrier oils have lubricating properties, but which oil or oils you choose to work with may depend also on other specific properties of the individual oils. The following are brief descriptions of some of the most popular carrier oils used for aromatherapy.

Almond Oil

Sweet almond oil is good for all skin types, and is especially good for making aromatherapy products to treat eczema. It helps to relieve itching, irritation, and inflammation, and also softens, soothes, and smooths dry skin. Almond oil is very lubricating but not very penetrating, making it good for massage and for protecting the surface of the skin. Use blends made with almond oil immediately, if possible; it goes rancid quickly.

Apricot Kernel Oil

Apricot kernel oil is rich and nourishing, and is particularly helpful for dehydrated, delicate, mature, or sensitive skin. It soothes and smooths dry or inflamed skin. Apricot kernel oil has a high vitamin A content.

Avocado Oil

Avocado oil nourishes and restores dry, dehydrated, and mature skin. It is a rich, heavy oil that is best blended with other carrier oils. Skin problems, especially eczema and psoriasis, respond to its high content of vitamins A and E. It goes rancid quickly.

Borage Oil

Borage oil stimulates skin cell activity and encourages skin regeneration. It penetrates the skin easily and benefits all types of skin, particularly dry, dehydrated, mature, or prematurely aging skin. Add borage oil to other carrier oils to promote healthy skin and hair and for added protection. Borage oil goes rancid quickly.

Calophyllum Inophyllum Oil

Calophyllum inophyllum oil is rich and thick, with a delicate nutty or spicy smell. It stimulates cell regeneration. It is good for fragile or broken capillaries. It helps wounds to heal and is soothing for eczema and skin irritations such as burns, rashes, and insect bites.

Camellia Oil

Camellia oil is good for preventing keloids, or unsightly thickening of the skin in scar tissue.

Canola Oil

Canola oil penetrates the skin quickly and softens skin. It is a light oil that has a high content of linoleic acid, which promotes skin health. It works well in massage or skin oils. Canola oil resists rancidity.

Evening Primrose Oil

Evening primrose oil has a high gamma-linolenic acid (GLA) content that promotes healthy skin and helps the skin repair itself. It soothes skin problems and inflammation, making it a good choice for people with psoriasis or any type of dermatitis. Evening primrose oil discourages dry skin and premature aging of the skin. It goes rancid easily, however.

Flaxseed Oil

Flaxseed oil is high in vitamin E, making it useful for preventing scarring and stretch marks. This rich, golden oil smells similar to melted butter. It nourishes the skin and promotes cell regeneration. It goes rancid quickly.

Grapeseed Oil

Grapeseed oil is a light oil that has no perceptible odor. The skin absorbs it easily. It is good to use as a skin oil or body oil on all types of skin. It is slightly astringent and tightens and tones the skin. Grapeseed oil does not aggravate acne.

Hazelnut Oil

Hazelnut oil lubricates and nourishes all types of skin. It tones and tightens the skin and helps to maintain firmness and elasticity. It also helps to strengthen capillaries. Add hazelnut oil to facial oils to encourage cell regeneration. A word of warning: Hazelnut oil that is low in price may be adulterated with other oils.

Jojoba Oil

Jojoba oil is very similar in composition to human sebum, or natural skin oils. It penetrates the skin rapidly to nourish it. It softens and moisturizes mature and dry skin. Jojoba oil helps to heal inflamed skin conditions such as psoriasis or any form of dermatitis; it also helps control acne, oily skin, and an oily scalp. Jojoba has antioxidant properties and can keep other oils from going rancid as quickly as they otherwise would. Use jojoba oil in fragrances and facial oils, and add it to massage oils, body oils, and hair treatments.

Olive Oil

Olive oil has very therapeutic properties that benefit both skin and hair. It soothes, heals, and lubricates the skin. Olive oil has a strong odor, however, making it most suitable for use with stronger smelling essential oils, such as basil, rosemary, tea tree, and thyme. You can add small amounts of olive oil to other carrier oils as well.

Peanut Oil

Peanut oil is a heavier oil with a heavier odor. It is therefore best used as a carrier oil for stronger smelling essential oils. It is very lubricating and does not penetrate the skin rapidly, making it useful in massage oils. It can be used by all skin types.

Rose Hip Seed Oil

Rose hip seed oil, also called rosa mosqueta oil, reduces scarring, heals burns, and softens scars and keloids. It is reputed to reduce fine lines and retard premature aging by promoting the regeneration of skin cells. It can help diminish broken capillaries. Rose hip seed oil may aggravate acne or blemished skin, however, and it goes rancid quickly.

Safflower Oil

Safflower oil is light, odorless, and inexpensive. However, it turns rancid very rapidly, and although it was frequently used in the past, it is no longer recommended for aromatherapy purposes. Use one of the other carrier oils discussed here instead.

Sesame Oil

Sesame oil is a thick oil with a heavy odor. Use it for massage oils containing stronger smelling essential oils such as basil, eucalyptus, rosemary, tea tree, and thyme. Sesame oil is good for all skin types and especially benefits eczema, psoriasis, and prematurely aging skin. Some people claim it helps arthritis.

Soy Oil

Soy oil is light, with a mild scent. It can be used on any type of skin. It nourishes dry skin and is readily absorbed by the skin. It does not aggravate acne or oily skin.

Sunflower Oil

Sunflower oil is easily absorbed and can be used on all skin types. Its high vitamin E content makes it especially helpful for delicate and dry skin.

Vitamin E Oil

Vitamin E oil is an antioxidant that extends the shelf life of other carrier oils and aromatherapy blends. It promotes skin healing and cell regeneration. It can prevent scarring and may fade existing scars with regular use. Because it is very thick, it is usually blended with other carrier oils. When buying vitamin E oil, look for 100-percent alpha-tocopherol oil. Avoid d-alpha-tocopherol, which is synthetic vitamin E.

Wheat Germ Oil

Wheat germ oil is a thick, sticky antioxidant oil that is high in vitamin E. It nourishes dry or cracked skin and soothes skin problems such as eczema and psoriasis. It helps to prevent or reduce scarring, and may prevent stretch marks. All skin types benefit from wheat germ oil, particularly mature skin.

PART TWO

An Introduction to 36 Essential Oils

Introduction

Of the estimated 350,000 species of plants on earth, relatively few produce essential oils. Only between 150 and 300 essential oils are currently available with the existing methods of extraction. Many of these essential oils are readily available and easily affordable. Others are harder to obtain, but with patience—and for the right price—you can find them. Some are extremely rare and quite costly. Still others I have only heard or read about and have yet to see or smell.

This section features a discussion of thirty-six different essential oils. Selecting these oils was not an easy task. I have enjoyed every essential oil I have ever used and have profited from each one. I feel, however, that these thirty-six are among the most useful and valuable essential oils and that they will bring the greatest benefits to the most people. These essential oils have a broad range of activities for health, beauty, and emotional well-being. They are fairly common and are easy to obtain. Any of them can be purchased from one or more of the suppliers listed in the Aromatherapy Resource Guide at the back of this book. Most are relatively affordable.

Three of the oils discussed here—jasmine, neroli, and rose—are rather expensive, but I have included them because they are three of the best essences for treating emotional problems. They also have tremendous value in skin care and the treatment of skin disorders. When you consider the value that just one drop of these oils can bring, it far outweighs the cost. Besides, they are three of the most delightful smells on earth.

Each of the sections in this part of the book is devoted to a single essential oil. The section begins with an introduction that describes the plant that is the source of the essential oil and tells you its botanical name, its botanical family, its native habitat, and the countries in which it is currently cultivated. Information about the physical characteristics, the aroma, and the extraction of the essential oil is also included. Each section is then subdivided into five parts: Folklore and Herbal Heritage, Medicinal Uses, Beauty Benefits, Emotional Effects, and Primary Actions, and, where appropriate, Cautions. Folklore and Herbal Heritage traces the plant's colorful history and tells about some of the ways people have used it in the past. Some plants have been used since the beginning of recorded history; in many cases, you will see how modern aromatherapy applications began. Some essential oils are still being used as remedies for the same ailments that our ancestors used them for hundreds or thousands of years ago.

Medicinal Uses focuses on the role of the essential oil today in maintaining health and treating physical problems. Much of the information in this section comes directly from medical research done in Europe. Many European physicians regularly prescribe essential oils for their patients. In fact, some use essential oils and other plant extracts exclusively, rather than prescription drugs. Beauty Benefits explains how a particular essential oil can be used to improve your appearance through skin, body, and hair care treatments. Aromatherapy skin care is one of the most natural and effective forms of skin care. Skin and hair care specialists across America and abroad are using essential oils to achieve results that satisfy their clients.

Emotional Effects discusses the impact that the essential oil can have on the emotions. Many psychotherapists in Europe treat their patients with essential oils and report being impressed with the results. Finally, Primary Actions and Cautions summarize the main actions of the essential oil and point out reasons for caution about using it, if any.

This part of the book will provide you with enough background information on each essential oil so that you can decide which oils you want to use, and so that you will feel comfortable and confident using them. Essential oils can make a great difference in your daily life, as well as being enjoyable to use. They are a great gift from nature that can open a gateway to healing and guide you on a path toward improved health.

Basil

Sweet basil is a tender annual herb with dark-green pointed oval leaves that may be fuzzy. It bears whorls of green, white, or pink flowers. The entire basil plant, *Ocimum basilicum,* emits a fresh, sweet, herbaceous scent. Steam-distilling the flowering herb produces a oil that can be colorless, pale yellow, or pale green. Basil oil has a light, spicy smell with a balsamic or camphor-like undertone.

Native to tropical Asia and Africa, this member of the Lamiaceae family is cultivated throughout Europe, the Mediterranean, on islands in the Pacific, and in North and South America. Brazil, Bulgaria, Egypt, France, Hungary, Indonesia, Italy, Morocco, South Africa, and the United States all produce basil oil.

FOLKLORE AND HERBAL HERITAGE

The word "basil" stems from the Greek words *basilokos,* meaning "royal," and *basileus,* meaning "king." The ancient Greeks considered basil the "king of plants." It was an important ingredient in a regal oil for anointing kings. The Greeks also prized the herb for its medicinal and culinary properties.

Hindus believed basil to be sacred to the deities Vishnu and Krishna. They placed sprigs of basil on the chests of deceased loved ones to protect them from evil and provide safe passage into the next life. Ayurvedic doctors prescribed basil to relieve respiratory problems such as asthma, bronchitis, colds, coughs, and emphysema.

Ancient Chinese doctors treated digestive and kidney ailments with basil. They also used it to cure epilepsy. Basil was a popular antidote for poisonous insect or snake bites. It was also used to fight fevers, epidemics, and malaria. Herbalists have recommended basil to alleviate headaches and to comfort colds. It has been used to soothe irritated skin conditions, nervous disorders, and the pain of rheumatism as well.

Many people have considered basil an aphrodisiac and it has been closely linked to love. Italian women placed basil plants on their balconies to alert suitors to their availability; a man would give a woman a sprig of basil in the hope that she would fall in love with him and remain forever faithful.

MEDICINAL USES

Today, European physicians treat a variety of respiratory ailments with basil oil. It can restore a lost sense of smell, relieve sinus congestion, and avert attacks of asthma, bronchitis, and emphysema. It can ward off colds and the flu and relieve whooping cough. Digestive disorders respond to basil oil's stomach-soothing properties. It aids digestion, dispels gas, prevents constipation, and relieves nausea, stomach cramps, and vomiting.

Basil oil opens and clears the head, and can ease headaches, including migraines. It helps overcome the nasal stuffiness of colds and the flu, while at the same time fighting infection. It can revive someone who has fainted. Basil oil also eases the discomfort of earaches, soothes mouth ulcers, and fights gum infections. It stimulates circulation and reduces muscle spasms and cramping. It reduces the pain of menstrual cramps and promotes menstrual flow. Basil oil helps relieve the pain of arthritis, rheumatism, muscular aches and pains, injuries, and physical overexertion. It acts as an insect repellent and can soothe the sting of mosquito bites and wasp stings. It also provides relief for many of the symptoms of chronic fatigue syndrome.

BEAUTY BENEFITS

Because basil oil has the ability to stimulate circulation, it enlivens dull-looking skin, improves skin tone, and gives the complexion a rosy glow. It helps to control acne. It also adds luster to dull hair.

EMOTIONAL EFFECTS

Basil oil possesses both sedating and stimulating actions. Its sedative action wards off anxiety attacks and nervous tension, and helps to vanquish insomnia; its stimulating action fights mental fatigue and strengthens mental functions. Basil oil increases concentration, sharpens the senses, clarifies thoughts, and clears the head. As a nerve tonic, basil oil can calm nervousness. In Europe, psychologists and physicians use it to treat melancholy and depression. Basil oil can minimize fear and sadness while fortifying weak nerves.

PRIMARY ACTIONS

Basil oil fights infection, clears the head, expels excess mucus, and cools fevers. It improves circulation and general bodily functions. Basil oil relieves muscle spasms and cramps and soothes digestive disorders. It stimulates menstrual flow and, in nursing mothers, it promotes the flow of milk. Basil oil maintains nerve health and decreases depression.

CAUTIONS

Because basil oil stimulates menstrual flow, it should be avoided during pregnancy. It can also trigger epileptic seizures in susceptible individuals, so if you suffer from a seizure disorder, it is wise to avoid it. The overuse of basil oil may have a sedative or stupefying effect. Basil oil may irritate sensitive skin.

Benzoin

Fragrant clusters of silky white blossoms adorn the benzoin tree, *Styrax benzoin*, which can attain an imposing height of up to 115 feet. When workers slash triangular cuts into the bark of benzoin trees that are over seven years old, the trees secrete a thick sap. The sap flows forth in tears, or lumps, that harden into a yellow to reddish-brown resinous mass. During an average productivity cycle of one decade, each tree yields a total of about thirty pounds of benzoin resin.

Native to Java, Sumatra, Thailand, and other tropical areas of Asia, this member of the *Styraceae* family produces a thick, exotic-smelling resin. The resin of the Siam benzoin tree (*Styrax tonkinensis*), which comes from Cambodia, Laos, Thailand, and Vietnam, is yellowish-red; that of benzoin Sumatra (*Styrax paralleloneurus*), which comes from Java, Malaysia, and Sumatra, is reddish- or grayish-brown. Both resins are thick and viscous, with a vanillalike aroma, although benzoin Sumatra has an undertone suggestive of cinnamon. Benzoin is also called gum benzoin, gum benjamin, and styrax benzoin. Because the gums or crude tears produced by these trees are so thick, they are either melted by heat or extracted with alcohol or a chemical solvent such as hexane before they are used.

For aromatherapy purposes, only solid benzoin tears or benzoin dissolved in alcohol should be used. Also, while for the sake of simplicity benzoin is often considered together with the essential oils, it is more accurate to refer to it as benzoin resin.

FOLKLORE AND HERBAL HERITAGE

Ancient peoples incorporated benzoin into incense for its sweet, soothing smell. They believed it could drive away evil spirits. Ayurvedic doctors treated shingles, ringworm, and other skin disorders with benzoin. Southern Asians used it to heal sores on their feet.

Benzoin was often added to cosmetics to keep skin clear and youthful. People in many different cultures have appreciated its ability to soothe and stimulate the skin. By adding benzoin to the animal fats used in making jasmine and tuberose enfleurage, perfumers protected those precious oils from turning rancid. Benzoin was also an important fragrance component in pomanders, potpourris, sachets, and soaps.

Tincture of benzoin, also known as friar's balsam, was used to help warm chills, fight the flu, and soothe sore throats, coughs, and laryngitis. By encouraging the movement of fluids through the body, it improved circulation, promoted urination, relieved congestion, and dispelled gas. Ballerinas applied friar's balsam to heal their battered feet.

MEDICINAL USES

Physicians in Europe still use benzoin resin for respiratory ailments such as asthma, bronchitis, colds, coughs, laryngitis, sinusitis, sore throats, and tonsillitis. Its soothing action tones the lungs, while its expectorant qualities reduce congestion and help the body expel phlegm. Benzoin resin helps improve physical strength, endurance, and energy, and is especially helpful during convalescence.

Benzoin resin increases circulation, eases the aches and pains of arthritis and rheumatism, and relieves sore muscles and stiff joints due to overexertion or physical activity. It improves digestion, calms the digestive tract, and alleviates flatulence. As a diuretic, benzoin resin increases urination, which can relieve the discomfort of urinary tract infections where urination is difficult or scant. Because of its antibacterial activity, it is often used to fight leukorrhea and yeast infections. Benzoin resin can also relieve some of the symptoms of premenstrual syndrome (PMS).

Benzoin resin soothes rashes and speeds the healing of wounds and sores. It soothes inflamed and irritated skin and relieves the redness and itching of psoriasis as well as eczema and other forms of dermatitis.

BEAUTY BENEFITS

Cosmetic chemists often add benzoin to protective skin care products because it helps chapped or blistered skin to heal. Its rejuvenating action repairs dry, cracked skin, especially on the hands and heels. Benzoin resin helps to maintain skin's elasticity and preserve its suppleness. Regular application can soften scar tissue over time.

EMOTIONAL EFFECTS

Benzoin's warming and soothing qualities extend to the emotions. It is mentally calming and pacifying and it eases nervous tension, stress, and anxiety. It calms the central nervous system. When you are feeling drained or emotionally exhausted, benzoin can soothe your frazzled nerves. It offers comfort in times of sadness or loneliness and its uplifting effect helps to overcome depression and restore confidence. Benzoin resin dispels anger, diminishes irritability, and reduces worrying. Its sweet scent is slightly sensuous, exotic, and euphoria-inducing. Some people say that it helps overcome sexual problems, especially impotence and premature ejaculation.

PRIMARY ACTIONS

Benzoin resin fights bacteria, inflammation, and

infection. It promotes urination, dispels gas, and releases mucus. Benzoin also tightens and tones tissue and encourages new cell production. It clears the head, tones the heart, and calms nerves.

CAUTIONS

For aromatherapy, only solid benzoin tears or benzoin resin that has been dissolved in alcohol should be used. If benzoin has been diluted with solvents, these can penetrate the skin and enter the bloodstream.

Bergamot

Lush green leaves and tiny white star-shaped flowers cover the branches of the bergamot tree, which can attain a height of sixteen feet. It bears a pear-shaped yellow fruit that is smaller than an orange and was once called the bergamot pear. The bergamot tree is the result of the crossbreeding of the lemon tree and the bitter orange tree, which created the bergamot hybrids *Citrus bergamia* and *Citrus aurantium,* subspecies *bergamia.*

A member of the *Rutaceae* family, bergamot originated in tropical Asia. Farmers in most countries have had little or no success in cultivating the tree commercially. Today, bergamot grows in the Ivory Coast in Africa, in the Calabria region of Italy, and in Sicily.

A simple pressing or expression of the rinds of the sour green fruit renders a pale emerald-green oil. It has a flowery lemon-orange smell with a slightly sweet, balsamic undertone. The best quality oil is hand pressed. Peels from 1,000 bergamot fruits yield about thirty ounces of oil.

FOLKLORE AND HERBAL HERITAGE

Some controversy exists about the origin of the word "bergamot." According to one story, the name originates from the Turkish word *beg-ar-mudu,* meaning "prince's pear." Another account claims that it comes from the name of the small town of Bergamo in northern Italy, supposedly the site of the original distribution of bergamot oil in Italy. Early tales credit Christopher Columbus with transporting bergamot from the Canary Islands to Italy, where it has been cultivated ever since. Since bergamot was virtually unknown to the rest of the world until relatively recently, most of the folklore concerning bergamot comes to us from Italy. Italians used it to cool and relieve fevers and protect against malaria. They took it internally to expel intestinal worms. Bergamot also gives Earl Grey tea its delightful flavor and distinctive aroma.

MEDICINAL USES

Bergamot oil possesses strong antiseptic properties, making it useful against urinary tract infections such as cystitis and urethritis. Using it in sitz baths can help prevent bacterial infections from spreading from the urethra to the bladder. Bergamot oil's antiseptic properties also alleviate respiratory ailments. It cools fevers, subdues the symptoms of colds and flu, and soothes sore throats, tonsillitis, and laryngitis. As a digestive aid, bergamot oil calms stomach cramps and stimulates the appetite.

Applied topically, bergamot oil can minimize the discomfort and hasten the healing of cold sores and other herpes infections, as well as mouth ulcers. It alleviates the pain of shingles and chickenpox, which are also caused by a herpes virus, varicella-zoster. It can heal dry, chapped, and irritated skin, making it an excellent choice for relieving symptoms of eczema and psoriasis.

Bergamot is useful in treating chronic fatigue syndrome. Used in a lamp or diffuser or as an inhalant, bergamot oil has been reported to help people who are trying to break the smoking habit. Bergamot oil fights fatigue from stress, helps restore physical and emotional strength, and is useful for restoring immunity in a person convalescing from a long illness.

BEAUTY BENEFITS

Bergamot oil's antiseptic action makes it useful for the treatment of acne and skin infections. Its astringent quality helps regulate excessive oiliness of the skin or scalp. Its deodorizing action can freshen your body, your home, or your office. Bergamot oil compresses help draw out the inflammation of blemishes or boils and promote rapid healing. Bergamot also repels insects and soothes insect bites. Along with neroli, orange, and rosemary, bergamot was a component of the original *eau de cologne*. Modern perfumers prize it for the fruity-floral bouquet it imparts to their creations.

EMOTIONAL EFFECTS

Bergamot oil is refreshing and uplifting. It acts as a stimulant and tonic to balance the emotions. Research conducted in Italy indicates that bergamot oil relieves feelings of fear and anxiety, diminishes depression and sadness, and calms anger. Studies show that it equalizes emotions and moods by balancing the activity of the hypothalamus. Smelling bergamot oil can stabilize a person in a shaky emotional state. Bergamot oil evokes feelings of happiness and joy and can restore self-confidence. During times of sadness or grieving, bergamot oil helps to heal emotional wounds and can inspire or restore loving feelings.

PRIMARY ACTIONS

Bergamot oil reduces pain and relieves muscle spasms. It fights infection, cools fevers, and kills insects. Bergamot oil calms nerves and diminishes depression. It clears excess mucus, tones the heart, aids digestion, and dispels gas. Bergamot oil encourages the growth of new tissue and the formation of healthy scar tissue.

CAUTIONS

Bergamot oil promotes sensitivity to the sun. Avoid wearing it outdoors in sunlight, as this can lead to severe burning or uneven darkening of the skin.

Black Pepper

A woody perennial crawling vine, the black pepper plant has heart-shaped leaves, small white flowers, and red berries that turn black when mature. The plant can climb up to twenty feet. The dried, crushed berries—or peppercorns—of *Piper nigrum* produce a clear to pale-green oil when steam-distilled. Its fragrance is fresh, dry, and warm, with woody, spicy, and sweet notes.

Native to southwest India, this member of the *Piperaceae* family is now cultivated and distilled in many tropical areas, primarily China, India, Indonesia, Madagascar, and Malaysia. Europe and America also produce some black pepper oil from imported peppercorns.

FOLKLORE AND HERBAL HERITAGE

Ayurvedic and Chinese doctors have used pepper for thousands of years to treat malaria and cholera and to relieve digestive difficulties such as dysentery and diarrhea. Indian monks ate black pepper every day to sustain their endurance and increase their energy.

MEDICINAL USES

Because black pepper oil stimulates circulation and improves muscle tone, it can relieve the discomfort of arthritis, muscular aches, rheumatism, sports injuries, and sprains. When massaged onto muscles before exercising, it prevents stiffness and soreness. Black pepper oil also relieves pain and stiffness following strenuous physical activity.

Black pepper oil helps to ward off and speed recovery from colds and the flu. It warms chills, clears congestion, and fights infection. As a digestive aid, black pepper oil increases the appetite and stimulates sluggish digestion. It soothes stomach cramps and reduces intestinal gas, and can help reduce colic, diarrhea, heartburn, and nausea. It also boosts red blood cell production in the spleen and may help overcome anemia.

BEAUTY BENEFITS

Applied to the skin, black pepper oil can be extremely stimulating and even potentially irritating. As a result, it is not usually used for skin care purposes. However, some women use it to eliminate cellulite because it stimulates circulation.

EMOTIONAL EFFECTS

Black pepper oil increases alertness and improves concentration. It stimulates mental energy, especially blocked energy. Black pepper oil can motivate people into action when they feel "stuck." It encourages feelings of courage and bravery, particularly about speaking in public. It is a very settling and stabilizing oil and provides a sense of

protection for vulnerable people. Some people use black pepper oil as an aphrodisiac.

PRIMARY ACTIONS

Black pepper oil fights infection. It relieves pain, cools fevers, and reduces muscle spasms. Black pepper oil stimulates the appetite, improves digestion, promotes bowel movements, dispels gas, and encourages urination. It increases circulation and improves overall body functions. It also increases sexual desire.

CAUTIONS

Black pepper oil may irritate the skin.

Cedarwood

Three types of cedar trees produce essential oils for aromatherapy purposes. The most common is red cedar, or *Juniperus virginiana*. Native to North America, this slow-growing tree attains a regal height of up to 100 feet. It grows primarily in the mountainous regions east of the Rocky Mountains. Distillation of its reddish heartwood and seed-bearing cones renders a yellow to orange oil with a sweet, balsamic scent.

Texas cedarwood, or *Juniperus mexicana,* is a smaller tree that grows up to twenty-one feet tall. It is native to the southwestern United States, Mexico, and Central America. Its viscous dark-orange or brown oil has a sweet, smoky, and woody aroma and is distilled from the tree's stiff green needles and twisted branches.

The Atlas cedar, *Cedrus atlanticus,* grows atop the Atlas mountains of North Africa. This member of the *Pinaceae* family reaches heights of 100 feet. Steam distillation of wood chips and sawdust from the Atlas cedar yields a thick yellow to honey-colored oil with a soft and sweet, warm and woody, pinelike odor.

About twenty-nine pounds of plant material is used to produce one pound of cedarwood oil. To obtain the oil of the red cedar, the tree must be felled; the other two cedar trees remain intact during the harvesting of their plant material. Some cedars can live for 1,000 to 2,000 years.

FOLKLORE AND HERBAL HERITAGE

During Biblical times, the famed cedars of Lebanon (*Cedrus libani*) provided one of the world's earliest perfumes. Visitors sought solitude in this holy forest, praying and seeking spiritual guidance. Although the oldest surviving cedar tree is 2,500 years old, most *Cedrus libani* trees were destroyed long ago.

Noah is said to have burned an offering of cedarwood and myrtle incense to show his gratitude for surviving the great flood. Tibetans likewise burned cedarwood incense in their temples; they also used it as a medicinal remedy. The Temple of King Solomon was built of cedarwood to symbolize strength, nobility, and dignity. In Greek mythology, Artemis was given the surname *Cedreatis* because images of her were hung high atop the cedar trees.

Cedarwood oil was an important ancient antidote for poisoning. The ancient Egyptians included cedarwood oil in their embalming preparations and they also constructed sarcophagi from cedarwood. Many of these 3,000-year-old coffins are still in good condition. Egyptian incense, perfumes, and cosmetics often contained cedarwood. When they discovered that the reddish-brown wood repelled insects, the Egyptians built ships and furniture from cedarwood. Each pharaoh owned his own ceremonial cedarwood barge.

A coating of cedarwood oil was used to protect papyri.

Native Americans in what is now New Mexico treated skin rashes, arthritis, and rheumatism with Texas cedarwood. Other Native Americans burned cedar leaves as incense, and used red cedarwood to fight respiratory ailments, tuberculosis, kidney infections, skin disorders, gonorrhea, venereal warts, and delayed menstruation. Cedar was also used to repel insects and vermin.

For centuries, people have used cedar-lined closets and chests to protect valuable clothing and personal belongings from moths and other insects. At one time a popular commercial insecticide contained cedarwood and citronella oils as active ingredients. Cedarwood chips were often added to sachets and potpourris to release a fresh, clean aroma into the atmosphere and to combat insects.

MEDICINAL USES

Like the oils from other coniferous trees, cedarwood oil makes an excellent choice for treating respiratory problems. Cedarwood oil eases coughs and decreases the discomforts of colds or the flu. As an expectorant, it helps expel mucus from the lungs; it also decreases the congestion common with bronchitis and sinusitis. Cedarwood oil promotes urination and is useful against urinary tract infections and prostate problems. Its antiseptic action assists in combatting infection, particularly cystitis and urethritis. It helps to control the pain and swelling of arthritis and rheumatism. Cedarwood oil heals skin rashes, soothes the discomfort and irritation of dermatitis and psoriasis, and fights fungal infections.

BEAUTY BENEFITS

Cedarwood oil contributes to clear skin by healing skin rashes and clearing blemishes. It reduces excessive secretions of sebum, or oil, and normalizes both dry and oily skin and hair. Cedarwood oil controls dandruff and seborrhea, improves the condition of the hair, and stimulates the scalp and hair follicles. It can minimize hair loss, and some men claim it even promotes hair growth.

EMOTIONAL EFFECTS

Cedarwood is a calming oil that eases anxiety, nervous tension, and stress-related conditions. It helps diffuse aggression, anger, and fear. It also helps stabilize energy imbalances. Cedarwood oil can comfort and strengthen you during difficult times, reinforcing resolve and independence. It can help you see situations more objectively and remain emotionally composed. Many people claim that cedarwood oil is an aphrodisiac as well.

PRIMARY ACTIONS

Cedarwood oil fights infection. It stimulates menstrual flow, increases urination, and clears excess mucus. It also calms the nerves and can stimulate sex drive. Cedarwood oil soothes and softens skin and strengthens bodily functions, particularly circulation.

CAUTIONS

Because cedarwood oil can stimulate menstrual flow, it should be avoided during pregnancy.

Chamomile

Three different species of chamomile—German chamomile, Roman chamomile, and chamomile mixta—are cultivated for their essential oils. All are members of the *Asteraceae* family and share similar properties.

The fine, feathery leaves of the Roman chamomile plant (*Chamaemelum nobile* or *Anthemis nobilis*) surround tiny daisylike flowers that are white with bright-yellow centers. This perennial plant attains a height of nine to twelve inches. Native to southern and western Europe, Roman chamomile is now cultivated in many different countries, including Belgium, Bulgaria, England, France, Hungary, and Italy. Steam distillation of the flowers renders a yellow essential oil with a sweet, warm, herbaceous odor.

German chamomile (*Matricaria chamomilla* or *Matricaria recutita*) is similar in appearance to Roman chamomile, except that it is taller (it grows about two feet tall) and its flowers have smaller heads and fewer petals. German chamomile is an annual. Once native to Europe and parts of Asia, it now grows in eastern Europe, Egypt, North America, and in areas of the former Soviet Union. German chamomile oil has a characteristic deep-blue or bluish-green color, and for this reason is sometimes referred to as blue chamomile. It gets its color from its high content of azulene, a chemical component that is produced during the distillation process and that also has a strong anti-inflammatory action. Stronger in smell than Roman chamomile oil, German chamomile oil has a sweet, slightly fruity, slightly spicy scent that is almost intoxicating.

Chamomile mixta, or Moroccan chamomile (*Anthemis mixta*), is a distant relative of the other two chamomiles and bears no physical resemblance to either. The chamomile mixta plant is characterized by hairy leaves and tubular yellow flowers. This native of northwestern Africa and southern Spain also grows in Egypt, Israel, and Morocco. Its oil smells spicy and fresh, with a balsamic undertone.

FOLKLORE AND HERBAL HERITAGE

The ancient Egyptians offered chamomile to Ra, their sun god, to honor and appease him. They also massaged chamomile into their skin to cool fevers, to alleviate aches and pains, and to relieve muscle soreness and spasms.

It was the ancient Greeks who gave chamomile its name. They called it *kamai melon,* which means "ground apple." Although the chamomile plant looks nothing like an apple tree, its sweet scent is reminiscent of fresh-cut apples. In Spanish, the herb and a chamomile-flavored sherry share the name *manzanilla,* meaning "little apple." Greek herbalists and physicians prescribed chamomile baths and poultices to relieve headaches and to dissipate disorders of the kidneys, liver, and bladder.

During the Middle Ages, Europeans scattered chamomile flowers on their floors. Stepping upon the flowers released a sweet fragrance into the atmosphere. Chamomile purportedly possessed the power to replenish a person's energy when he or she was confronted with adversity. In Beatrix Potter's famous children's story *Peter Rabbit,* Peter's mother gave him a dose of chamomile tea to calm and comfort him after a day of mischief in the garden. Chamomile tea has long been a popular nighttime beverage because it helps to induce restful sleep.

For centuries, herbalists have recommended chamomile for colic, gout, headaches, heartburn, indigestion, and loss of appetite, as well as to promote urination and relieve diarrhea. They have also suggested it to prevent nightmares or to help calm a person who has suffered from a nightmare. Chamomile poultices were applied for abscesses, swelling, and pain. Chamomile has long been a favorite of English country gardeners. Besides adding color and fragrance to the garden, this hardy plant repels insects. In fact, chamomile was nicknamed the "plant's physician" because it supposedly cured any ailing plant placed near it.

MEDICINAL USES

Modern European doctors prescribe chamomile to treat many of the same conditions for which traditional herbalists recommended it. Doctors regularly prescribe it as a sedative, stress-reducer, and digestive aid, as well as for healing skin problems. Chamomile oil reduces any kind of inflammation. Azulene, the chemical component that gives German chamomile oil its characteristic blue color, is largely responsible for chamomile's anti-inflammatory action. By reducing swelling and calming irritated skin, chamomile oil relieves the discomfort of psoriasis, eczema, dermatitis, and sunburn. In addition to reducing inflammation, chamomile fights infection and irritations, and speeds up the healing process. Chamomile oil relieves injuries such as bruises, inflamed tendons, sprains, and swollen or overexerted muscles. It soothes muscle pain and inflamed joints, and reduces the discomfort of arthritis and rheumatism.

Many Germans believe chamomile oil is capable of healing almost any problem. Medical practitioners in Germany recommend it for female disorders such as painful or irregular periods, scanty periods, vaginitis, menopausal problems, and premenstrual syndrome (PMS). Its diuretic properties reduce the fluid retention that often accompanies PMS, while its antidepressant action helps alleviate feelings of depression, irritability, and stress. Chamomile oil minimizes the pain of headaches, including migraines. It is often effective in treating symptoms of chronic fatigue syndrome.

Chamomile oil is mild enough to use on infants and children. For centuries, mothers have used chamomile to calm crying children, ease earaches, fight fevers, soothe stomachaches and colic, and relieve toothaches and teething pain. Chamomile oil can safely and effectively reduce irritability and minimize nervousness in children, especially hyperactive children.

BEAUTY BENEFITS

Scientific studies have shown that chamomile reduces dryness, itching, redness, and sensitivity in irritated and inflamed skin. Chamomile oil soothes dry or sensitive skin. With regular treatment, it can reduce the redness of fragile or broken capillaries. Chamomile oil conditions the hair and scalp and adds shine, silkiness, and luster to hair.

EMOTIONAL EFFECTS

Chamomile oil's subtle sedative action is much milder than that of harsh and potentially habit-forming prescription tranquilizers. Because it is calming and relaxing, it can combat depression, insomnia, and stress. It eliminates some of the emotional charge of anxiety, irritability, and nervousness. Chamomile oil can dispel anger, stabilize the emotions, and help to release emotions linked to the past. Applied over the throat, it can help a person express his or her true feelings.

PRIMARY ACTIONS

Chamomile oil calms nerves, promotes nerve health, and decreases depression. It softens and soothes skin, encourages cell regeneration, and soothes inflamed skin. Chamomile oil cools fevers and fights infection. It reduces muscular aches, pains, and spasms. It aids digestion, dispels gas, and settles the stomach. Chamomile oil increases urination and stimulates menstrual flow.

Clary Sage

From May to September, the clary sage plant displays hardy whorls of pale blue, purple, or pink blossoms atop long spikes. Heart-shaped green leaves with soft and fuzzy crinkled surfaces surround the flowers. This stout biennial or perennial is a member of the *Lamiaceae* family and attains a height of three to five feet.

Steam distillation of the flowering tops and leaves of *Salvia sclarea* yields a colorless or pale yellowish-green oil. The aroma of clary sage oil is sweet, fresh, and clean, with warm, herblike, nutty, and balsamic undertones.

Native to southern France, Italy, and Syria, clary sage is now cultivated worldwide, especially in Mediterranean climates, central Europe, England, Morocco, Russia, and the United States. Superior oils come from England, France, and Morocco.

FOLKLORE AND HERBAL HERITAGE

Herbalists throughout the ages have used clary sage to treat digestive disorders, kidney diseases, respiratory infections, and sore throats. It was also used to cool and calm inflammation and bring relief for abscesses, skin disorders, swelling, and wounds. The herb was a common remedy for female complaints.

Clary sage derives its name from the Latin *clarus,* meaning "clear," and was famous for its ability to clear eye problems such as tired or strained eyes or blurred vision. In fact, its nickname during the Middle Ages was "clear eyes." Mucilage from clary sage seeds would be inserted into the eye to expel a foreign object.

Germans called clary sage muscatel sage due to its similarity in taste to muscatel wine. Some wine merchants adulterated cheap wines with clary sage to impart the taste of the more expensive muscatel wine. When added to or taken with any alcoholic beverage, clary sage tends to exaggerate drunkenness and increases the discomfort of the hangover that follows.

MEDICINAL USES

The oil of common sage (*Salvia officinalis*) is often toxic, making clary sage a safer choice for aromatherapy. Clary sage oil possesses many of the same attributes and healing properties of common sage oil without the danger.

Clary sage oil contains hormonelike components that can balance female hormones. In Europe, physicians prescribe it to diminish menopausal discomfort, ease menstrual cramps, encourage delayed or scant periods, minimize the symptoms of premenstrual syndrome, and regulate menstrual cycles. It can cool hot flashes and ease migraines that are related to menopause or menstruation. Clary sage oil relaxes abdominal and lower back muscles and reduces the pain of menstrual cramps. It also relaxes muscular aches and pains resulting from mental or emotional stress and nervous tension.

Clary sage oil strengthens the immune system and is helpful in treating chronic fatigue syndrome. It restores and invigorates the body during convalescence from illness. Clary sage helps regulate blood pressure; high blood pressure often decreases after clary sage baths and inhalations. As a muscle relaxant, clary sage oil helps soothe spasms and tightness in the muscles surrounding the bronchial tubes of asthma sufferers. In addition, it alleviates the anxiety and emotional tension that frequently accompany asthma attacks. Clary sage oil relieves respiratory ailments such as colds, bronchitis, sore throats, laryngitis, and tonsillitis. It encourages better digestion by soothing the muscles of the digestive tract, and can calm such digestive disorders as colic, gas, and stomachache.

Psoriasis responds well to clary sage's ability to reduce inflammation, as do eczema and other types of dermatitis. Clary sage oil also helps cuts, wounds, and burns to heal. It minimizes the pain, itching, and irritation of herpes and candida outbreaks.

BEAUTY BENEFITS

Clary sage oil promotes the regeneration of skin cells, helping to ward off wrinkles and keep skin looking healthy and youthful. It helps oily skin and hair by controlling excessive oil secretions. It also improves acne and seborrhea. It is equally effective in treating dandruff, dry skin, and dry hair. Used as a scalp massage, clary sage oil reputedly encourages hair growth and minimizes hair loss.

EMOTIONAL EFFECTS

Clary sage oil balances the extremes of emotions and restores emotional equilibrium. It alleviates melancholy and lifts depression. As a nervous system tonic, it eases fear and nervousness. Clary sage oil helps both men and women become more aware of their feminine qualities. It can increase concentration and stimulate mental activity without being overstimulating. Clary sage oil inspires creativity and awakens intuitive powers. Many people report that they have very vivid dreams after using it. Clary sage oil makes an ideal companion in times of personal challenge or change, especially when there is external stress and extreme pressure. In situations of midlife crisis, clary sage oil can exert a balancing, inspiring, and revitalizing influence.

In stressful situations, clary sage oil reduces deep-seated tension, slows a racing mind, and calms nerves. By restoring inner tranquility, clary sage oil minimizes the debilitating effects of stress and stress-related disorders. It reduces irritability, anxiety, and feelings of panic as it revives frazzled nerves. Clary sage oil can even create a state of euphoria, and many people consider it an aphrodisiac. European physicians and psychotherapists have successfully treated cases of frigidity and impotence with clary sage oil.

PRIMARY ACTIONS

Clary sage oil restores nerve health, calms nerves, and diminishes depression. It fights infection, reduces inflammation, and relieves muscle spasms. Clary sage oil regulates the oiliness of the skin and hair and has a rejuvenating effect on the skin. It also aids digestion, regulates the menstrual cycle, and can heighten sexual desire.

CAUTIONS

Clary sage oil should be avoided during pregnancy because of its ability to stimulate menstrual flow. Also, you should avoid alcohol when using it. Clary sage oil can exaggerate the effects of alcohol and intensify drunkenness and hangovers. It can also cause drowsiness.

Coriander

The bright-green, feathery leaves of the coriander plant are delicately lobed. After its tiny, lacy white or pale-pink flowers bloom, they turn into green seeds that eventually become brown or brownish-gray. At maturity, the plant reaches a height of two to three feet.

Steam-distilling the crushed ripe seeds produces a colorless or pale-yellow oil with a fresh, spicy fragrance that is sweet, woody, and slightly balsamic. It takes about forty-five pounds of seeds to produce one pound of coriander oil.

Known also as Chinese parsley or cilantro, *Coriandrum sativum* is a member of the *Apiaceae* family.

Coriander is indigenous to Morocco and the Middle East, and is now grown commercially in India, North Africa, Russia, South America, southern Europe, and western Asia. Romania, Russia, and the other former Soviet republics produce the majority of coriander oil. Coriander leaf oil is also available. It smells similar to the seed oil but is stronger, greener, and not as sweet.

FOLKLORE AND HERBAL HERITAGE

Coriander is one of world's oldest flavorings and has been cultivated for over 3,000 years. The ancient Egyptians called it the "spice of happiness" and used it as an aphrodisiac. They also presented coriander seeds as funeral offerings to deceased pharaohs.

The ancient Greeks and Romans flavored wines with coriander and also used it as a medicinal herb. The Chinese incorporated coriander into their medical practice as long ago as 207 B.C., and believed that coriander could bestow immortality. Coriander was said to have grown in the Hanging Gardens of Babylon; the Hebrews supposedly used it as one of the bitter herbs in Passover rites.

After coriander was mentioned as an aphrodisiac in the *Arabian Nights,* numerous love potions containing coriander appeared. In India, coriander was used as a remedy for constipation and insomnia as well as to ease the pain of childbirth. In magical and religious ceremonies, Indians offered the seeds as gifts to their deities. Women consumed the seeds regularly and claimed they promoted fertility.

Coriander was a popular potted plant in England. During the Elizabethan era, candy-coated coriander seeds were served as a sweet after meals and to guard against gas. Besides being an integral part of many ethnic cuisines, coriander adds a distinctive flavor to Benedictine and Chartreuse liqueurs and a savory scent to many tobacco blends.

MEDICINAL USES

Like many other culinary herbs and spices, coriander improves digestion and alleviates such disorders as colic, diarrhea, gas, indigestion, stomach cramps, and nausea. Coriander oil stimulates the appetite; it can be useful for anorexics seeking to overcome eating disorders. Chinese physicians prescribe it for dysentery and nausea. Chewing on the seeds after a meal prevents indigestion and freshens the breath. Coriander oil can also stop hiccups.

As a circulatory stimulant, coriander oil encourages the release of toxins from the body, thereby improving conditions such as arthritis, chronic fatigue syndrome, gout, and rheumatism. It also helps regulate breathing. Coriander oil's antispasmodic and analgesic actions relieve muscular aches and pains and stiffness in the joints. It can diminish facial tension from stress and relax the facial muscles, and is therefore effective in relieving facial neuralgia and nervous facial cramps. In general, coriander is very cleansing and toning for the body and improves physical energy when it is low.

Chinese doctors recommend coriander for hemorrhoids, hernias, measles, and toothaches. European physicians use coriander oil to treat fatigue, flu, physical exhaustion, and migraines and other headaches. It is an overall tonic for the glands and can encourage estrogen production, helping to regulate the menstrual cycle and alleviate symptoms of premenstrual syndrome (PMS) and menopause. It also helps to reduce fluid retention.

BEAUTY BENEFITS

Coriander oil is a natural deodorant. Coriander oil is also frequently used in perfumery, particularly in men's fragrances. Because it stimulates circulation and fights fluid retention, it is helpful for cellulite.

EMOTIONAL EFFECTS

Coriander oil stimulates the central nervous system and relieves lethargy, mental fatigue, and nervousness. Some people say it decreases dizziness. It improves the memory and mental functions. Coriander oil can even inspire creativity.

Coriander oil refreshes and energizes, yet it is also relaxing and calming for anxiety, irritability, and stress. It is especially revitalizing during recovery from illness. Coriander oil brings comfort in times of emotional shock or fear. Due to its estrogenlike component, it balances female hormones and can stimulate erotic feelings. It also reputedly helps overcome impotence.

PRIMARY ACTIONS

Coriander oil relieves pain and muscle spasms, particularly if they result from arthritis. It stimulates the appetite and aids digestion. Coriander oil fights bacteria and fungi. It boosts circulation and stimulates the heart and the nervous system. It encourages menstrual flow and arouses sexual desire.

CAUTIONS

Because coriander oil can promote menstruation, it should not be used during pregnancy.

Cypress

Pointing upward toward the heavens, the cone-bearing cypress maintains an erect shape even at heights of over eighty feet. This evergreen, *Cupressus sempervirens,* has slender horizontal branches that bear small, round gray-brown cones, dark-green needles, and small flowers. Originally from southern Europe and western Asia Minor, this member of the *Cupressaceae* family now grows wild in France, Italy, North Africa, Portugal, Spain, and some of the Balkan countries. France, Italy, Morocco, and Spain are the primary producers of cypress oil.

Cypress oil is clear, light yellow, or greenish yellow in color. Its fragrance is sharp and smoky, warm and woody, resinous and spicy, with a lemony and balsamic undertone. Steam-distilling about thirty pounds of cypress needles, twigs, and cones yields one pound of oil.

FOLKLORE AND HERBAL HERITAGE

Ancient civilizations valued cypress for both medicinal and religious reasons. The Egyptians dedicated the cypress tree to the gods of death; the Greeks dedicated it to Pluto, the god of the underworld. In one Greek myth, when Cyparissus, a beloved of Apollo and Zephyrus, accidentally killed his favorite stag, his grief transformed him into a cypress tree. The evergreen branches of the cypress tree were considered symbolic of life after death. In fact, *sempervirens* means "ever-living." People in many cultures have planted cypress trees in cemeteries.

The ancient Egyptians treated urinary problems with cypress. They also used cypress to control problems involving excessive secretions of bodily fluids, such as heavy menstrual flow, perspiration, and diarrhea. The Chinese found cypress beneficial for the liver and respiratory system, and ate cypress nuts for their nutritional value. In the early twentieth century, one brand of French cough lozenges contained cypress.

MEDICINAL USES

Cypress oil stimulates circulation and has a detoxifying effect on the entire body. It relieves conges-

tion and eases coughing. It can also stop cuts and wounds from bleeding. Cypress oil soothes bleeding gums and periodontal disease. It provides relief from hemorrhoids. A cypress foot bath will ease tired, swollen feet and reduce foot odor and perspiration. Cypress oil can decrease any excessive flow of fluids, whether a runny nose, diarrhea, excessive menstrual flow, or perspiration.

Cypress oil releases muscle spasms and can avert an attack of asthma or bronchitis when used in a diffuser or as an inhalant. Cypress oil also relieves muscular cramps and sore muscles. It balances female hormones, eases heavy menstrual flow, relieves cramping, and reduces hot flashes during menopause. Massaged over the area above the ovaries, it reportedly can inhibit the growth of cysts. Used in a sitz bath, it speeds recovery from cystitis.

BEAUTY BENEFITS

Cypress oil regulates oil production, making it a useful treatment for oily skin, oily hair, acne, and dandruff. Its deodorizing action and its ability to control excessive bodily secretions make it beneficial as a deodorant. Cypress oil acts as a styptic and is ideal for stopping the bleeding of nicks and cuts from shaving. Broken capillaries and varicose veins respond well to cypress oil's stimulating properties and its ability to constrict blood vessels. It makes an effective treatment for cellulite because it strengthens weak connective tissues, improves circulation, and helps release toxins. It also repels insects.

EMOTIONAL EFFECTS

Cypress oil helps revitalize a nervous system that is overloaded with stress. It calms the mind and increases objectivity. It soothes upset emotions and helps stop crying fits. Cypress oil also improves concentration and helps focus thoughts. It helps to provide support and a sense of structure during major transitions, such as a career change, changes in relationships, divorce, loss of a loved one, or a change in residence. It gives comfort, strength, and endurance in times of grief or mourning.

PRIMARY ACTIONS

Cypress oil relieves pain and muscle spasms. It fights infection. Cypress oil constricts blood vessels, tightens tissues, and inhibits bleeding. It can reduce the excessive flow of bodily fluids. It soothes the emotions and subdues stress.

Elemi

As it sprouts new leaves, the elemi tree exudes a white resin with a pungent aroma. When exposed to the air, the resin hardens and turns yellow. Steam distillation of this resin yields a clear or light-yellow oil with a fresh, slightly sweet aroma that is citrusy and spicy. Sometimes the oil is called Manila elemi or gum elemi.

The elemi tree, *Canarium luzonicum,* is a member of the *Burseraceae* family and is a relative of the plants that produce frankincense and myrrh. The tree, which reaches heights of up to ninety feet, originated in the Philippines and the Moluccas, a group of islands in Indonesia. It is now cultivated commercially also in Brazil and Central American countries.

FOLKLORE AND HERBAL HERITAGE

In Arabic, *elemi* means "above and below," which has spiritual connotations. Ancient Turks and Arabs used elemi as an ingredient in incense, probably because it can heighten a meditative state. The ancient Egyptians used elemi in embalming because of its preservative properties.

Beginning in the fifteenth century, Europeans incorporated elemi into medicinal balms, liniments, and unguents. They also used it to treat respiratory problems. A topical plaster of elemi was used to help knit broken bones. Soldiers suffering from sword wounds supposedly found speedy relief by applying elemi to their wounds. Skin care products and cosmetics also frequently contained elemi for its skin-healing qualities.

MEDICINAL USES

Elemi oil activates the immune system. In Europe, physicians and aromatherapists use it to treat and tone the thymus gland, a key organ of the immune system. A good general stimulant for the entire body, elemi oil reinforces the body's ability to resist disease and restores physical strength, especially after an illness.

Elemi oil possesses many of the same properties that its relatives, frankincense and myrrh, have. It helps fight respiratory ailments such as bronchitis, colds, coughs, and the flu. It eases congestion and helps the body to expel excess mucus. Elemi oil tones the urinary tract and helps to cure cystitis. Massaging elemi oil onto the area where a bone has broken or fractured will hasten healing and minimize aches and pains, especially if it is applied before the bone is set in a cast. Continued treatment with elemi will help prevent rheumatic arthritis from developing in the area of the break. Elemi oil also hastens the healing of cuts, sores, and wounds, and encourages the development of new skin cells. It cools inflamed skin and can help clear chronic skin conditions such as eczema, especially weeping eczema, and other types of dermatitis. Fungal infections such as athlete's foot, candida infections of the skin, and fungal infections of the fingernails also respond well to elemi oil.

BEAUTY BENEFITS

Elemi oil's cell-regenerating action benefits dry or mature skin. It makes a rejuvenating treatment for wrinkled or sagging skin. By balancing sebum secretions, elemi oil helps to normalize either oily or dry skin. It can also control heavy perspiration.

EMOTIONAL EFFECTS

Elemi oil balances the nerves. It calms nervousness and promotes harmony within oneself and with others. It revitalizes a mind overwhelmed by mental fatigue or stress. Its sedative effect helps in overcoming stress-related disorders. Elemi oil strengthens, centers, and focuses the mind and emotions. It brings peacefulness and clarity, and acts as an aid to meditation.

PRIMARY ACTIONS

Elemi oil fights infection. It promotes cell regeneration and regulates the skin's oil production. Elemi oil relieves pain and calms nerves. It clears excess mucus. It tones the body and improves immune function.

CAUTIONS

Elemi oil may irritate sensitive skin.

Eucalyptus

As eucalyptus trees mature, their young round, silvery blue-green leaves turn into long, swordlike, deep-green leaves that emit the characteristic camphoraceous odor of eucalyptus. Woody seed pods dangling down from the creamy-colored branches almost completely cover the budding blossoms; hence the tree's name, which comes from the Greek word *eukalyptos*, meaning "covered" or "wrapped."

Eucalyptus oil has a refreshing, penetrating, and stimulating aroma that smells somewhat medicinal. About fifty pounds of eucalyptus leaves yields one pound of clear or pale-yellow eucalyptus oil.

Australia is the original homeland of eucalyptus, the tallest deciduous tree on earth. Some species of eucalyptus stretch skyward nearly 500 feet. Over 75 percent of all the trees in Australia are eucalyptus; in all, there are over 500 varieties of eucalyptus worldwide. They thrive in the Mediterranean-like climates of Algeria, California, Egypt, Hawaii, India, Portugal, South Africa, and Spain. Eucalyptus trees are also cultivated in India, Latin America, South Africa, southern Europe, and Tahiti.

Eucalyptus globulus is the most common species employed in aromatherapy, although over a dozen others—including *Eucalyptus australiana, Eucalyptus bakeri, Eucalyptus citriodora, Eucalyptus dives, Eucalyptus polybrachtea, Eucalyptus radiata,* and *Eucalyptus smithii*—also yield essential oils. The oil of *Eucalyptus citriodora* has a citruslike aroma; *Eucalyptus dives* yields an oil with a smell reminiscent of peppermint. All of these trees are members of the *Myrtaceae* family.

FOLKLORE AND HERBAL HERITAGE

Many mothers have massaged away their children's cold symptoms with rubs containing medicinal-smelling eucalyptus. Inhaling its fresh, camphorlike smell opens up sinuses and clears congestion. Eucalyptus' action in fighting colds, coughs, and other respiratory conditions is well known. During the 1940s and 1950s, cold and cough medicines commonly contained eucalyptus for its strong antibacterial, expectorant, and cough-suppressant properties.

Australian aborigines bound eucalyptus leaves around serious wounds to prevent infection and expedite healing. Water stored in the roots of eucalyptus trees provided liquid for native peoples and early European settlers in Australia. The settlers cultivated the trees for their hardwood and for their ability to fight malaria. The trees' massive root systems absorb large amounts of water, so they were able to drain the mosquito-infested marshes that fostered malaria. In addition, insects dislike the strong camphorlike smell emitted by eucalyptus leaves, which may explain the tree's success as an insect repellent. Veterinarians have administered eucalyptus to horses with influenza, dogs with distemper, and a variety of animals with parasitic skin afflictions.

MEDICINAL USES

Eucalyptus oil fights bacterial and viral infections that can cause colds, coughs, the flu, laryngitis, sinusitis, sore throats, and tonsillitis. It loosens and expels mucus and reduces inflammation. Eucalyptus oil eases nasal congestion and hay fever, and can prevent asthma attacks. It increases the blood's oxygen supply so that more oxygen and nutrients can be delivered to cells throughout the body. Eucalyptus oil also stimulates the regeneration of lung tissue. Dispersed through the air in a spray, diffuser, or vaporizer, it can inhibit the spread of infection.

Many popular topical medications rely on eucalyptus oil to relieve the joint pains, muscular aches, and swelling that accompany arthritis, rheumatism, and injuries. Eucalyptus oil can reduce the pain of headaches, including migraines. It kills germs and disinfects skin abscesses and wounds. It fights fevers by cooling down the body.

Used in sitz baths, eucalyptus oil can treat urinary tract infections such as cystitis. It encourages urination and fights bacteria that contribute to infection. It also helps improve immunity. Reports from Europe state that eucalyptus oil, especially when used together with geranium oil and juniper oil, can help to lower or regulate blood sugar levels. Used alone or with bergamot, eucalyptus oil minimizes the pain and hastens healing of cold sores, herpes outbreaks, chickenpox, and shingles. It speeds the process of recovery from burns and wounds, particularly slow-healing ones, and fights fungal infections such as athlete's foot or fungal infection of the fingernails. Eucalyptus oil repels insects and helps to reduce the sting of insect bites. Many commercial air fresheners and insecticides contain eucalyptus oil.

BEAUTY BENEFITS

Eucalyptus oil clears acne and skin blemishes by reducing excessive oiliness. It promotes the regeneration of skin tissue and can also soothe the pain of sunburn.

EMOTIONAL EFFECTS

Eucalyptus oil's stimulating and refreshing nature helps overcome sluggishness. During times of emotional overload, it can restore balance, improve concentration, and increase intellectual capacity. Eucalyptus oil can cool the heat of anger. After a fight or conflict, diffusing eucalyptus oil through the room will cleanse the environment.

PRIMARY ACTIONS

Eucalyptus oil fights bacterial, viral, and fungal infections. It eases respiratory congestion and cools fever. It relieves muscular aches and pains. Eucalyptus oil promotes cell regeneration and regulates the oiliness of the skin. It increases circulation and helps stabilize blood sugar.

CAUTIONS

Eucalyptus oil can irritate sensitive skin.

Fennel

Umbrellas of delicate yellow flowers rise above the gray-green feathery fronds stemming from the celerylike stalks of the fennel plant. After blooming, the flowers turn into grayish-brown seeds with a licoricelike flavor.

At maturity, fennel stands about four feet tall. Fennel oil, steam-distilled from the crushed seeds, smells similar to anise. It has a sweet and zesty, sharp and spicy, fresh and warm aroma.

Indigenous to the Mediterranean area, fennel flourishes in environments near the sea. Sweet fennel, or *Foeniculum vulgare dulce,* is a member of the *Apiaceae* family and is now cultivated in China, France, Germany, India, Iran, and Russia.

FOLKLORE AND HERBAL HERITAGE

The ancient Chinese used fennel to cure snakebite. The ancient Egyptians and Romans ate it after meals to tone their digestive tracts and release toxins from their bodies. Garlands of fennel were customarily awarded as praise to victorious warriors because fennel was believed to bestow strength, courage, and longevity.

The word fennel is derived from the Latin *fenuculum,* which means "hay." The plant probably got its name from fennel's frequent use as fodder. The ancient Greeks called it *marathon,* meaning "to grow thin." Wealthier Greeks supposedly ate fennel as a slimming aid because of the feeling of fullness it gave. For the same reason, poor people chewed fennel seeds to hush their growling stomachs and Roman soldiers chewed the seeds to stave off hunger during long marches when meals were sporadic. Devout Christians often used fennel for the same reason when fasting.

Fennel has been used for thousands of years for its toning effect on the female reproductive system. Physicians and herbalists have treated earaches, eye problems, insect bites, kidney complaints, and lung infections with fennel. It has also been used to expel worms. Medieval Europeans often hung bunches of fennel over doorways or stuffed it into keyholes to ward off evil spirits and block spells cast by witches.

MEDICINAL USES

Fennel oil helps rid the body of accumulated toxins, particularly after overindulgence in foods, spirits, or drugs. Its detoxifying properties are helpful for controlling cellulite and for dieting. Fennel also suppresses the appetite. European doctors have successfully treated gout with fennel oil. They also use it to prevent and cure arthritis and rheumatism because it prevents the buildup of toxins in the body, especially in the joints.

Fennel oil fights infection in the urinary tract. Its diuretic action prevents the retention of urine and aids in eliminating bladder infections by flushing toxins from the body. Eating fennel seeds reputedly prevents the development of kidney stones. Fennel oil also soothes a variety of digestive difficulties. It tones the stomach, improving digestion and easing stress-related indigestion. It relieves colic, gas, hiccups, nausea, and vomiting. By toning the smooth muscles of the intestines, fennel oil strengthens peristalsis and counteracts constipation.

Fennel contains a substance that is similar to estrogen and helps to regulate menstrual cycles, minimize symptoms of premenstrual syndrome

(PMS), and reduce fluid retention. Fennel can increase scant menstrual flow and heighten low libido. It is also helpful for menopausal distress. Estrogen helps maintain good muscle tone, skin elasticity, good cirulcation, and strong bones—all of which deteriorate with degenerative aging. Perhaps the ancients claimed that fennel promoted longevity because of its similarity in action to estrogen. Athletes use fennel oil in baths or massage oils to tone their muscles. It restores muscle tone and vitality to people convalescing after illness.

Bronchitis, colds, and coughs all respond well to fennel oil. It also helps fight gum infections. Fennel oil can pull poisons from insect and snake bites. In Europe, it is frequently used for its detoxifying action in the treatment and rehabilitation of alcoholics and drug abusers, and it can counteract alcohol poisoning. Fennel oil has a toning influence on the liver, kidneys, and spleen.

BEAUTY BENEFITS

Fennel oil's muscle-toning effect helps maintain youthful facial muscles. It reputedly wards off wrinkles and minimizes puffiness around the eyes. In addition, it restores moisture to dry and dehydrated skin. Some aromatherapists say that regularly massaging fennel oil into the breasts helps to keep them firm and attractive.

EMOTIONAL EFFECTS

Fennel oil has an overall calming effect on the emotions. It reduces stress and nervousness. Fennel oil provides a sense of protection, strength, and courage during vulnerable or emotionally low times. It can also increase sexual desire.

PRIMARY ACTIONS

Fennel oil reduces inflammation and relieves muscle spasms. It fights infection, kills insects, and clears excess mucus. Fennel oil stimulates appetite, promotes healthy bowel function, and increases urination. It regulates the menstrual cycle. It eliminates toxins and improves overall bodily functions.

CAUTIONS

Fennel oil should be used with caution by persons with seizure disorders, because it can trigger epileptic seizures in susceptible individuals. If you have a history of seizures, consult with a health care professional before using fennel.

Frankincense

The small, shrubby frankincense tree bears abundant foliage and white or pale-pink blossoms. Gatherers gash and peel back the bark, which exudes a milky white juice. When it comes into contact with air, this sap solidifies into tear-shaped lumps that are amber or burnt orange in color and range from about one-quarter inch to one-and-one-half inches in size. Steam distillation of the gum resin of *Boswellia carteri* or *Boswellia thurifera* renders a clear, pale-yellow, or yellowish-green oil. It has a warm and woody, sweet and spicy, rich and resinous aroma, with a light, lemony undertone. Some frankincense oil is extracted with alcohol or a chemical solvent such as hexane. Only steam-distilled or alcohol-extracted frankincense resin should be used for aromatherapy purposes.

A member of the *Burseraceae* family, frankincense is native to areas in the Middle East around the Red Sea, as well as to China, Iran, Lebanon, and Oman. It grows wild throughout northeast Africa, primarily in Ethiopia and Somalia. Most of the distillation takes place in Europe. There is some distillation of frankincense oil in India as well.

FOLKLORE AND HERBAL HERITAGE

Since the beginning of recorded history, frankincense has been associated with spirituality. The sensuous, spicy fragrance of burning frankincense wafted through temples in ancient Egypt. During religious rituals, Egyptians offered it to their gods in hopes of expelling evil spirits.

Since antiquity, frankincense has been incorporated into incense in China, Egypt, and India. Worshippers in these cultures inhaled it to achieve deeper levels of meditation. Today the tradition of burning frankincense continues in some churches.

Frankincense was a prized possession in ancient times, as valuable as many precious gems and metals. As a result, it exerted an influence on the political activities of many countries, and crises developed when various governments attempted to monopolize the frankincense market. It was the major economic resource of some Arabic countries. The queen of Sheba, which was a main supplier of frankincense in ancient times, reportedly undertook a perilous journey to visit King Solomon in Israel to ensure his business.

Camel caravans voyaged through treacherous terrain and extremes of weather to deliver this beloved botanical from Arabia to other parts of the known world. Both the Egyptians and the Hebrews spent fortunes importing it from the Phoenicians. Egyptians mixed it with cinnamon to soothe aching muscles and limbs. Babylonians and Syrians dedicated abundant amounts of frankincense to their gods. Besides burning frankincense for religious purposes, the Romans relied on it for government ceremonies as well as for its many medicinal properties. According to the Bible story, it was given as a gift to the baby Jesus, probably because it was so cherished and valuable, and also because of its association with spirituality.

The ancient Chinese used frankincense to treat leprosy and tuberculosis. Both Eastern and Western medical practitioners treated such conditions as digestive disorders, nervous complaints, respiratory problems, rheumatism, skin diseases, syphilis, and urinary tract infections with frankincense. Frankincense was one of the first cosmetic "miracle" ingredients; it proved so successful when Egyptian embalmers used it to preserve the bodies of dead royalty and rulers that people decided to take advantage of its rejuvenating and restorative properties while they were still alive. They began formulating cosmetics with frankincense to maintain soft and supple skin. One of its most popular applications was in a rejuvenating facial mask. Facial oils, ointments, and perfumes also contained frankincense.

MEDICINAL USES

Medical professionals in Europe and England today prescribe frankincense oil to treat many of the same disorders as the ancients did. It has a soothing and healing effect on mucous membranes, wounds, and inflammations. As an expectorant, it can clear congestion in the lungs. Frankincense oil reduces swollen lymph glands in the neck. It soothes respiratory problem such as colds, coughs, bronchitis, and laryngitis; it eases shortness of breath and helps avert asthma attacks.

Frankincense oil soothes stomach distress and eases digestive difficulties. It is frequently used in Europe to treat reproductive and urinary tract maladies. Medical practitioners say that it alleviates the discomforts of cystitis, genital infections, and kidney complaints. Inflammation of the breast responds well to applications of frankincense oil. Some doctors use it to tone the uterus and relieve uterine hemorrhaging and heavy menstrual flow.

Frankincense oil can also ease labor pains and decrease postnatal depression.

BEAUTY BENEFITS

Although well known to ancient peoples, for centuries frankincense oil's skin-beautifying properties were practically forgotten. Its restorative, regenerating, and rejuvenating actions are especially useful for dry, mature, and sensitive skins. It smooths lines and wrinkles, and soothes and softens raw, chapped skin. Frankincense oil's astringent properties help balance oily skin. It accelerates the healing of blemishes, inflammations, sores, scars, skin ulcers, and wounds. Frankincense was one of the first botanical essences to be used in fragrances. It has a powerful fixative quality and is still used to add "staying power" to perfumes.

EMOTIONAL EFFECTS

Frankincense oil can help to fortify a mind burdened with mental anxiety, nervous tension, or stress. It reduces anxiety and revitalizes the body and mind when a person is mentally or physically exhausted. It comforts and soothes the emotions and heals emotional wounds. Frankincense oil can help you sever ties with the past that are hampering your personal growth. By slowing respiration, frankincense oil produces a sense of serenity and calms restlessness. It is a stabilizing and centering oil and helps to focus energy.

PRIMARY ACTIONS

Frankincense oil reduces inflammation, fights infection, and clears excess mucus. It tightens and tones skin, and stimulates cell regeneration. Frankincense oil aids digestion. It increases urination, stimulates menstruation, and tones the uterus. It also calms nerves.

Geranium

Of over 700 varieties of geranium, only a few—*Pelargonium roseum, Pelargonium graveolens, Pelargonium odorantissimum,* and *Pelargonium radula*—produce essential oils. The entire plant, including leaves, stalks, and flowers, is steam-distilled to produce a pale greenish-yellow oil with a green, sweet scent that is sometimes rosy, sometimes minty.

Originally native to southern Africa, these members of the *Geraniaceae* family now flourish in many countries. China, Egypt, Morocco, Russia, and the island of Réunion, in the southwestern Indian Ocean, specialize in the commercial cultivation of geraniums. Many authorities believe the world's finest geranium oil comes from Réunion.

FOLKLORE AND HERBAL HERITAGE

For centuries, geraniums have adorned window boxes, walkways, gardens, and homes around the world with splashes of brilliant red, lavender, pink, and white blossoms. Both the showy flowers and serrated-edged leaves of these tender perennial plants can emit delightful fragrances. Dutch sailors transported geraniums to Europe from Africa during the 1600s. Europeans appreciated them for their delightful fragrance and their adaptability to the European climate. Many gardeners planted geraniums to ensure that no evil spirits would enter their homes. Colonial American housewives lined baking pans with rose geranium leaves to impart a delicate rose flavor to their cakes.

Herbalists and doctors treated such maladies as dysentery, hemorrhoids, inflammations, and heavy menstrual flow with geranium. Some folkloric sources even claimed geranium as a cure for cancer; others say it has been used as a remedy for bone fractures, tumors, and wounds. Nineteenth-century perfumers discovered to their delight that inexpensive rose geranium oil smelled similar to costly rose oil. Few of their customers could detect the difference in the final fragrances.

MEDICINAL USES

European physicians today prescribe geranium oil to treat such ailments as diarrhea, gallstones, kidney stones, and urinary tract infections. It relieves respiratory problems, particularly sore throats and tonsillitis. Geranium oil can balance hormones; it stimulates the adrenal cortex, which regulates the balance of hormones secreted by other organs. Some European physicians recommend it for treating diabetes. Geranium oil improves immune function and is helpful for relieving some of the symptoms of chronic fatigue syndrome.

Geranium oil provides many European women with relief from female problems such as painful periods, premenstrual syndrome (PMS), and menopausal difficulties. It normalizes fluctuating hormones during menopause. In addition, geranium oil is a diuretic and diminishes fluid retention, a common source of discomfort with PMS. It can ease inflammation of the breast and reduce breast engorgement. Geranium oil stimulates the lymphatic system and the circulatory system, making it useful for boosting circulation and for reducing or eliminating edema. It helps to ease skin disorders such as eczema and other forms of dermatitis, herpes infections, and seborrhea, and accelerates the healing of bruises, burns, cuts, skin ulcers, and other wounds.

BEAUTY BENEFITS

Geranium oil helps almost any skin type or skin condition. Its stimulating action promotes the regeneration of skin cells and speeds the healing of acne and blemishes. It also soothes dry, sensitive skin. Geranium oil imparts a healthy glow to the complexion, making the skin appear radiant and more youthful. It improves the appearance of broken capillaries and varicose veins. Because it stimulates both the lymphatic and circulatory systems, geranium oil helps to combat the kind of sluggish circulation and waste accumulation present with cellulite, and it clears skin that is blemished or dull and dry as a result of the accumulation of toxins. Geranium oil also helps control excessive oiliness of the skin.

EMOTIONAL EFFECTS

Inhaling geranium oil eases the anxiety and tension of mentally and physically demanding days. Like most flower oils, geranium oil acts as an antidepressant. Its uplifting effect frees the mind from negative or depressing thoughts. Almost any stress-related condition responds to a few whiffs of geranium oil. As an added bonus, geranium oil can stimulate feelings of sensuality.

Geranium oil encourages self-expression, improves communication, and helps overcome the fear of speaking. It promotes harmony between the sexes and balances aggressive and passive tendencies. Some people respond to geranium oil's sedative, somewhat analgesic effect; others say it stimulates them. For most people, it simultaneously calms and energizes.

PRIMARY ACTIONS

Geranium oil relieves pain and fights infection. It stops the bleeding of cuts and wounds. It stimulates new cell growth and tones and tightens tissue. Geranium oil diminishes depression and lowers blood sugar levels. It increases urination and reduces fluid retention.

CAUTIONS

Geranium oil can lower your blood sugar level. Use it with caution or avoid it if you have hypoglycemia (low blood sugar).

Ginger

The glossy grasslike spears of this tropical perennial protrude upward two to four feet from thick, spreading tuberous roots called rhizomes. Erect reedlike spikes with compact white, yellow, or yellow-green conical flowers stem directly from the rhizomes, which look like white or beige hands with multiple fingers.

Sharp and spicy, peppery and pungent, warm and wonderful, the aroma of golden-yellow or amber ginger oil has slightly woody and lemony undertones. Ginger oil is steam-distilled from the unpeeled dried ground roots of the plant.

Native to southern Asia, China, India, and Java, *Zingiber officinale* is a member of the *Zingiberaceae* family. Ginger is now cultivated in the tropical regions of China, India, Jamaica, Japan, Nigeria, and the West Indies. Many experts claim the finest ginger grows in Jamaica. Most ginger oil comes from China, England, and India.

FOLKLORE AND HERBAL HERITAGE

For thousands of years, ginger has been treasured as a spice and medicinal remedy. Over 4,000 years ago, the enticing aroma of warm gingerbread emanated from Greek ovens. The Greeks treated stomach disorders with ginger and administered it as an antidote to poison. The ancient Egyptians incorporated ginger into their cuisine to ward off epidemics, and it was a staple in Arabian pharmacies. Romans took advantage of its aphrodisiac powers and added it to wine. Indians drank ginger tea to soothe upset stomachs.

Chinese doctors prescribed ginger as a tonic to strengthen the heart, to relieve head congestion, and to fortify the constitution. They treated any illness associated with cold, damp conditions—such as colds and flu—as well as rheumatism, headaches, and muscle tension with ginger.

Hawaiians scented their clothing with ginger root. They also cooked with ginger and used the fresh root to cure indigestion. They made shampoos and massage oils from the secretions of ginger flowers.

During the Middle Ages, ginger found its way to Europe via the spice route. From there it crossed the Atlantic Ocean with Spanish explorers headed for South America and the Caribbean.

MEDICINAL USES

Today, European physicians prescribe ginger oil for ailments ranging from digestive disorders to respiratory ailments, jet lag to motion sickness, sore throats to menstrual cramps. Ginger oil increases immunity and often can ward off colds and the flu. It warms chills caused by dampness and it reduces fevers and cools down the body by inducing sweating. Ginger oil soothes the pain of sore throats and tonsillitis. It also reduces the drainage of a runny nose and eases respiratory infections.

Ginger helps to calm an upset stomach and alleviate nausea. It can avert the discomfort and queasiness of a hangover, motion sickness, or morning sickness. Ginger promotes better digestion by stimulating the secretion of digestive juices. It also increases appetite, relieves gas and diarrhea, and soothes cramps, whether intestinal or menstrual. The *British Herbal Pharmacopoeia* indicates ginger for gas and colic.

As an analgesic, ginger relieves the pain of arthritis and soothes sprains and muscle spasms, especially in the lower back. It stimulates circulation and is useful for treating varicose veins. Chinese doctors use fresh ginger to treat a wide variety of conditions, including chills, colds, coughs, congestion, diarrhea, dysentery, the flu, malaria, rheumatism, sinusitis, and toothaches. Ginger oil can also speed the healing of bruises, sores, and blemishes.

BEAUTY BENEFITS

Ginger oil is widely used in perfumery to impart a sharp green, spicy note to fragrances, particularly men's colognes. It is rarely used in skin care because of its tendency to irritate sensitive skin, but because it increases circulation, ginger oil is sometimes used to treat varicose veins and cellulite.

EMOTIONAL EFFECTS

Ginger oil's warming tendency can heat up a cold, dull, or fearful emotional nature. It warms the heart and opens up feelings, helping to improve communication. Ginger oil sharpens the senses, improves memory, and aids in recall. It stimulates energy, yet at the same time it is helpful in cases of nervous exhaustion. Its aphrodisiac qualities may help in cases of impotence, especially when ginger is combined with coriander and rosemary.

PRIMARY ACTIONS

Ginger oil diminishes digestive discomfort, stimulates appetite, and eases nausea. It promotes bowel movements and dispels gas. Ginger oil fights infection and relieves pain. It cools fevers and warms chills. Ginger stimulates circulation and improves the functions of the body. It can increase sexual appetite.

CAUTIONS

Ginger oil can be irritating to sensitive skin.

Helichrysum

Shiny golden daisylike flowers sit atop the ball-shaped flower heads of the helichrysum plant, which is also known as Italian strawflower. These papery flowers emit an enticing, almost intoxicating fragrance with the essence of honey. The pale-yellow or yellowish-green essential oil they yield has a sweet, warm, and woody scent, with spicy and rosy undertones.

Due to its dry nature, helichrysum produces a limited quantity of oil. Several species of the flowering tops of helichrysum may be codistilled to increase yields of this essential oil.

Indigenous to Africa and Australia, helichrysum—also called immortelle—will grow almost anywhere, even in poor soil conditions, although it prefers a hot, dry climate with abundant sunlight. *Helichrysum angustifolium, Helichrysum gymnocephalum, Helichrysum orientale, Helichrysum italicum,* and *Helichrysum kilimandjarum* are all members of the *Asteraceae* family, and they prosper in Italy, Spain, the south of France, and other Mediterranean countries, both in the wild and as cultivated crops.

FOLKLORE AND HERBAL HERITAGE

Early herbalists recommended helichrysum for many respiratory conditions, such as asthma, bronchitis, and whooping cough; as a relief for headaches; and as a cure for liver ailments and skin disorders. Helichrysum is more popular, and probably more familiar to many people today, as an ornamental dried flower. Commonly called everlasting, it lives up to its name by retaining its fragrance, color, and shape almost forever.

MEDICINAL USES

European physicians prize helichrysum oil as a treatment for any skin disorder or irritation because of its ability to reduce inflammation and fight bacterial infection. Helichrysum is also recommended for abdominal or stomach cramps, bronchitis, colds, coughs, gallbladder infections, menstrual cramps, and sinus infections. Helichrysum oil stimulates digestion and improves the function of the liver and the pancreas. It can ease digestive, facial, or pulmonary spasms, as well as other muscle spasms. It also reduces the swelling and inflammation of arthritis.

Helichrysum oil has virtually unlimited value in treating dermatitis and other skin disorders. Its ability to reduce inflammation exceeds that of any other essential oil. It improves the itching, redness, scaliness, and puffiness of psoriasis as well as that of eczema and other forms of dermatitis. Helichrysum also relieves the pain and redness of sunburn.

BEAUTY BENEFITS

Helichrysum helps to decrease the inflammation of acne. In addition, helichrysum oil encourages regeneration of the skin and helps it adapt to stress. Mature skin responds especially well to helichrysum oil's restorative properties.

EMOTIONAL EFFECTS

Helichrysum oil helps clarify thought processes and opens the mind to new concepts and ideas. During times of transition, it helps to instill self-confidence and provide the illumination necessary to accept change. Helichrysum oil activates the right side of brain, elevating awareness, awakening intuitive and creative processes, and inspiring personal growth. It also helps improve meditation and visualization. Some people report that helichrysum oil increases their dream activity and helps them to remember their dreams, which sometimes deliver important messages to them.

PRIMARY ACTIONS

Helichrysum reduces inflammation and relieves muscle spasms. It fights bacteria, fungi, and viruses. Helichrysum softens and soothes skin, tightens and tones tissues, and stimulates new cell growth. It improves the function of the liver, spleen, and gallbladder. It also calms nerves.

Jasmine

Delicate white star-shaped jasmine flowers fragrance the air with their exotic, erotic, and nearly narcotic aroma. Shiny green leaves cover the large evergreen shrub *Jasminium officinalis* or *Jasminium grandiflorum,* which can reach twenty to thirty feet in height. Jasmine can also grow along the ground or cascade downward in vines. Native to China, India, and Iran, this member of the *Oleaceae* family is chiefly cultivated in China, India, the Mediterranean countries, and northern Africa.

Working at night, gatherers pick these flowers by hand, making the production of jasmine essence very labor-intensive. About 1,000 pounds of flowers—or over 3.5 million blossoms—yields just one pound of precious jasmine essence.

While jasmine is commonly considered together with the essential oils, because of the way in which it is extracted it is more accurate to refer to it as jasmine enfleurage or jasmine absolute. For simplicity's sake, however, jasmine enfleurage and jasmine absolute are referred to as jasmine essence in this section.

Jasmine essence is a thick, mahogany-colored oil that has a rich warm, floral scent with tealike undertones. This intensely sweet "king of essential oils" smells of mystery and magic. Its long-lasting fragrance has a pheromonelike quality, perhaps due to its chemical similarity to human perspiration, which some scientists speculate may contain pheromones.

FOLKLORE AND HERBAL HERITAGE

In India, jasmine was called the "queen of the night" and "moonlight of the grove," and was used as both an aphrodisiac and an aid to spiritual growth. For millennia, women have adorned their bodies with perfumes and cosmetics made with jasmine. In many religious traditions, the jasmine flower symbolizes hope, happiness, and love.

The Chinese treated hepatitis, cirrhosis of the liver, and dysentery with jasmine. They also used it to help overcome nervous system disorders, including depression and nervousness, and to ease coughs and improve breathing. For centuries, the Chinese have enjoyed drinking jasmine tea. Jasmine was a favorite fragrance of the Japanese for both perfumes and incense. The Japanese used jasmine as a remedy for reproductive problems, and to stimulate uterine contractions in pregnant women as childbirth approached.

MEDICINAL USES

In Europe, many physicians use jasmine essence to ease labor pains and encourage contractions. It helps to speed the expulsion of the afterbirth and overall recovery from giving birth. It also helps to relieve postnatal depression. Jasmine essence stimulates the production of milk, tones the uterus, and can induce menstrual flow. It can also soothe and comfort women going through menopause.

Jasmine is helpful for men as well as women. It strengthens the male reproductive system and can relieve the discomfort of an enlarged prostate gland. As an aphrodisiac, jasmine helps overcome impotence and frigidity.

Jasmine essence also helps to soothe muscle spasms and sprains. It can calm coughs, ease hoarseness and laryngitis, and act as an expectorant to help the body clear excess mucus. Jasmine essence calms skin inflamed as a result of a skin disorder such as dermatitis, or as a consequence of stress or an emotionally related disorder.

BEAUTY BENEFITS

The hormone-balancing action of jasmine essence affects the condition of the skin. Jasmine benefits any skin type—whether dry, oily, irritated, or sensitive. It inhibits bacteria and regulates oil production, thereby helping acne and oily skin. Jasmine essence also helps to moisturize dry, dehydrated, or mature skin. Jasmine has played an important part in all grand perfumes, softening and smoothing out any harsh notes.

EMOTIONAL EFFECTS

Jasmine essence benefits almost any nervous condition. It decreases anxiety, depression, nervous exhaustion, and stress. It elevates spirits and balances moods. Jasmine essence encourages optimism and self-confidence while diminishing fear. It is both emotionally and physically relaxing.

Jasmine essence warms the emotions and helps counteract apathy and indifference. It spurs creativity, inspires artistic expression, and awakens intuition. It arouses an appreciation of the beauty in the world and helps dissolve emotional blocks that hinder personal growth. The sensual and inspirational aroma of jasmine essence creates a sense of euphoria that engenders trust and true love. As a sensual stimulant, jasmine promotes feelings of attractiveness and allure.

PRIMARY ACTIONS

Jasmine essence diminishes depression, calms nerves, and stimulates sexual feelings. It relieves pain and eases muscle spasms. Jasmine essence reduces inflammation, fights infection, and clears excess mucus. It softens and soothes skin, tones the uterus, eases delivery during childbirth, and promotes the flow of milk in nursing mothers.

CAUTIONS

Because jasmine can stimulate menstruation, it should be avoided during pregnancy until childbirth is imminent.

Juniper

Of over fifty species of juniper, only one—*Juniperus communis*—yields the berries that produce juniper oil. This evergreen member of the *Cupressaceae* family bears green needles, yellow flowers, and round bluish-green berries that turn black upon maturity. Juniper may sprawl near the ground as a prickly shrub two to four feet high or stand erect as a bush of six to twelve feet tall. Some wild junipers grow as high as thirty feet.

Fresh ripe, black berries, when steam-distilled, produce a clear or yellowish-green oil. The oil has a pinelike aroma with spicy, peppery, and earthy undertones. Juniper trees, which are native to Europe, have become naturalized throughout the Northern Hemisphere. They flourish in the forests of Canada, Korea, and Sweden, and atop mountains in Hungary and Scotland. Austria, Canada, France, Germany, Italy, Slovakia, and Spain produce the most juniper oil.

FOLKLORE AND HERBAL HERITAGE

Ancient Egyptians anointed their bodies with juniper and used it to embalm the bodies of the dead. They burned juniper incense for physical and spiritual purification. During biblical times, juniper was often used to banish evil spirits. According to one traditional story, Mary hid the baby Jesus under a juniper tree to protect him from King Herod, earning the juniper the reputation of affording protection against harm.

Because black pepper was expensive and difficult to obtain, ancient Romans used juniper berries in place of pepper to flavor their food. They added the crushed berries to wine and drank it to treat liver complaints and for its diuretic action. The ancient Greeks burned juniper berries to discourage epidemics.

Juniper has been used in many parts of the world to fight the spread of plagues, epidemics, and contagious diseases. As late as 1870, French hospitals burned juniper wood for this purpose during a smallpox epidemic. During the Middle Ages, people found multiple uses for juniper: as a cure for headaches, kidney, and bladder problems, as a treatment for pulmonary infections, and as a fever reducer. Bundles of juniper berries were hung over doors to ward off witches, and burning juniper wood supposedly deterred demons. Many medieval Europeans considered juniper a panacea.

The Dutch are said to have been the first to flavor gin with juniper berries. Native Americans ate juniper berries alone or added them to their food. They drank tea made from the stems and leaves of the plant to relieve arthritis and urinary tract infections. They also applied juniper topically to cleanse infections and heal wounds, and burned the needles and branches for purification.

MEDICINAL USES

For centuries, juniper's primary medicinal application has been for urinary tract problems. Juniper oil encourages urination, fights infection, and helps the body to eliminate wastes, especially after indulgence in rich foods and/or alcohol. It is useful for menstrual difficulties; it eases painful menstrual cramps, promotes menstruation for women with scant or late periods, helps to regulate the menstrual cycle, and reduces fluid retention. Juniper oil is also useful in treating leukorrhea. Juniper oil sitz baths can ease the pain of hemorrhoids.

Juniper can minimize the pain of muscle spasms and the aches of arthritis. It speeds the healing of bruises, skin ulcers, and wounds. Respiratory problems such as bronchitis, colds, and coughs respond to inhalations of juniper oil. Juniper oil tones the digestive tract, stimulates or regulates appetite, and combats sluggish elimination, especially when one is recovering from illness. By encouraging the elimination of wastes and stimulating circulation, juniper oil helps to improve such conditions as arthritis and fluid retention. It accelerates healing, particularly of slow-healing wounds, and is helpful for psoriasis and dermatitis.

BEAUTY BENEFITS

Juniper oil is good for any kind of skin inflammation. Because juniper oil promotes the elimination of cellular wastes and stimulates circulation, varicose veins and cellulite conditions often respond to it. Juniper oil enlivens dull skin and helps to

clear acne. It can regulate oiliness, making it useful in treating acne, oily skin, oily hair, and seborrhea. Juniper is frequently added to fragrances, cosmetics, after-shaves, and men's colognes.

EMOTIONAL EFFECTS

Juniper oil helps to fight anxiety, nervous tension, and stress. It can clear mental clutter and confusion, revive exhausted emotions, and strengthen nerves. Juniper oil helps to neutralize negative emotions, particularly anger or confusion, and imparts a feeling of emotional cleanliness and purity.

PRIMARY ACTIONS

Juniper oil relieves muscle spasms and pain. It stimulates new cell growth. Juniper oil promotes the elimination of wastes, increases urination, and stimulates menstrual flow. It also kills germs and fights infection.

CAUTIONS

Juniper should be avoided during pregnancy because it can stimulate menstrual flow. Also, juniper activates the kidneys, so persons with kidney problems should consult with a health care professional before using it.

Lavender

Beautiful blue-violet or deep-purple blossoms resembling tiny purple pine cones grow in whorls around a single lavender stalk. The abundant branches have long, narrow pale silvery-green leaves. This woody evergreen shrub grows three or four feet tall.

Lavender smells clean and fresh and permeates the air with a delightful aroma that simultaneously stimulates and relaxes. Steam-distilling the flower tops and stalks produces a colorless, pale-yellow, or yellow-green oil. It has a sweet, floral, and herbaceous scent with a balsamic, woody undertone. An acre of lavender plants will yield about fifteen to twenty pounds of essential oil. Distilling only the blossoms produces a superior oil. Of the over thirty different species of lavender, *Lavandula officinalis*, *Lavandula angustifolia*, and *Lavandula vera* are the most popular varieties for producing essential oils. French lavender (*Lavandula stoechas*) is also used in aromatherapy.

A member of the *Lamiaceae* family, lavender thrives high atop the dry, rocky, sun-drenched mountain slopes in its native France, Persia (now Iran), the Mediterranean countries, and Tasmania. It is now also cultivated commercially in Bulgaria, England, Greece, Italy, Russia, Spain, and Turkey. France is the primary producer of lavender oil.

FOLKLORE AND HERBAL HERITAGE

The ancient Greeks and Romans prized lavender as a perfume and for its cleansing properties. They lavished it upon their bodies in scented soaps and baths. The Romans are credited with naming it, although there are two different theories of the name's derivation. One theory holds that "lavender" comes from the Latin word *lavare*, meaning "to wash," while according to the other, it derives from the Latin word *lividula*, which means "bluish in color." It is known that ancient Romans added lavender to their baths to relieve fatigue and stiff joints. Despite their enjoyment of lavender, however, the plant symbolized mistrust to them, probably because they believed lavender bushes were inhabited by the deadly asp.

Medieval Europeans considered lavender an herb of love. Many claimed it had aphrodisiac

properties; others touted its ability to keep the wearer chaste. England's Queen Elizabeth I supposedly ate lavender conserves most mornings. Lavender flowers freshened sickrooms and were added to potpourris for their fragrance. They were commonly strewn on floors so that when stepped upon, the flowers would release their essence into the air. This tradition continues today in Portugal and Spain.

For centuries, lavender was used as a remedy for ailments as diverse as insect bites, lice, muscular aches and pains, nervous disorders, scabies, sprains, and toothaches. Herbalists frequently prescribed it to fight fatigue, relieve respiratory ailments, and soothe stomachaches. Women relied on lavender to keep their skin clean, clear, soft, and supple.

Early twentieth century medications for colic, coughs, headaches, hoarseness, nervous palpitations, sore joints, and toothaches contained lavender oil. It was also used as an ingredient in smelling salts. In homes throughout Europe, delicate lavender sachets lined linen closets, scented lingerie drawers, and protected clothing from moths and insects. During World Wars I and II, soldiers and medics carried lavender oil with them on battlefields for disinfecting wounds.

MEDICINAL USES

European health professionals prescribe lavender oil for an array of ailments—digestive disorders, earaches, respiratory illnesses, skin disorders, and sore throats. Lavender oil clears the congestion and stuffiness of sinusitis and other respiratory ailments; it soothes sore throats, laryngitis, and tonsillitis. Lavender oil eases the pain and discomfort of muscular aches, spasms, and injuries, and helps to heal bruises, cuts, and insect bites. It relieves the pain of migraines and tension headaches. It is also useful in reducing some of the symptoms of chronic fatigue syndrome, and helps to boost immunity.

Lavender oil soothes the inflammation of skin disorders, including psoriasis, eczema, and other types of dermatitis. It cools burns and provides relief for cold sores and herpes. Lavender oil can treat many common childhood maladies. Because it is very mild, it is safe for infants and children.

BEAUTY BENEFITS

Lavender oil calms and soothes the skin. It balances oil production, helps heal blemishes, and stimulates circulation to the skin. Lavender oil reduces the inflammation of acne and soothes the pain of sunburn. It regulates the oil secretions of the scalp and helps repair damaged or overprocessed hair.

EMOTIONAL EFFECTS

Throughout Europe, physicians and psychologists recommend lavender oil for emotional difficulties such as depression, fear, insomnia, irritability, melancholy, mood swings, nervousness, and stress. They say that it strengthens the nervous system. Lavender oil clears thinking, dissipates fears, minimizes anger, and reduces worry. By balancing extremes of emotion, it contributes to emotional equilibrium. It relaxes the mind and promotes physical and mental well-being. Lavender oil can neutralize sensory overload and balance either a racing or sluggish mind. Used at bedtime, it helps overcome insomnia.

PRIMARY ACTIONS

Lavender oil stimulates new cell growth. It lifts depression, calms nerves, and promotes nerve health. Lavender oil fights infection, reduces inflammation, and eases congestion. It relieves pain

and muscle spasms. Lavender oil lowers blood pressure.

Lemon

The small, evergreen lemon tree has serrated-edged oval leaves, stiff thorny branches, and fragrant white or pale-pink flowers. The round or oval green fruits of *Citrus limon* or *Citrus limonum* turn sunshine-yellow when ripe. A native of India and Asia, this member of the *Rutaceae* family grows about eighteen feet tall. Lemon trees grow wild in Mediterranean climates and are cultivated in Guinea, Israel, Italy, and North and South America.

Cold expression of the fresh peels of the fruit renders a pale greenish-yellow oil. Its scent is fresh and light, slightly sharp but sweet, with the tart and tangy smell of fresh lemons. About 1,000 lemons will yield one pound of oil.

FOLKLORE AND HERBAL HERITAGE

The ancient Egyptians used lemons to fight food poisoning and typhoid epidemics. Inhabitants of Spain and some other European countries regarded lemon as a panacea for infectious illnesses. Europeans used it to resist malaria and typhoid fever. Lemons and limes were carried on English ships to control scurvy on long voyages. Credit goes to Christopher Columbus for carrying lemon seeds to the New World.

Historically, herbalists have used lemons to lower blood pressure and suggested fresh lemon juice for internal cleansing, for clearing excess toxins from the liver, and for relief from arthritis and muscular aches and pains.

MEDICINAL USES

French physicians treat such disorders as diabetes, gonorrhea, high blood pressure, malaria, syphilis, tuberculosis, and typhoid with lemon oil. It fights the infection of bronchitis, coughs, and sore throats, and relieves the discomfort of colds, fevers, and the flu. It can also avert asthma attacks. Because lemon oil can kill bacteria and other germs in minutes, many European hospitals use it to sanitize hospital rooms and kill airborne germs.

Lemon oil enhances immunity by stimulating white blood cell production and improving the body's ability to combat infection. It helps in treating disorders that may be related to a weakened immune system, such as chronic fatigue syndrome. As a digestive aid, lemon oil counteracts acidity in the body, calms an upset stomach, and helps heartburn. It encourages the elimination of wastes, reduces constipation, and eases arthritis. It tones the heart, kidneys, and liver. Lemon oil helps lower blood pressure and stimulates circulation.

Lemon oil can stop the bleeding of cuts and wounds. It helps with shaving nicks, nosebleeds, and bleeding gums from gingivitis or tooth extractions. Lemon oil also diminishes the pain of cold sores, herpes, and mouth ulcers. It relieves some of the symptoms of eczema and other types of dermatitis, and can help relieve headaches.

BEAUTY BENEFITS

Lemon oil balances overactive sebaceous glands that lead to oily or blemished skin, helps clear acne, and controls oily hair and dandruff. It revitalizes underactive and mature skin and helps with cellulite by improving circulation and encouraging the elimination of wastes. Lemon oil encourages the exfoliation of dead skin and enlivens the complexion. Long-term treatment with lemon oil reduces broken capillaries and varicose veins, softens scar tissue, and minimizes warts and corns. Lemon oil can also strengthen brittle nails.

EMOTIONAL EFFECTS

Lemon oil is cooling, refreshing, and uplifting. It encourages clarity, concentration, and recall. It can calm or prevent emotional outbursts. It fights depression, eases fear, strengthens resolve, and assists in communication and decision-making.

PRIMARY ACTIONS

Lemon oil fights infection, cools fever, and stops bleeding. It tightens and tones tissues and softens and soothes skin. Lemon oil promotes bowel movements and increases urination. It lowers both blood sugar and blood pressure. Lemon oil stimulates the immune system.

CAUTIONS

Lemon oil may be irritating to sensitive skin. It may also promote photosensitivity, leading to sunburn or uneven darkening of the skin.

Marjoram

Marjoram is a bushy tender perennial that grows up to one foot in height. Its many branches have square stems and tiny oval gray-green leaves that may be fuzzy. Knotlike buds borne on spikes open to form clusters of white or pink flowers. When in full bloom, marjoram branches are steam-distilled to produce an oil with a warm, woody, spicy, slightly peppery, camphorlike, and nutty aroma that is calming and comforting.

Thymus mastichina is commonly called Spanish

marjoram or Spanish wood marjoram. As the name implies, it grows primarily in Spain. Its oil is pale orange to amber in color and has a distinctive eucalyptuslike aroma. Sweet marjoram (*Origanum majorana* or *Majorana hortensis*) is native to the Mediterranean, North Africa, and southwest Asia. It produces a bright-yellow oil that often darkens with age.

Marjoram, a member of the *Lamiaceae* family, is grown in gardens around the world and is a favorite in English country gardens. Most of the marjoram oil used for aromatherapy is produced in Bulgaria, Egypt, France, Germany, Hungary, Morocco, and Tunisia.

FOLKLORE AND HERBAL HERITAGE

The ancient Romans called marjoram the "herb of happiness"; the Greeks called it "joy of the mountains." In both cultures, newlyweds were crowned with garlands of marjoram to bless them with marital bliss. Wreaths and garlands of marjoram served as decorations at weddings and funerals. Marjoram was used to warm both the body and the emotions. Greek physicians treated rheumatism, muscle spasms, and fluid retention with marjoram. They also used it to ease breathing and as an antidote for poisoning.

In many cultures, marjoram was believed to increase longevity. Growing it on a gravesite was meant to comfort the departed one buried there. In the Elizabethan era, the English would brew a blend of marjoram, rosemary, and sage with wine to treat blackened teeth. Women carried nosegays of marjoram to mask unsavory smells. Those curious about their futures anointed themselves with marjoram at bedtime so that they might dream of their future mates.

MEDICINAL USES

Physicians in Europe today use marjoram oil to treat high blood pressure and heart conditions. Marjoram oil dilates blood vessels, reducing the strain on the heart and creating warmth beneath the skin. It eases the pain of arthritis, tense muscles, and muscle spasms. Its warming action increases flexibility and range of motion, and it can prevent or reduce the pain of sports injuries. By improving circulation, marjoram oil encourages the removal of wastes from the muscles following physical exertion. It also relaxes overworked muscles and soothes sprains and strains.

Marjoram oil can counteract the symptoms of premenstrual syndrome (PMS), ease menstrual cramps, and stimulate menstrual flow. It improves digestion, reduces intestinal cramps from colic, and soothes an upset stomach. By strengthening peristalsis, it reduces gas and relieves constipation. Marjoram oil eases asthma, bronchitis, colds, and sinusitis. It calms coughs and soothes sore throats. Its calming and sedative actions help to alleviate migraines, tension headaches, and insomnia. Marjoram oil also reduces some of the symptoms of chronic fatigue syndrome.

BEAUTY BENEFITS

Marjoram facilitates the drainage of blood from bruised areas, helping to minimize bruising and speed healing time. It also helps release tension from facial muscles.

EMOTIONAL EFFECTS

Marjoram oil relaxes the body and mind and helps relieve insomnia. It calms emotions and minimizes emotional upsets, making it useful for anxiety, emotional exhaustion, nervous tension, and stress. Marjoram oil provides comfort during times of grief, loneliness, and sadness. It strengthens willpower. Marjoram oil gives greater control over sexual desire; regular use can permanently numb erotic sensations and impair sex drive and sexual function.

PRIMARY ACTIONS

Marjoram oil relieves pain and muscle spasms. It fights infection and lowers blood pressure. Marjoram oil improves digestion and promotes elimination. It stimulates menstrual flow. Marjoram oil calms nerves and decreases sexual desire.

CAUTIONS

Marjoram oil can cause drowsiness, so you should avoid driving or operating machinery when using it. It should also be avoided during pregnancy as it stimulates menstruation. Long-term use may permanently inhibit sex drive.

Mint

See PEPPERMINT.

Myrrh

Myrrh has a sweet, smoky, slightly musky, slightly spicy aroma with a warm, rich, timeless quality. To some people, the incenselike odor smells medicinal; others consider it spiritual. Its taste may explain the origin of its name, which comes from an Arabic word meaning "bitter."

Myrrh oil comes from a thorny, sparse, and scraggly shrub or tree, known as either *Commiphora* *myrrha* or *Balsamodendron myrrha*. There are several different varieties, growing to heights of about nine to fifteen feet in dry climates. The trees' sturdy branches are knotted with aromatic leaves and small white flowers.

Also called true myrrh or herrabol myrrh, this member of the *Burseraceae* family is native to Arabia, northern Africa, southwestern Asia, and the region around the Red Sea, especially Ethiopia, Somalia, and Yemen. Historians believe that myrrh grew in the Tigris and Euphrates valleys, now thought to be the site of the biblical Garden of Eden. Today, most myrrh is obtained from the Middle East, particularly Iran. It is collected by making incisions into the gray bark of the trunks of myrrh trees. This encourages the exudation of its gum resin, a pale yellowish-white fluid that hardens into reddish-brown tears.

Steam-distilling the resin renders a pale-yellow or amber oil. Myrrh oil may also be extracted from the tears of resin by means of alcohol or a chemical solvent such as hexane. Only steam-distilled or alcohol-extracted myrrh oil should be used in aromatherapy.

FOLKLORE AND HERBAL HERITAGE

From antiquity, ancient cultures made myrrh an integral part of religious rituals, medical practice, beauty treatments, and perfumery. Writings from over 2,700 years ago mention myrrh and its uses in embalming, perfumery, and incense. Originally, myrrh was collected from the beards of goats that grazed on the tasty leaves of myrrh bushes. Myrrh was used as a cure for cancer, leprosy, and syphilis. Over 2,000 years before the Magi were said to have presented myrrh, frankincense, and gold to the baby Jesus, myrrh was a precious commodity along the spice route. Demand far exceeded supply, making myrrh one of the most expensive items in the world.

References in the Bible, the Vedas, ancient Egyptian papyri, and the Koran link myrrh to religious rituals. The Egyptians burned myrrh incense in their temples. They burned Kyphi, an incenselike substance that contained myrrh, every day at noon in sun-worshipping rituals; during evening ceremonies they offered myrrh as a consecration to the moon. The Egyptians believed that in addition to appeasing the gods, Kyphi incense quelled fear and anxiety, improved meditation, and induced restful sleep with pleasant dreams.

The Egyptians employed myrrh in mummification because it kept skin and body tissues intact. Embalmers would smear a thin coat of myrrh resin over the skin to preserve it before wrapping the body in cloth. Such expensive treatments were usually reserved for pharaohs and high officials. Eventually, when clever "cosmetic chemists" realized that myrrh would work similar wonders on living skin, they incorporated it into balms, facial masks, pomades, and unguents.

Young Persian girls, preparing for court, used myrrh as part of a ritual purification. The ancient Hebrews created a holy anointing oil from myrrh, cinnamon, calamus, cassia, and olive oil; Moses consecrated his priests with it. Israelite women wore myrrh sachets next to their bodies, probably to have their body heat release myrrh's fragrant aroma and mask body odor. An unguent of myrrh, coriander, and honey was used to treat herpes. Prior to his crucifixion, Jesus was offered a drink of myrrh mixed with wine, probably as a form of sedative.

In Greek mythology, Aphrodite forced the goddess Myrrha into an incestuous relationship with her father, Cinyras. Cinyras avenged the act by turning his daughter into a myrrh tree. When the tree sprouted its blooms, their child Adonis was born. The resinous drops that exude from cuts in the tree's bark were said to be Myrrha's tears.

Myrrh held a prominent place as one of the most important aromatic materials in ancient perfumery.

Alexander the Great became enamored of myrrh and burned myrrh incense incessantly in his court. Greek and Roman perfumers created myrrh resins that were the longest lasting perfumes of the day. Regarded highly for its fixative properties, myrrh could last for up to ten years, often improving with age. Myrrh continues to lend its fixative powers and its smoky, balsamic undertones to about 7 percent of the perfumes produced today, particularly ones with exotic or heavy floral fragrances.

MEDICINAL USES

In Europe, physicians prescribe myrrh oil for arthritis, inflammation, gum disorders, and menstrual difficulties. Myrrh oil boosts immunity by stimulating the production of white blood cells. It fights infection and speeds recovery from illness. It tones the digestive tract, stimulates appetite, reduces stomach gas and acidity, and alleviates diarrhea. European gynecologists use myrrh oil to treat scanty menstrual periods, leukorrhea, and thrush, and to cleanse obstructions in the womb. Chinese doctors treat arthritis, hemorrhoids, menstrual problems, and wounds with myrrh.

Doctors prescribe myrrh oil for such respiratory ailments as bronchitis, colds, and coughs. It clears excess mucus, eliminates congestion, and soothes inflamed membranes. Myrrh oil relieves the itching and irritation of weeping eczema and fights the fungal infection of athlete's foot, candida, jock itch, and ringworm. The *British Herbal Pharmacopoeia* lists myrrh as a treatment for gingivitis and mouth ulcers. Many health care practitioners claim that myrrh oil is the best treatment for oral ulcers, gingivitis, periodontal disease, and other gum disorders. It can also prevent bad breath.

BEAUTY BENEFITS

Myrrh oil maintains healthy skin and reputedly

prevents premature aging of the skin. Many people claim it wards off wrinkles. Myrrh oil soothes and softens rough, cracked, or chapped skin. It stimulates the regeneration of skin cells, reduces inflammation, fights infection, and helps to heal wounds. It improves circulation, imparting a healthy glow to the complexion and helping skin look smoother and more youthful. Myrrh oil also helps heal blemishes, skin ulcers, and wounds.

EMOTIONAL EFFECTS

Myrrh oil fortifies the nerves and emotions. It replaces feelings of apathy, weakness, and lack of initiative with motivation, power, and strength. Myrrh oil provides the clarity, focus, and strength to pull through troubled times. Its cooling and calming effect subdues angry or inflamed emotional states.

PRIMARY ACTIONS

Myrrh oil fights bacterial and fungal infections and reduces inflammation. It encourages new cell growth and promotes wound healing. Myrrh oil expels mucus and tones the lungs. It aids digestion and reduces gas. It restores and maintains healthy gums.

CAUTIONS

Because of its ability to stimulate menstrual flow, myrrh oil should be avoided during pregnancy.

Neroli

Pale-yellow neroli oil emits a sweet, full-bodied citrus aroma with a slightly spicy, slightly bitter undertone. Neroli oil is produced from the delicate white blossoms of the bitter orange or Seville orange tree. This evergreen tree bears glossy, dark-green oval leaves, and in May and October, an abundance of small white flowers appear. One ton of hand-picked blossoms from *Citrus aurantium,* *Citrus bigaradia,* or *Citrus vulgaris* yields only one quart of neroli oil, or orange blossom oil. This makes neroli oil comparatively expensive. Unfortunately, distillers and suppliers often adulterate neroli due to its high cost.

The bitter orange tree, which grows to heights of twenty to thirty feet, belongs to the *Rutaceae* family. Once native to central Asia and China, these trees now grow in subtropical regions of California, Mexico, and South America, as well as in areas surrounding the Indian Ocean and the Mediterranean. Farmers in Egypt, Italy, Morocco, Sicily, southern France, Spain, Tunisia, and the Comoro Islands, located off the southeast coast of Africa, cultivate commercial crops of bitter orange trees. Many experts claim the best neroli oil comes from Tunisia.

FOLKLORE AND HERBAL HERITAGE

So enamored of the smell of orange blossoms was Anna Maria de la Trémoille, a seventeenth-century princess of Nerola (in what is now Italy), that she adorned herself and almost everything in her environment with its fragrant oil. Elite members of the court followed her lead, making orange blossom oil the most sought-after scent of the time. In praise of the princess, orange blossom oil was said to have been given the name *neroli* (although another account suggests that the name is derived from that of the Roman Emperor Nero).

Throughout history, brides have crowned their heads with garlands of orange blossoms and woven the blossoms into bridal bouquets. Orange blossoms symbolized chastity; brides wore them to signify that their purity was equal to their loveliness. Neroli's ability to calm the nerves probably helped many brides to be composed on their wedding nights.

On the other hand, neroli purportedly possessed aphrodisiac and euphoria-inducing properties, and prostitutes once supposedly wore it to distinguish themselves. Prospective customers could easily detect a prostitute by the unique smell of neroli emanating from her body.

Herbalists often recommended orange flower water, a byproduct of the steam distillation of neroli, to aid digestion. For centuries, people in North Africa and the Middle East have added orange flower water to various foods, both to impart a delightfully sweet flavor and to increase their digestibility. Mothers would give babies a spoonful of orange flower water to induce sleep or overcome insomnia. People drank orange flower tea for its enjoyable flavor, to fight off fevers, and to protect against plagues.

Neroli was a component in Hungary water, reputedly created by Queen Elizabeth of Hungary. The queen claimed that the formula healed her of crippling, disfiguring arthritis; afterwards she won the love of a man many years her junior. The original *eau de cologne*, formulated in the eighteenth century, also contained neroli, along with bergamot, lavender, lemon, and rosemary.

MEDICINAL USES

Pharmacies still sell orange flower water as a digestive aid and sedative. European physicians and aromatherapists use neroli oil to settle heart palpitations and gently calm a person suffering from shock. Some health care practitioners use it to lower blood pressure. Neroli oil is helpful for diarrhea, especially diarrhea that is related to nerves or stress. It soothes tense muscles and muscle spasms.

It can bring relief for menstrual cramps and premenstrual syndrome (PMS). Neroli also soothes the irritation and itching of psoriasis, eczema, and dermatitis.

BEAUTY BENEFITS

Neroli oil increases circulation and stimulates new cell growth. It can prevent scarring and stretch marks. It is useful in treating skin conditions linked to emotions or stress, as it calms the emotions as well as the skin. Any type of skin can benefit from neroli oil, although it is particularly good for dry, irritated, or sensitive skin. It regulates oiliness and minimizes enlarged pores. Neroli oil helps to clear acne and blemished skin, especially if the skin lacks moisture. With regular treatment, it can reduce the appearance of fragile or broken capillaries and varicose veins.

EMOTIONAL EFFECTS

Neroli oil soothes emotional upsets and eases anger, depression, grief, hysteria, mood swings, nervousness, and shock. Health care practitioners and aromatherapists in Europe use it to bring quick relief for anxiety attacks and to treat chronic anxiety. Neroli oil subdues stress and tension. Its hypnotic effect helps to induce sleep. It encourages confidence, courage, joy, peace, and sensuality. Neroli oil can provide the strength and support to get through difficult or trying times.

PRIMARY ACTIONS

Neroli oil calms nerves, lifts depression, and increases sexual desire. It fights infection and inflammation. It relieves muscle spasms. Neroli oil stimulates new cell growth and softens and soothes skin. It aids digestion and dispels gas.

Orange

Smooth and shiny oblong leaves, fragrant white flowers, and sweet-tasting, nutritious fruit adorn the bounteous orange tree. The bitter orange tree, *Citrus aurantium,* yields orange oil from its fruit, neroli oil from its flowers, and petitgrain oil from its foliage. The sweet orange tree, *Citrus sinensis,* yields orange oil from its fruit and occasionally an oil called neroli Portugal from its blossoms.

Cold-expressing either whole oranges or orange peels, by hand or machine, yields a yellow or orange oil with a zesty, refreshing, slightly green-smelling, and very citrusy aroma. Some orange oil is steam-distilled from fresh orange peels. Approximately fifty oranges render one ounce of orange oil.

Native to China and India, the orange tree belongs to the *Rutaceae* family. Oranges grow abundantly in the Americas, Israel, and Mediterranean countries. Brazil, Cyprus, Israel, Mexico, and the United States are the primary producers of orange oil.

FOLKLORE AND HERBAL HERITAGE

From early times, oranges have been associated with generosity and gratitude. Once called "golden apples," oranges symbolized innocence and fertility. According to tradition, Mary fed the baby Jesus, Joseph, and herself with three oranges from a tree inhabited by a sleeping eagle. The original pomanders were oranges pierced with clove buds.

The word "orange" comes from the Persian *narang* by way of the Arabic word *narandj.* Early Spanish missionaries transported oranges to California, which now has a thriving orange industry.

Orange peels are the key ingredient in orange marmalade, and they flavor curaçao, a West Indian liqueur.

MEDICINAL USES

Orange oil relieves the discomfort of bronchitis and the flu. It aids in the absorption of vitamin C, boosts immunity, helps prevent colds and flu, and relieves some of the symptoms associated with chronic fatigue syndrome. Orange oil heals mouth ulcers and gingivitis. It also soothes painful muscles and joints. The Chinese treat anorexia nervosa, colds, coughs, and malignant breast sores with dried orange peels.

Orange oil calms an upset stomach, especially if nerve or stress related, and can aid in digestion and restore appetite. It regulates the bowels and relieves diarrhea and constipation. Orange oil encourages the elimination of wastes and promotes urination, making it helpful in treating obesity, fluid retention, and premenstrual syndrome (PMS). It can lower body temperature and either cool a fever or warm chills. Orange oil soothes inflammation from psoriasis as well as eczema and other types of dermatitis.

BEAUTY BENEFITS

Orange oil restores balance to dry or oily skin. It maintains healthy, youthful skin by promoting the production of collagen. It reduces puffiness and discourages dry, wrinkled skin. Orange oil stimulates circulation to the skin surface and softens rough skin. It also clears blemishes and improves acne-prone skin. It tends to increase perspiration, thus assisting the release of toxins from dull or blemished skin. Orange stimulates the circulation of lymphatic fluids and helps relieve tissue swelling and fluid retention. It improves cellulite, which is sometimes called "orange-peel skin."

EMOTIONAL EFFECTS

Orange oil balances the emotions, either relaxing or stimulating as needed. It revitalizes and energizes when boredom and lethargy set in. Orange oil has a warm, happy, and light influence that prevents extreme seriousness. It calms the nerves and can combat anxiety and insomnia. Orange oil brightens gloomy feelings, dissipates depressing thoughts, and subdues tension and stress, particularly in wintertime or if the stress is related to premenstrual syndrome or menopause. It eases fear of the unknown and encourages a more adventuresome attitude. It brings a more positive outlook, replacing sadness with warmth and happiness. Orange oil awakens creativity, inspires harmony, and promotes self-awareness.

PRIMARY ACTIONS

Orange oil fights infection, reduces inflammation, and relieves muscle spasms. It aids digestion and eases digestive disorders. It cools fevers and warms chills. It stimulates lymphatic circulation and improves immunity. Orange oil calms nerves and diminishes depression.

CAUTIONS

Orange oil may irritate skin and promote photosensitivity, leading to sunburn and uneven darkening of the skin. Avoid using it if your skin will be exposed to sunlight.

Palmarosa

Palmarosa is a sweet-smelling grass that grows wild in tropical climates. Clusters of bluish-white flowers rise out of its long, slender leaves. As they mature, the flowers turn dark red.

Harvesting, drying, and steam-distilling palmarosa grass before the flowers mature assures a higher yield of superior palmarosa oil. This pale yellowish-green oil has floral notes reminiscent of roses or geraniums.

Originally from central and northern India, *Cymbopogon martini* is a member of the *Poaceae* family. It now grows in Africa, Java, Madagascar, and the Seychelles.

FOLKLORE AND HERBAL HERITAGE

Since the eighteenth century, the Turks have distilled palmarosa oil to adulterate costly Turkish rose oil. Palmarosa was once known as Turkish or Indian geranium oil because of its geraniumlike odor. Indian doctors prescribed palmarosa to prevent infections and fight fever. Palmarosa was also added to Indian curry dishes and some West African meat dishes to kill bacteria and aid digestion.

MEDICINAL USES

Indian doctors use palmarosa oil to fight bacteria and infection. Palmarosa oil cools fevers and eases the discomforts of colds or the flu. It can hasten recovery from illness and bring relief of general malaise. It accelerates the healing of cuts and wounds. Palmarosa oil can also help the body restore healthy intestinal flora. It stimulates the appetite and can help in cases of anorexia nervosa.

BEAUTY BENEFITS

Palmarosa oil enhances any skin type. It regulates the production of sebum, or oil, helping to normalize oily skin; in dry or mature skin, it stimulates sebum production and helps replenish moisture. It helps clear acne and blemishes; with regular application, it can fade old acne scars. It stimulates the regeneration of cells, discourages wrinkles, heals wounds and sores, and soothes inflamed or irritated skin. Palmarosa oil also minimizes the appearance of broken capillaries with long-term use.

EMOTIONAL EFFECTS

Palmarosa oil promotes recovery from nervous exhaustion or stress. It calms and uplifts the emotions while refreshing the mind and clarifying thoughts. It reduces stress and tension.

PRIMARY ACTIONS

Palmarosa oil fights infection and cools fevers. It stimulates new cell growth, regulates oil production, and speeds wound healing. Palmarosa oil improves digestion and circulation.

Patchouli

Patchouli oil is pungent and powerful, mossy and musty, earthy and exotic, sweet and spicy. It is steam-distilled from the dried and fermented fuzzy young leaves of *Pogostemon patchouli* or *Pogostemon cablin,* a three-foot-tall perennial bush with white flowers that have a purplish or mauve hue. Age enriches the heavy herbal odor of its viscous amber, orange, or dark-brown oil.

A member of the *Lamiaceae* family, patchouli is native to tropical Asia and is cultivated in India, Indonesia, Malaysia, the Philippines, and Singapore. Patchouli oil is produced in Burma, India, Malaysia, and a number of South American countries.

FOLKLORE AND HERBAL HERITAGE

For centuries, the people of China, India, Japan, and Malaysia have relied on patchouli for various medicinal purposes. They used it to fight infection and cool fevers and to tone the skin—and, indeed, the entire body. It was also used as an antidote for insect and snake bites. It is the combination of patchouli and camphor that gives India ink its characteristic smell.

During the Victorian era, British manufacturers imported patchouli oil to fragrance machine-made cashmere shawls, in the hope that buyers would then be unable to distinguish between their wares and authentic handmade cashmere shawls from India, which had a lingering odor of patchouli. In India, patchouli sachets were used to scent fabrics and protect them against insects. Patchouli perfume also provided the persistent and unforgettable fragrance associated with the "flower power" movement of the 1960s and 1970s.

MEDICINAL USES

Patchouli oil helps with weight loss: It curbs the appetite and it tones and tightens skin to prevent sagging after weight is lost. By increasing urination, it discourages the water retention associated with premenstrual syndrome (PMS). It may also reduce hot flashes during menopause. Patchouli diminishes the distress of diarrhea. It fights fungi and is useful in treating athlete's foot, jock itch, and fungal infections of the skin, such as candida. Patchouli oil reduces the inflammation of skin disorders such as acne, psoriasis, sunburn, skin allergies, and eczema and other forms of dermatitis.

BEAUTY BENEFITS

Patchouli oil regenerates skin cells and is reputed

to ward off wrinkles. It also tightens and tones sagging skin. Patchouli oil speeds the healing of sores and wounds and helps to fade scars. It cools and calms inflamed skin and sunburn; it soothes and smooths rough, dry, and cracked skin. At the same time, it regulates the oiliness of skin and hair and helps control acne and scalp disorders such as dandruff and seborrhea. It also repels insects. By reducing fluid retention and tightening saggy skin, patchouli oil helps combat cellulite. It acts as a deodorant and helps control perspiration.

EMOTIONAL EFFECTS

Patchouli oil diminishes depression and eases anxiety. It helps recovery from nervous exhaustion, stress, and stress-related conditions. It reduces mental fatigue and banishes lethargy. In low doses, it acts as a sedative, while in larger quantities it is stimulating. It can sharpen intelligence, improve concentration, and provide insight. It cools and calms during physically or emotionally hot situations. It is a stabilizing and balancing oil with aphrodisiac attributes that can heighten libido.

PRIMARY ACTIONS

Patchouli oil calms nerves, lifts depression, and stimulates sexual desire. It reduces inflammation and fights infections and fungi. It repels insects. Patchouli oil stimulates new cell growth, tightens and tones tissues, and speeds healing of sores and wounds. It reduces body odor and cools fever.

Pepper

See BLACK PEPPER.

Peppermint

Compact, serrated-edged leaves on short, square stems contrast with the long, spearlike spikes bearing the tiny purple, pink, or white flowers of the peppermint plant. Originally native to Asia and Europe, this member of the *Lamiaceae* family is now grown commercially in humid regions of Australia, Brazil, China, England, France, Japan, Morocco, Spain, and the United States, which is the primary producer of peppermint oil.

Steam-distilling 1,000 pounds of mature *Mentha piperita* plants in full bloom will produce about one pound of peppermint oil. This clear or pale-yellow oil emits a strong, sharp menthol aroma that is pungent and powerful, even overwhelming.

FOLKLORE AND HERBAL HERITAGE

In Roman mythology, when Pluto professed his love for the nymph Mentha, his wife Persephone, afire with jealousy, crushed Mentha into dust on the ground. Pluto, unable to change her back, transformed her into a peppermint plant and gave her a fresh fragrance so that she would smell sweet whenever stepped upon.

The ancient Hebrews added peppermint to perfumes, possibly for its aphrodisiac attributes. Peppermint played a prominent part in Greek and Roman religious rites. For thousands of years, Asians, Egyptians, and Native Americans have soothed digestive difficulties with peppermint and used it to freshen their breath.

During the eighteenth century, peppermint became a well-known medicine throughout Europe and North America. It was used to relieve such common complaints as colic, gas, headaches, heartburn, and indigestion. Today's pharmacists still suggest peppermint oil for upset stomach and indigestion. Overindulgent diners sip peppermint tea to soothe bloated bellies, stimulate sluggish digestion, and reduce heartburn and gas. For decades, peppermint has added a refreshing punch to numerous commercial products, including breath mints, chewing gums, toothpastes, toothpicks, after-dinner mints, and mouthwashes. In addition, the food industry utilizes its invigorating taste and strong aroma to enliven foods, teas, candies, and pastries.

MEDICINAL USES

Peppermint oil stimulates the central nervous system and counteracts drowsiness and fatigue by increasing alertness and promoting clear thinking. It calms and soothes muscles, particularly those of the digestive tract when they are affected by stress and poor diet. It eases motion sickness and nausea, and can revitalize someone suffering from jet lag. Chronic fatigue syndrome also responds to peppermint's stimulating action.

Peppermint oil relaxes tense muscles and muscle spasms. It eases painful menstrual cramps, cools hot flashes and fevers, and reduces the inflammation and swelling of muscular aches, pains, sprains, and strains. Peppermint oil relieves the itching and swelling of dermatitis and sunburn. It also relieves headaches, whether from tension or migraine. It clears sinuses, and can improve breathing.

BEAUTY BENEFITS

Peppermint oil fights bacterial infection and reduces the oiliness present with acne and blemishes. It stimulates circulation and helps enliven dull, dry skin. Peppermint oil leaves skin feeling soft and silky. It also regulates and normalizes oily skin and

hair. It constricts capillaries and minimizes the redness of broken capillaries and varicose veins.

EMOTIONAL EFFECTS

Peppermint oil cools emotions and dissipates anger, hysteria, and nervousness. It energizes and relieves mental fatigue. It diminishes depression. Peppermint oil increases alertness and improves concentration. It awakens the central nervous system, stimulates the brain, and clarifies thought processes.

PRIMARY ACTIONS

Peppermint oil relieves pain, eases muscle spasms, and reduces inflammation. It fights infection, clears congestion, and opens the sinuses. It tightens and tones tissues and regulates oiliness. Peppermint oil aids digestion. It stimulates the brain, clears the head, and promotes nerve health. It cools fevers.

CAUTIONS

Peppermint oil may irritate sensitive skin. It can stimulate menstrual flow and stop the flow of milk, so women who are pregnant or nursing should avoid it. Peppermint oil can counteract homeopathic remedies. If you are using both peppermint oil and a homeopathic remedy, allow at least one hour between the two.

Pine

Majestic, aromatic Scotch pine trees tower above the forest, reaching heights of 65 to 115 feet. Deep fissures mark the reddish-brown bark of this large evergreen, *Pinus sylvestri,* also known as the Norway pine. Yellow-orange flowers and pointed amber, green, or brown cones cluster around gray-green or blue-green needles.

Native to Europe and Asia, this member of the *Pinaceae* family is now found in northern Europe, northeastern Russia, Scandinavia, and the eastern United States. The tree's needles, twigs, and cones are steam-distilled to produce pine oil. This colorless or light-yellow oil emits an earthy, resinous, and medicinal odor that is strong, fresh, and balsamic. Trees grown in more northerly climates produce superior oils.

FOLKLORE AND HERBAL HERITAGE

The ancient Greeks dedicated pine trees to the sea god, Neptune, because pine wood was used to build the first Greek ships. They also honored the gods Bacchus and Pan with it. In Greek mythology, Pitys, one of Pan's many nymphs, escaped the embraces of Boreas by becoming a pine tree. According to folklore, the sayings "pining for" and "pitying" someone may have come from that incident.

One Christian tradition holds that the cross on which Jesus was crucified was made from a pine tree. In some cultures, mourners placed pine branches on the coffins of loved ones to signify immortality. To the Japanese, pine trees symbolized constancy and fidelity because they are always green.

Native Americans stuffed pine needles into their mattresses to repel lice and fleas. Arabs treated pneumonia and other lung infections with pine. Pine branches have been bruised and floated in baths to revitalize people suffering from mental or emotional fatigue and nervous exhaustion. Pine was also used to improve circulation and relieve aching muscles; in the nineteenth century, pine was a popular diuretic. It could induce perspiration and helped break fevers. Pine-tar ointments have been used to relieve skin disorders such as psoriasis and eczema and to heal sores. Pine was also a remedy for constipation.

MEDICINAL USES

Pine oil fights any type of respiratory infection, especially bronchitis, colds, the flu, laryngitis, and sore throats. It encourages the release of mucus; it relieves congestion and clears the sinuses; it eases coughing and makes breathing easier. Pine oil can either warm chills or cool a fever, depending on what the body needs. It soothes muscle aches and pains and stiffness in joints, providing relief for arthritis, gout, rheumatism, and sciatica. Pine also stimulates circulation, raises blood pressure, and activates the adrenal glands. It acts as a kidney and liver cleanser and can help treat cystitis and prostate problems. It soothes the itching and inflammation of eczema and psoriasis, and helps to heal cuts and sores. Pine oil has a revitalizing effect on the entire body.

BEAUTY BENEFITS

Pine oil encourages the elimination of toxins from the skin, making it useful for clearing dull, dry skin as well as acne. It improves oily scalp conditions, dandruff, and seborrhea. As an insect repellent, it protects against bug bites. It also reduces excessive perspiration.

EMOTIONAL EFFECTS

Pine oil is refreshing and revitalizes a body and mind suffering from general malaise or mental fatigue. It restores strength after physical weakness or during convalescence.

PRIMARY ACTIONS

Pine oil fights infection and repels insects. It relieves muscle and joint pain. It releases mucus, clears congestion, and increases urination. Pine oil increases blood pressure and stimulates the adrenal glands and the circulatory system.

CAUTIONS

Because pine oil can increase blood pressure, you should avoid using it if you have high blood pressure. Pine oil may also be irritating to sensitive skin.

Rose

Of the estimated 5,000 or more species of roses that grace our environment, the damask rose (*Rosa damascena*) and the cabbage rose (*Rosa centifolia*) are the most fragrant, and they are the two primary roses that produce essential oils for aromatherapy. At one time, the red rose (*Rosa gallica*) supposedly yielded rose oil as well, but it is so rare as to be essentially unavailable today.

Native to the Orient, Persia (now Iran), and Syria, these members of the *Rosaceae* family are now cultivated in the temperate regions of Bulgaria, China, France, India, Italy, Morocco, Russia, Tunisia, and Turkey. These bushy deciduous shrubs grow three to six feet tall or taller. Their sweet-scented blossoms range in color from white to pink to red.

Steam-distilling over 60,000 fresh-picked roses will yield only one ounce of rose oil. Pale-yellow or deeper yellow rose oil, or *rose otto*, has a rich, sweet, and spicy floral fragrance. *Rose absolute*, a reddish-orange oil with a heavier, sweeter scent, is extracted with solvents. Because residues of solvent may remain in rose absolute, rose oil is more desirable for aromatherapy purposes.

FOLKLORE AND HERBAL HERITAGE

Fossil records reveal that roses have been in existence for 32 million years. Over 3,000 years ago, the rose was christened the "queen of flowers."

Throughout history, roses have been the subject of art, literature, poetry, medicine, and love. There are many myths and legends surrounding the rose. In Roman mythology, the goddess Venus was presented with a rose as she arose from the sea; according to Greek mythology, the blood of Aphrodite, who pricked her finger on a thorn of the rosebush while helping Adonis, colored roses red. The rose was sacred to both Aphrodite and Eros.

One tradition holds that thorns appeared on rosebushes only after the Fall, when Adam and Eve were expelled from the Garden of Eden. Another myth attributes the thorns to Cupid's arrow, which accidentally punctured the rosebush, permanently endowing it with thorns.

In ancient times, roses meant confidence. The practice of hanging a rose over a meeting table signified that everything said would be held in strictest confidence; hence the term *sub rosa*. Other meanings attributed to roses included beauty, enjoyment, fertility, joy, love, and pleasure. In addition, each color of rose was supposed to have its own special meaning: red for passion and desire; pink for simplicity, happiness, and love; white for innocence and purity; yellow for jealousy or achievement. Egyptian art and architecture contained depictions of roses; Cleopatra's cosmetics contained actual roses. She supposedly employed the seductive powers of the rose when entertaining Mark Antony by carpeting her floors—knee-deep—with red rose petals.

Roses became an integral part of Roman culture. Lavish displays of roses decorated banquet tables and rose petals covered floors at feasts. Romans crowned newlyweds with garlands of roses. They planted gardens of roses in conquered lands for use in bathing, confectionery, cosmetics, medicine, and perfume, and as a cure for hangovers. Rose petals floated atop rose water in canals in the Shalimar Gardens for the wedding of Shah Jahan and his bride, in whose honor the shah later built the Taj Mahal. Legend has it that when his wife noticed the rose oil particles surfacing on the water, she ordered them collected for her perfume.

Roses were used for centuries to soothe the pain of fever blisters and cold sores. Until the Middle Ages, roses were a chief cure for digestive disorders, eye infections, headaches, menstrual difficulties, nervous tension, and skin disorders, and were used to treat respiratory ailments and asthma. In Elizabethan England, many foods were flavored with roses. Middle Eastern cuisine still employs rose water in some dishes.

MEDICINAL USES

Physicians in Europe prescribe rose oil to fight coughs and mouth sores and to heal wounds. Rose oil clears congestion and soothes inflammation. Rose water relieves conjunctivitis, helps heal herpes outbreaks, and soothes gingivitis. Rose oil strengthens the digestive system and helps overcome constipation, nausea, and vomiting. It can also relieve the pain of migraine and other headaches.

Rose oil helps balance female hormones. It regulates the menstrual cycle, reduces menstrual cramps, and eases the discomforts of premenstrual syndrome (PMS) and menopause. It is also helpful in treating genitourinary conditions. Sexual difficulties such as frigidity and impotence respond to rose oil, particularly if they are stress related. Rose oil stimulates circulation and tones the capillaries. It soothes and comforts psoriasis, eczema, dermatitis, and other skin disorders by reducing inflammation.

Rose oil is gentle enough to use on babies and children.

BEAUTY BENEFITS

Rose oil benefits all skin types, especially mature, sensitive, dry, or damaged skin. It helps restore the moisture balance and smooths wrinkles. It constricts tiny blood vessels, thus helping to diminish the redness of broken capillaries.

EMOTIONAL EFFECTS

Rose oil soothes the emotions. It lifts depression, eases anxiety, elevates spirits, and reduces stress and tension. It stabilizes mood swings, particularly if they are related to postnatal depression. It calms the nerves and helps to overcome insomnia. Rose oil can ease grief and subdue sadness. It helps to eliminate feelings of disappointment, jealousy, and resentment, and can help dissolve emotional blocks standing in the way of happiness. Rose oil symbolizes purity and innocence, yet it is a sensual and stimulating aphrodisiac. It promotes feelings of love and may help in overcoming impotence or frigidity.

PRIMARY ACTIONS

Rose oil fights infection, reduces inflammation, and relieves muscle spasms. It calms nerves, decreases depression, and stimulates sexual desire. It increases urination, encourages bowel movements, aids digestion, and helps to regulate menstrual cycles.

Rosemary

Cascades of rosemary emit a pungent, pinelike aroma with a woody, camphoraceous note. This aromatic shrub, *Rosmarinus officinalis*, has scaly bark and dense leathery, needlelike leaves. Tiny pale-blue blossoms abound from December through spring. Rosemary can grow to heights of five to six feet.

Steam distillation of 100 pounds of rosemary in bloom will yield one pound of strong, clean, and potent rosemary oil. Rosemary oil from varieties grown in Spain and North Africa smell similar to eucalyptus oil, while the scent of oil from plants grown in France are reminiscent of frankincense. Rosemary has several *chemotypes,* or plants that differ in the chemical composition of the essential oil they produce but not in physical appearance. *Moroccan rosemary, Spanish rosemary, rosemary Provence,* and *rosemary verbenone* are four common chemotypes of rosemary used in aromatherapy.

A member of the *Lamiaceae* family, rosemary is native to the Mediterranean regions of Europe. The Dalmatian islands, France, Spain, and Tunisia produce the majority of rosemary oil.

FOLKLORE AND HERBAL HERITAGE

Rosemary, whose name comes from the Latin *ros marinus,* meaning "dew of the sea, was one of the first plants used for medicine, food, and religious rituals. In ancient times, it was a part of almost all feasts and festivals. Rosemary was seen as a reminder of the cycle of life and death.

In flower lore, rosemary means "remembrance," possibly because of its ability to improve memory. In fact, to reinforce recall, students in ancient Greece wore garlands of rosemary on their heads while studying. Both the Greeks and the Romans associated rosemary with love and marriage. On her wedding day, a bride would wear a wreath woven with sprigs of rosemary and scented with rosemary oil. Rosemary flowers were carried in bridal bouquets. At a Greek or Roman funeral, friends and family members would toss rosemary into the grave to express the hope that the departed would be remembered.

During the sixteenth century, refreshing rosemary incense was a luxury of the wealthy, who paid perfumers to scent their homes with it. Hospitals burned rosemary to purify the air and prevent the spread of infection. People placed sprigs of rosemary under their pillows to ward off demons and prevent bad dreams during the night. Rosemary was used extensively in exorcisms to expel evil spirits. One of rosemary's most famous uses was in a therapeutic formula called Hungary water, named for Queen Elizabeth of Hungary. After bathing in this formula, drinking it, and having it massaged it into the joints of her paralyzed limbs, the queen—then in her seventies—supposedly recovered from her many ailments, and soon thereafter, she won the heart of a man many decades her junior.

Herbalists have long recommended rosemary to stimulate the activity of the stomach, the liver, and the gallbladder, as well as to improve circulation. Elizabethan physicians used rosemary to treat headaches, brain disorders, and toothaches. Philippus Aureolus Paracelsus, the sixteenth-century German physician who first introduced the disease theory of illness, regarded rosemary as a most essential component in his medicines. He and other healers of his time used rosemary to treat disorders affecting the brain, heart, eyes, and liver. Arab herbalists used it to restore memory, speech, and strength. Rosemary was also used to improve the condition of the hair and scalp.

MEDICINAL USES

European doctors use rosemary oil in medical treatments for arthritis, colds, coughs, depression, diabetes, headaches, the flu, memory loss, migraines, and muscle spasms. British physicians prescribe rosemary oil to lower blood cholesterol levels and strengthen people with cardiovascular weaknesses. They also use rosemary oil to treat colic, cirrhosis of the liver, gallbladder infections, gallstones, and hepatitis. Digestive disorders such as colitis, gas, and indigestion often improve with rosemary, as do liver problems and jaundice. Rosemary oil also relieves respiratory ailments such as asthma, bronchitis, colds, sinusitis, and whooping cough. It fights infection and helps the body to expel excess mucus.

Rosemary oil stimulates circulation and helps raise low blood pressure. It relieves the pain and swelling of arthritis, muscle spasms, injuries, and sprains. It encourages cellular metabolism and assists in the drainage of lymphatic fluid. Rosemary oil tones the entire body and is helpful in treating chronic fatigue syndrome and weakened immunity. It soothes the itching and inflammation of psoriasis, eczema, and other types of dermatitis.

BEAUTY BENEFITS

Rosemary oil stimulates cell renewal. It improves dry or mature skin, eases lines and wrinkles, and heals burns and wounds. It can also clear acne, blemishes, or dull, dry skin by fighting bacteria and regulating oil secretions. It improves circulation and can reduce the appearance of broken capillaries and varicose veins. Rosemary oil nourishes the scalp and keeps hair looking healthy and shiny. Many users claim that it promotes hair growth. It normalizes excessive oil secretions and improves most scalp problems, particularly dandruff and seborrhea. Rosemary oil is also helpful in treating cellulite.

EMOTIONAL EFFECTS

Rosemary oil helps to overcome mental fatigue and sluggishness by stimulating and strengthening the central nervous system. It enhances mental clarity while aiding alertness and concentration. Rosemary oil can help you cope with stressful conditions and see things from a clearer perspective. It relaxes nerves and restores nerve health, especially after long-term nervous or physical ailments.

Rosemary oil balances intense emotions and controls mood swings. It lifts spirits and counters depression. It assists in managing stress and overcoming stress-related disorders and nervous exhaustion. Rosemary oil can open the heart and bring the wisdom and discrimination necessary to establish healthy boundaries in relationships. Rosemary oil arouses ambition and drive, inspires the desire to achieve, and strengthens willpower. It also reputedly helps in overcoming impotence.

PRIMARY ACTIONS

Rosemary oil tightens and tones tissues, promotes new cell growth, and regulates oil secretion. It fights infection, relieves joint pain, and eases muscle spasms. Rosemary oil eases digestive disorders. It improves the functioning of the heart and the nervous system and promotes nerve health. Rosemary oil stimulates the activities of many internal organs and systems, including the adrenal glands, circulatory system, liver, and gallbladder.

CAUTIONS

Rosemary oil elevates blood pressure, so you should avoid using it if you have high blood pressure. It may be irritating to sensitive skin. Rosemary oil can also trigger epileptic seizures in susceptible individuals.

Rosewood

Rosewood oil's subtle smell is soft, sweet, and spicy, with fresh floral notes. It is reminiscent of rose, citrus, and wood. This colorless or pale-yellow oil is distilled from the heartwood of the evergreen rosewood tree, *Aniba roseaodora*. Reaching heights of 125 feet, this member of the *Lauraceae* family has reddish bark and yellow flowers. It is native to the tropical areas around the Amazon River.

Rosewood trees grow and are harvested in the rain forests of South America. During the yearly flood season, huge rosewood tree trunks float downstream headed for the distilleries. Peru and Brazil supply most of the world's rosewood oil. So that the harvesting of rosewood trees does not lead to their extinction or to deforestation of ecologically sensitive areas, Brazilian legislation now requires that one new tree be planted for each one cut down.

FOLKLORE AND HERBAL HERITAGE

The original site of production of *bois de rose,* as the French called rosewood, was French Guiana, on the northern coast of South America. So great was the demand among the French for rosewood oil, which was used to create lily of the valley and lilac type fragrances, that they depleted the colony's rosewood forests. Carvings and chopsticks were commonly made from rosewood; the rose-scented heartwood was frequently used in cabinetmaking and to make handles for cutlery and hairbrushes. As an aphrodisiac, rosewood oil reputedly could restore a lost or diminished sex drive and overcome frigidity and impotence.

MEDICINAL USES

Rosewood oil is an overall tonic for the body; it is neither too stimulating nor too sedating. By boosting the immune system, it deters colds and the flu, subdues coughs, and fights fever. It clears the head and eases headaches, especially those caused or accompanied by nausea. Rosewood oil promotes alertness and can diminish jet lag. It helps to heal cuts and wounds, and reduces the itching and inflammation of psoriasis, eczema, and other forms of dermatitis.

BEAUTY BENEFITS

Until relatively recently, rosewood oil was used primarily in perfumery. When used in skin care, it stimulates new cell growth, regenerates tissue, and minimizes lines and wrinkles. Rosewood oil can balance either dry or oily skin. It soothes sensitive and inflamed skin; it also clears blemishes and improves acne. With regular application, it helps to diminish scars.

EMOTIONAL EFFECTS

Rosewood oil calms and relaxes the nerves and helps relieve anxiety and stress. It strengthens the nervous system, steadies nerves, and balances the emotions. Rosewood oil arouses alertness, especially under stressful circumstances. It encourages self-acceptance and the appreciation of others. As a subtle aphrodisiac, it stirs positive sensual feelings, especially in persons whose past sexual experiences were traumatic.

PRIMARY ACTIONS

Rosewood oil diminishes depression and stimulates sexual feelings. It relieves pain and fights infection. Rosewood oil stimulates the brain and clears the head. It improves immunity, soothes skin disorders, and maintains healthy skin.

Sage

See CLARY SAGE.

Sandalwood

An abundant array of small blossoms, ranging in color from red to yellow to pinkish-purple, sprout forth from the leathery leaves and the yellowish limbs of the sandalwood tree. This slow-growing evergreen, *Santalum album*, grows to a height of twenty-four to thirty feet over the course of thirty to sixty-four years. These heavy, somewhat parasitic members of the *Santalaceae* family obtain much of their nourishment by sending out suckers that tap into roots of other nearby trees.

Pale or golden-yellow sandalwood oil emits a sweet, woody, velvety fragrance that is warm, rich, and exotic. Steam-distilling twenty-five pounds of crushed heartwood yields about one to one and one-half pounds of thick, viscous oil.

Sandalwood is native to tropical Asia; India is the main producer of sandalwood oil. The finest sandalwood comes from the area of Mysore, in southern India. The Indian government now permits the harvesting only of mature trees that are approaching the end of their long lives. Once the trees are felled, ants eat away the outer bark and leave the heartwood exposed. It is the heartwood that contains the essential oil.

FOLKLORE AND HERBAL HERITAGE

Sweet, sacred-smelling sandalwood oil has played an integral part in Indian religion and culture for millennia. Furniture and even entire temples were built from the heartwood of sandalwood trees because it resisted attack by insects.

Sandalwood incense permeated Indian temples, helping worshippers to relax and achieve higher states of meditation. Sandalwood was closely associated with yogic, tantric, and other spiritual practices. It purportedly awakened *kundalini*, or the latent life force energy, of anyone who breathed it during meditation. At funerals, sandalwood incense was burned to free the soul of the deceased.

Indians anointed their bodies with the seductive scent of sandalwood. Sandalwood oil's sultry smell has an erotic quality that earned it a reputation as an aphrodisiac. Many people claim that its aroma is similar to the masculine hormone androsterone. Indeed, for centuries men have worn sandalwood-based scents to elicit desired responses from women.

In ancient times, caravans carried sandalwood from India to Egypt, Greece, and Rome. The Egyptians used sandalwood in the embalming process. Sandalwood's popularity in religious ceremonies—especially in India and China—continues today, and many Eastern cultures still consider sandalwood sacred.

The Polynesians added powdered sandalwood to massage oils that they used to treat earaches, headaches, and skin ailments. Unfortunately, during the 1800s, greedy traders travelled to such places as India, Indonesia, and Hawaii, where flourishing forests of sandalwood trees embellished the local landscapes. These traders ravaged entire forests. This led to the extinction of some species of sandalwood and the endangered status of others.

MEDICINAL USES

Ayurvedic doctors in India still use sandalwood oil to fight infection and to treat urinary problems, such as cystitis, prostatitis, and urethritis. They rely on sandalwood to relieve diarrhea, earaches, and respiratory infections. Chinese doctors prescribe sandalwood to cure cholera, gonorrhea, stomachaches, and vomiting. Other health care practitioners also treat gastritis and nausea with sandalwood oil.

Sandalwood oil stimulates the immune system, benefitting the entire body. Respiratory ailments such as bronchitis, coughs, laryngitis, sinusitis, and sore throats respond to sandalwood oil treatments. Sandalwood oil also eases a variety of skin complaints. It helps to heal cuts and wounds, soothes skin, and relieves the itching and inflammation of psoriasis, eczema, and other types of dermatitis.

BEAUTY BENEFITS

Sandalwood oil moisturizes dry, dehydrated, and mature skin. It smooths and softens lines and wrinkles. It can balance either oily or dry skin and benefits any skin type or condition. Sandalwood oil helps to clear acne and blemishes by regulating oil production and fighting bacteria. It calms barber's rash, relieves itching and irritation after shaving, and inhibits the growth of bacteria that can cause infection of ingrown hairs. Sandalwood oil is mild enough even for sensitive skin.

EMOTIONAL EFFECTS

Sandalwood oil soothes emotions that are exhausted from a hectic lifestyle. It relaxes the body and mind and relieves stress, elevates spirits, and lifts depression. Sandalwood oil also subdues aggression and irritability. It helps to release confusion, fear, nervousness, and stress. Sandalwood oil promotes compassion, openness, and under-

standing. It can help an introverted person to become more sociable and outgoing. Sandalwood stimulates the senses and clears thought processes. During times of emotional turmoil, sandalwood oil strengthens resolve and is stabilizing. As an aphrodisiac, sandalwood oil helps overcome frigidity and impotence.

PRIMARY ACTIONS

Sandalwood oil fights infection, particularly of the urinary tract, and relieves muscle spasms. It softens and soothes skin and stimulates new cell growth. It releases mucus and clears congestion. Sandalwood oil calms nerves and stimulates sexual drive.

Tea Tree

The swampy, flood-prone marshlands in the subtropical coastal areas of northeastern New South Wales and southeastern Queensland, Australia, provide the perfect climate and growing conditions for tea trees, also called paper bark trees. Feathery bright-green leaves cover the branches of these small trees, which at maturity rarely reach over twenty feet in height. Clusters of yellow flowers sometimes embellish these trees.

Of the 300 varieties of tea trees, one variety, *Melaleuca alternifolia*, produces the tea tree oil that is most commonly used for aromatherapy. Australian scientists are currently researching the therapeutic properties of essential oils from other tea trees. All tea trees are members of the *Myrtaceae* family.

Distilling the needlelike tea tree leaves yields a colorless or pale-yellow oil with a characteristic camphorlike odor. The aroma is spicy, strong, and pungent. It smells similar to its aromatic relative, eucalyptus.

FOLKLORE AND HERBAL HERITAGE

For centuries, Australia's Bundjalung aborigines have applied poultices of tea tree leaves to cuts, wounds, and skin infections, and have inhaled crushed tea tree leaves to treat respiratory problems. The tree supposedly received its common name in the eighteenth century, when Captain James Cook, after drinking a refreshing herbal tea brewed from the leaves of these hardy, disease-resistant trees, christened it "tea tree."

Modern science first acknowledged tea tree oil's medicinal properties in 1925. Laboratory experiments showed it was twelve times stronger than phenol (carbolic acid), then the standard for antiseptic compounds. In the 1920s, dentists and surgeons began using tea tree oil to disinfect wounds and incisions. It became a standard dental treatment for bleeding gums, gingivitis, and periodontal disease. Physicians prescribed it for cystitis, fungal infections, skin disorders, throat infections, and yeast infections. During World War II, Australian soldiers were issued first aid kits containing tea tree oil. Medics poured the oil directly into wounds to disinfect them and speed healing without damaging the surrounding tissues. The Australian government regarded tea tree oil as such an important contribution to the war effort that workers employed in producing it were exempt from military duty.

Prior to tea tree oil's current popularity, farmers tried (unsuccessfully) to destroy the trees, which they considered a nuisance. Tea trees exhibit extraordinary persistence; some authorities liken the tea tree's own powers of recovery to its strong immune-stimulating abilities. Today, people visit coves of coppery-colored water formed by the flooded wetlands surrounding tea trees, seeking therapeutic benefits from basking in the oily secretions floating atop the water.

MEDICINAL USES

Australians call tea tree oil a "first aid kit in a bottle." Their claims may sound far-fetched, but they are not. Tea tree oil exhibits a broad spectrum of uses. It is effective for the treatment of abscesses, acne, bites, blisters, burns, cuts, dandruff, skin disorders, and scalp problems. It cleanses and disinfects wounds and soothes and heals burns. Like its cousin, eucalyptus oil, tea tree oil aids respiratory ailments. It relieves the symptoms of asthma, bronchitis, colds, congestion, coughs, earaches, fevers, laryngitis, sinusitis, sore throats, tonsillitis, and whooping cough. It reputedly improves immunity and reduces the incidence of colds, fevers, the flu, and other infectious illnesses.

Reproductive and urinary tract infections, such as vaginitis and cystitis, respond to tea tree oil. It fights fungal infections such as athlete's foot, candida infections, and jock itch, and helps heal cold sores, herpes outbreaks, and hemorrhoids. It relieves the itching, redness, and scaling of psoriasis, seborrhea, and eczema and other types of dermatitis. Tea tree oil improves oral hygiene and relieves gingivitis, mouth ulcers, periodontal disease, and toothaches. Because it is nontoxic and nonirritating and exhibits powerful action against bacteria, fungi, and viruses, it has attracted the attention of medical researchers. Tea tree oil can also help relieve some of the symptoms of chronic fatigue syndrome.

BEAUTY BENEFITS

Tea tree oil works well on a wide range of skin problems, including blemishes, rashes, and warts. Clinical studies in Australia have shown that tea tree oil rivals benzoyl peroxide for effectiveness in fighting acne, but without causing dryness, itching, stinging, burning, redness of the skin, or other side effects. Men can prevent skin irritation from shaving and the infection of ingrown hairs by applying tea tree oil after shaving. Tea tree oil also provides an effective treatment for fungal infection of the fingernails, an increasing problem that may be linked to the growing use of artificial fingernails.

EMOTIONAL EFFECTS

Tea tree oil can restore energy depleted by everyday stress. It is calming and centering during times of emotional shock.

PRIMARY ACTIONS

Tea tree oil kills insects and fights infections and fungi. It soothes skin disorders and heals wounds. Tea tree oil releases mucus and relieves respiratory congestion. It increases immunity.

CAUTIONS

Tea tree oil may be irritating to sensitive skin.

Thyme

Thyme grows as a small, woody evergreen shrub with many branches that are covered with fragrant foliage. Common thyme, *Thymus vulgaris,* has tiny gray-green oval leaves and pink, lilac, or white flowers. *Thymus citriodoria,* or lemon thyme, has lemon-scented leaves and lavender-colored flowers. These perennial members of the *Lamiaceae* family grow about one foot tall. Native to Spain and other Mediterranean countries, thyme is now

cultivated in Algeria, central Europe, China, Israel, Russia, Turkey, Tunisia, and the United States.

The fresh or partially dried leaves and flowering tops of the plant are steam-distilled to produce thyme oil. The first distillation yields red thyme oil, which is red, brown, or orange in color and has an intense warm and spicy smell. Further distilling renders white thyme oil, a clear or pale-yellow oil with a sweet, fresh, and mild green aroma. White thyme oil contains fewer irritants than red thyme oil does. There are several different *chemotypes* of the thyme plant (plants with similar appearances whose essential oils have different chemical compositions) that produce oils with different therapeutic properties. Some of these, such as *thyme linalol* and *thyme citral,* are less irritating than common thyme. Spain is the primary producer of thyme oil, but Algeria, France, Germany, Greece, Israel, Morocco and the United States also produce some.

FOLKLORE AND HERBAL HERITAGE

Early inhabitants of Mediterranean countries used thyme for health and culinary purposes. Hippocrates, the ancient Greek physician known as the "Father of Medicine," spoke highly of thyme's healing properties. Thyme probably derives its name from one of two Greek words, either *thymos,* meaning "to fumigate" or "perfume," or *thymus,* meaning "courage."

According to Greek mythology, thyme developed from the teardrops of Helen of Troy. The Greeks created perfumes with thyme and fumigated against infectious diseases with it. They also used it to treat nervous disorders. Thyme incense burned at the altars of their gods. For millennia, thyme has enhanced foods with both its flavor and its digestive effects. Before refrigeration existed, thyme was added to meat to preserve it and prevent it from spoiling. The ancient Egyptians took advantage of thyme's preservative property in embalming.

In medieval Europe, sprigs of thyme were presented to chivalrous knights to reward them for courageous acts; judges carried thyme into their courtrooms for purification purposes. Sleeping on pillows stuffed with thyme reputedly relieved depression and epilepsy. Thyme was also supposed to cure leprosy, muscular atrophy, and paralysis. For centuries, herbalists treated colds, coughs, and sore throats with thyme. It was used to combat the infection of many European plagues and as a battlefield antiseptic during World War I.

MEDICINAL USES

The *British Herbal Pharmacopoeia* lists thyme as a remedy for asthma, bronchitis, diarrhea, dyspepsia, gastritis, laryngitis, and tonsillitis. European physicians use thyme oil to expel intestinal parasites. It combats infection and improves immunity by increasing the production of white blood cells. European physicians prescribe thyme oil for bronchitis, colds, coughs, the flu, laryngitis, sinusitis, sore throats, tonsillitis, and whooping cough. Lemon thyme oil is especially good for asthma and other respiratory conditions. Used in a mouthwash or gargle, thyme oil fights gum, mouth, and throat infections.

Thyme oil helps to reduce some of the symptoms of chronic fatigue syndrome. It counteracts general sluggishness, making it particularly valuable in convalescence. It restores energy depleted by physical fatigue or exhaustion. It also stimulates the appetite and expels gas. Thyme oil reduces fluid retention and helps with obesity, premenstrual syndrome (PMS), and edema. A thyme sitz bath relieves the discomforts of cystitis or urethritis.

Thyme oil stimulates menstrual flow. It increases circulation and is useful for low blood pressure. It relieves the pain of arthritis, sore mus-

cles, sprains, and injuries, and can ease the pain of headaches, including migraines. Thyme oil also helps fight athlete's foot and jock itch. It reduces the inflammation and irritation of skin disorders such as acne and psoriasis, as well as eczema and other types of dermatitis. It can accelerate the healing of bruises, burns, cuts, sores, or wounds, and it soothes the sting of insect bites.

BEAUTY BENEFITS

Thyme oil increases circulation to the skin and helps to improve sluggish and to regulate oily skin. It also encourages the elimination of wastes that contribute to cellulite.

EMOTIONAL EFFECTS

Thyme oil can strengthen your nerves when you are experiencing emotional fatigue. It eases nervousness, stress, and some stress-related complaints. It enhances memory and increases concentration. Thyme oil is stimulating, although when used in a bath, it helps overcome insomnia. It can balance you, either keeping you alert or helping you to sleep.

PRIMARY ACTIONS

Thyme oil fights infection and improves immunity. It eases muscle spasms and the pain of arthritis. It improves digestion and relieves urinary tract problems and respiratory ailments. Thyme oil improves circulation and elevates blood pressure. It helps overcome emotional fatigue, nervousness, and stress. Thyme oil regulates the oiliness of the skin and hair, and decreases the irritation of skin disorders.

CAUTIONS

Thyme oil can irritate or sensitize skin and mucous

membranes. Because it can stimulate menstrual flow, it should be avoided during pregnancy. It should also be avoided by persons with hyperthyroidism or high blood pressure.

Vetiver

Tall and tufted vetiver grass has long, narrow aromatic leaves and straight stems. This perennial member of the *Poaceae* family is related to citronella and lemongrass, and grows up to six feet tall. Washed and dried vetiver roots are steam-distilled to produce an amber or dark-brown oil with a viscous texture. It smells smoky and woody, earthy and musty, like a damp forest after heavy rain. It also has sweet and spicy undertones. About 200 pounds of vetiver roots yields about one pound of oil. The older the root, the better the oil; the oil itself also improves with age.

Vetiver (*Vetiveria zizanoides*, *Vetiveria odorata*, or *Andropogon muricatus*) is native to India, Indonesia, and Sri Lanka. It grows wild in the tropical climates of Haiti, India, Java, and Tahiti. Vetiver is cultivated commercially today in China, the Comoro Islands, Indonesia, Japan, Malaysia, the Philippines, the island of Réunion in the southwestern Indian Ocean, and countries in South America, western Africa, and the West Indies. Most of the vetiver oil used in aromatherapy comes from Java, Haiti, and Réunion. Many people consider vetiver oil from Réunion to be the best.

FOLKLORE AND HERBAL HERITAGE

Since antiquity, many civilizations have regarded vetiver as a fine fragrance. Vetiver's calming action earned it the name "oil of tranquility" in India and Sri Lanka. East Indian peoples constructed awnings, called *tatties*, and sunshades from vetiver grass, which is also known as *khus khus*. These shades were used to keep homes cool, to keep insects away, and, when wetted down, to emit an enticing aroma. Javanese servants waved ceremonial fans of woven vetiver to cool their rulers. Ancient Indians also used vetiver fans. When vetiver was transported to Louisiana, Creole belles quickly adopted this practice.

In India and Russia, sachets commonly contained vetiver roots. Because vetiver repels moths, it is also known as moth root. In tropical climates, the roots and leaves are woven into thatched roofs and huts. In many areas of the world, farmers and conservationists plant vetiver to counteract soil erosion; the plant's root system extends deep into the earth.

Many perfumes have included vetiver. One of these was the famous Mousseline des Indes, named for the scent of Indian muslin; the Indians used vetiver to protect muslin from insects. Today, vetiver adds an earthy, mossy note to approximately one third of all Western perfumes and one fifth of men's fragrances.

MEDICINAL USES

Vetiver oil stimulates the production of red blood cells, which transport oxygen throughout the body. This improves circulation and immunity. Vetiver oil relives the muscular aches, pains, spasms, and stiff joints of arthritis, rheumatism, sprains, and strains.

Vetiver oil calms nervousness and has proven helpful with anorexia nervosa. It is a natural tranquilizer and helps to induce restful sleep. It also helps balance female hormones and tone the reproductive organs. Because of its ability to induce relaxation, it may help overcome sexual dysfunction that is caused by nerves or stress.

BEAUTY BENEFITS

Vetiver oil balances the activity of the sebaceous glands, or oil glands, and helps to normalize oily skin and clear acne. It replenishes moisture in dry and dehydrated skin and has a rejuvenating effect on mature skin. It helps heal cuts and wounds and soothes irritated and inflamed skin. When used regularly during pregnancy, vetiver oil reportedly prevents stretch marks. It also has natural deodorizing properties.

EMOTIONAL EFFECTS

Vetiver oil strengthens the central nervous system. It is emotionally calming and is helpful in overcoming depression, insomnia, and nervousness. Vetiver oil reduces anxiety, stress, and tension. It settles nerves and can revive a person who is suffering from emotional exhaustion. Vetiver oil restores balance and harmony, brings thoughts and actions into focus, and helps to stabilize energy. It normalizes either extreme sensitivity or insensitivity. Some people use vetiver oil as an aphrodisiac.

PRIMARY ACTIONS

Vetiver oil fights infection and relieves muscle spasms. It calms nerves and stimulates sexual feelings. It stimulates circulation and improves immunity.

Ylang Ylang

Tall and willowy, the majestic ylang ylang or perfume tree displays clusters of large star-shaped flowers on downward-drooping branches. These unusual flowers range in color from white to pink to yellow to yellowish-green. Their fragrance is fresh and floral, sweet and seductive, exciting and exotic. This refreshing scent is relaxing, almost intoxicating.

Shortly after sunrise in either early summer or autumn, workers gather ylang ylang blossoms. Immediately afterwards, they begin the steam distillation process, which lasts several days. About fifty pounds of fresh-picked flowers yields one pound of ylang ylang oil.

Ylang ylang (*Cananga odorata*, variety *genuina*) is closely related to cananga (*Cananga odorata*). Both are members of the *Annonaceae* family, and both yield essential oils. Ylang ylang oil, however, is far superior to cananga oil. Also known as "poor man's jasmine," ylang ylang flowers can produce six different grades of syrupy yellowish oil. Experts contend that the yellow flowers produce the best oil. Whole ylang ylang oil is most desirable for aromatherapy purposes. The finest quality oil is purchased by the perfume industry, which includes small amounts of it in some expensive scents. Cosmetic manufacturers utilize the lower grade ylang ylang oil or cananga oil.

Originally native to Southeast Asia and the Philippines, the "flower of flowers"—the Malay meaning of *ylang ylang*—now thrives throughout the tropics. Blossoms of trees growing in the wild produce little fragrance, but when the trees are carefully tended, their scent intensifies. Ylang ylang is cultivated commercially in the Comoro Islands, Haiti, Java, Sumatra, and Zanzibar.

FOLKLORE AND HERBAL HERITAGE

In tropical climates, leis strung with ylang ylang flowers were worn around the neck. In Indonesia, the marriage beds of newlyweds would be covered with ylang ylang flowers. This tradition probably stems from ylang ylang's use as an aphrodisiac and sexual stimulant. For centuries, people in tropical cultures have scented coconut oil with ylang ylang for its beautifying benefits in skin treatments. They also smoothed it over their skin to soothe insect bites.

Tropical women—famous for their thick, shiny, lustrous hair—have used ylang ylang in hair preparations for hundreds of years. Ylang ylang reputedly helps control split ends. During the Victorian era, a hair treatment called Macassar oil contained ylang ylang. This preparation supposedly promoted hair growth by stimulating the scalp. In Samoa and Tonga, indigenous cultures used ylang ylang to treat colic, constipation, indigestion, and stomachaches. Throughout the tropics, many people have used ylang ylang to regulate the heartbeat and respiration.

MEDICINAL USES

In Europe, aromatherapists, massage therapists, and medical professionals prescribe ylang ylang to lower blood pressure, regulate respiration, and calm heart palpitations. They say that ylang ylang is soothing to the nervous system, eases muscle spasms, and relaxes tense muscles. Ylang ylang oil is often helpful in treating female disorders such as irregular periods, menstrual cramps, and premenstrual syndrome (PMS). It calms and comforts women going through menopause. It also soothes the inflammation and irritation of psoriasis, eczema, and other types of dermatitis.

BEAUTY BENEFITS

Ylang ylang oil benefits any type of skin but is most effective in treating oily skin. It balances oil production, reducing excessive oiliness. By fighting bacterial infection, it helps control acne and blemishes. Ylang ylang oil softens and smooths skin and stimulates new cell growth. It reportedly can ward off wrinkles and premature aging because it relaxes facial muscles and releases facial tension that can contribute to lines, wrinkles, and sagging skin.

EMOTIONAL EFFECTS

European psychotherapists treat depression, insomnia, and nervous tension with ylang ylang oil. It relaxes and calms excited emotional states. Ylang ylang oil subdues anxiety, stress, and stress-related disorders. It reduces worrying and tension and stabilizes moods. It minimizes anger, fears, and frustrations, while fostering feelings of love, security, and serenity. It stimulates enthusiasm and can provide comfort during times of change. Ylang ylang oil encourages positive emotions and feelings, helping to improve attitude. It awakens an appreciation of self and others, as well as of the beauty of life. It inspires creativity, intuition, and understanding, and helps both men and women to enjoy their feminine qualities. Some European medical and psychological professionals recommend ylang ylang oil for sexual difficulties such as frigidity, impotence, and feelings of sexual inadequacy, especially when these problems stem from stress. Ylang ylang oil arouses sensuality, creates erotic and euphoric moods, and induces deep relaxation.

PRIMARY ACTIONS

Ylang ylang oil calms nerves and lifts depression. It stimulates sex drive. Ylang ylang oil fights infection, improves circulation, and lowers blood pressure.

PART THREE

Common Conditions That Can Be Treated With Aromatherapy

Introduction

Long before man-made medicines lined the shelves of pharmacies, people sought relief from their physical and mental ailments with botanicals. Healing plants helped earth's earliest inhabitants maintain health and well-being and fight illness and disease. The first known physicians were priests and perfumers who used aromatic oils and ointments infused with the healing properties of plants to heal both body and soul. Since ancient times, herbalists, physicians, and healers have passed on their evolving knowledge of plants from generation to generation as herbal folklore.

For thousands of years, botanicals were the only kind of healing medicines available. Up until the beginning of the twentieth century, many European homes had their own "still rooms" for making essential oils and aromatic waters. Many people blended their own perfumes and medicines with essential oils. Apothecaries, or pharmacies, sold medicines made from essential oils and other botanicals.

As recently as the 1940s, the American medical community still officially recognized the germ-killing effects of many essential oils. Physicians treated gonorrhea with sandalwood oil. Thyme oil was prescribed to treat hookworm. Camphor, eucalyptus, and clove oils were administered as anesthetics; benzoin, eucalyptus, and peppermint oils were used to treat respiratory ailments; citronella oil was used to repel insects; and geraniol, a major component of such essential oils as geranium and palmarosa, was the key ingredient in an agricultural insecticide.

Essential oils were frequently employed to mask the unpalatable tastes of many medicines. Through World Wars I and II, the first aid kits that soldiers carried into battle contained essential oils such as lavender and tea tree for disinfecting and treating wounds.

With the advent of modern chemistry and modern medicine, most essential oils were relegated to the shelves of perfumery laboratories. However, even today many pharmacists and medical professionals recognize the therapeutic value of some essential oils. *Martindale: The Extra Pharmacopoeia* (Pharmaceutical Press, 1993) details the modern-day usage of many essential oils, including anise, bay, bergamot, cajeput, caraway, cassia, cinnamon, citronella, clove, coriander, dill, eucalyptus, fennel, geranium, juniper, lavender, lemon, lemongrass, mace, neroli, niaouli, nutmeg, orange, peppermint, pine, rose, rosemary, rue, sassafras, spearmint, and thyme. Eucalyptus helps to ease nasal congestion and coughs and is helpful for respiratory tract disorders. Rosemary dispels gas and is used in hair lotions and liniments. Thyme helps in the treatment of respiratory tract disorders because it acts as an expectorant and eases coughs. It also helps dispel gas.

Aromatherapy offers you new options for taking care of yourself and your health. Instead of running to the medicine cabinet for an aspirin to quell a headache, you can inhale the fragrant aroma of lavender or peppermint oil, or apply essential oil to the painful areas. Instead of clutching your bottle of antacid, you can massage your abdomen with a few drops of chamomile, fennel, marjoram, or peppermint oil. Instead of taking painkillers for a toothache, you can dab a drop of tea tree or chamomile oil on your gums. Aromatherapy gives you greater freedom to take care of your health in a natural way.

Each section in this part of the book is devoted to a common condition that can be helped with aromatherapy, either as a treatment or as a preventive measure. Following a description of the usual causes and typical symptoms of the condition, a section on Helpful Treatments outlines some alternative treatments, such as nutrition, exercise, and relaxation, that can be used together with aromatherapy. This is because, although the focus of this book is on aromatherapy, a combination of different treatments usually provides the best results. Each section also contains a list of essential oils that are helpful for the condition, as well as suggestions for ways to use aromatherapy.

Each section then includes one or more formulas for specific aromatherapy blends that are useful for the particular condition being discussed. These blends are easy to make and easy to use; simply follow the directions. You will notice that most of the suggested aromatherapy treatments in this book involve combinations of several essential oils. This is because a combination of different essential oils produces a synergistic effect, with each oil intensifying the actions of the others. Finally, if appropriate, each section concludes with a section on Cautions that discusses any reasons for caution when using essential oils to treat that particular condition.

Once you become more familiar with the essential oils, you may wish to experiment with creating your own blends. I suggest that you start by looking at the essential oils mentioned in the section for the condition you want to treat. Then reread the sections on each of those essential oils in Part Two. Select the three or four oils that seem most appropriate, and then decide which method or methods will work best for you (consult Part Four, Ways of Using Aromatherapy, for complete instructions on mixing blends for each method).

When mixing aromatherapy blends, you should always keep in mind that it is important to follow instructions regarding the amounts of essential oils and carrier oils. Essential oils are extremely concentrated, and using higher levels of essential oils or applying them directly to your body could irritate your skin. Also, be sure to use only pure essential oils—not synthethic imitations—for all your aromatherapy blends. Synthetics are made from petroleum byproducts and they simply do not have the therapeutic properties of pure essential oils. Worse, they may even be harmful when absorbed through the skin.

I hope you will find the aromatherapy blends as much fun to make and use—and as helpful—as have the many people who have used them successfully to treat these common conditions. I urge you to experiment with the blends and, in doing so, to discover a new world of natural remedies.

General Guidelines
for Using Essential Oils

To ensure that you obtain the best possible results from essential oils, always keep in mind the guidelines below. These apply whether you are using the aromatherapy blends suggested in this book or experimenting with essential oils on your own.

❏ Use only pure essential oils. Never substitute synthetics.

❏ Buy your essential oils from reliable sources that guarantee the purity of their oils. Consult the Aromatherapy Resource Guide in the Appendix for recommended suppliers.

❏ Always dilute essential oils in a carrier oil, such as almond, apricot kernel, canola, hazelnut, jojoba, or sunflower oil, before applying them to your body. Essential oils are highly concentrated—sometimes as much as 100 times stronger than the fresh plant or dried herb—so even one drop of pure essential oil applied directly to your skin can cause irritation.

❏ When using an essential oil, uncap the bottle for a few seconds only. Drop the oils from the dropper into the palm of your hand or into a clean container for blending. Keep the dropper and the rim of the container from touching your skin or anything else. Keep bottles tightly capped and away from sunlight and heat when not in use.

❏ Follow the directions for the aromatherapy blends carefully. Never add more than the recommended number of drops of an essential oil. You can use fewer drops if you wish.

❏ When using essential oils on infants or children, dilute them even more. Consult the instructions for different types of aromatherapy treatments in Part Four for the correct dilutions.

❏ Use glass containers for all blends consisting of essential oils only, and for all other aromatherapy blends whenever possible. Suitable glass bottles are available at some beauty supply stores, body care stores, and drug stores. Or ask your local pharmacist if you might purchase bottles through him or her. Many pharmacists will be willing to sell you some empty glass dropper bottles, but usually you have to ask for them.

❏ If you must use a plastic container for an aromatherapy blend, be sure to add the carrier oil or water to the container first and then add the essential oil or oils. Essential oils are very concentrated, and may damage a plastic container unless diluted.

❏ Do not shake bottles of essential oils, and do not shake an essential oil blend to mix it. Instead, turn the bottle upside down a number of times or gently roll the bottle between your hands for a few minutes to blend the ingredients.

❏ Trust your nose. If you dislike the smell of a certain oil, don't use it.

❏ Inhale essential oils for short periods only. If you are using a diffuser, run it for only five to ten minutes at a time.

❏ If you have doubts about using an essential oil or an aromatherapy blend, trust your instincts or check with a qualified aromatherapist or your health care professional.

❏   If you experience any irritation, sensitivity, or unpleasant reaction, discontinue use of the suspect oil.

❏   Never take essential oils internally, except as directed by a health care professional trained in the practice of medical aromatherapy.

❏   The essential oils and aromatherapy blends discussed in this book are safe for most people to use, provided they follow appropriate guidelines. However, people with certain medical conditions should be very cautious about using aromatherapy.

These conditions include asthma, cancer, epilepsy, high or low blood pressure, and pregnancy. Certain essential oils can trigger asthma attacks or epileptic seizures in susceptible people; cause harm to cancer patients; or elevate or depress blood pressure. If you have any of the conditions listed above, consult with a health care professional before using any essential oils. Essential oils can also counteract or diminish the effectiveness of homeopathic remedies, so if you are using any homeopathic preparations, you should check with a homeopathic physician.

Acne

Acne occurs when the sebaceous glands—the oil-secreting glands that lubricate the skin—secrete too much sebum, or oil. Normally, sebum flows from the sebaceous glands to the surface of the skin. But if dead skin cells accumulate inside the pores, they can clog the pores and prevent the normal flow of sebum. As a result, otherwise harmless bacteria that live beneath the surface of the skin and in the pores can multiply. This overgrowth of bacteria, together with the blocked sebum, causes pimples to form.

The skin mirrors internal health, and blemishes or acne can indicate internal problems. Acne sometimes signals a general toxic condition within the body. When the kidneys, lungs, and intestines become overloaded with more wastes than they can eliminate, the skin may be called upon to filter out wastes.

Other factors can make the skin more prone to develop pimples. These include allergies; a diet high in fats, preservatives, sugar, and pesticide and herbicide residues; dehydration; emotional problems; environmental pollution; too much exposure to the sun; heredity; hormones; oral contraceptives; poor hygiene; weakened immunity; and stress.

HELPFUL TREATMENTS

A nutritious diet rich in fresh vegetables and whole grains, an adequate intake of water, plenty of fresh air and exercise, and aromatherapy skin care can help clear acne. If you suspect you have a weak immune system, you may wish to consult a nutritionist to help you boost it with diet and supplements. Aromatherapy also can help you increase your immunity, in addition to helping you reduce stress. (See also WEAKENED IMMUNE SYSTEM and/or STRESS.)

Essential oils recommended for acne include anti-inflammatory oils, which reduce painful irritation and swelling; balancing oils, which normalize oil production while they improve the condition of the skin; and astringent oils, which help control oiliness. Anti-inflammatory essential oils that are effective against acne include benzoin, chamomile, clary sage, eucalyptus, frankincense, helichrysum, lavender, myrrh, orange, patchouli, peppermint, and sandalwood. Bergamot, eucalyptus, geranium, helichrysum, lavender, orange, palmarosa, rosemary, and sandalwood are good balancing oils. Recommended astringent oils are basil, cedarwood, cypress, elemi, frankincense, geranium, juniper, lavender, lemon, neroli, orange, palmarosa, patchouli, peppermint, rosewood, tea tree, thyme, vetiver, and ylang ylang. Recent tests in Australia showed that tea tree oil was as effective in clearing acne as benzoyl peroxide, the most common over-the-counter acne medication. And benzoyl peroxide causes numerous side effects, such as a burning sensation, dryness, flakiness, irritation, and redness, whereas tea tree oil does not.

If you have acne, resist the temptation to squeeze or pick at blemishes; this aggravates them and makes them last longer. It can also cause infection and lead to scarring. If blemishes are left alone and treated with essential oils, which fight the bacteria that cause pimples, they usually go away within a few days.

Proper skin care is crucial for clearing acne. Keeping your skin clean and your pores unclogged and reducing oil secretions can help clear up your complexion. Cleanse your skin twice a day, use a facial scrub several times a week, and spot-treat blemishes with essential oils to help control breakouts. In addition, apply a facial mask one or more times a week. This will help minimize oiliness and clear plugged pores. You can customize the skin care products you already use by adding any of the essential oils listed above. Or use the blends below, which are designed specifically for acne, as follows:

- Twice a day, cleanse your skin with Green Clay Cleanser. French green clay is very cleansing and healing for blemished skin. Follow this with an application of Skin-Clearing Toner, then Oily Skin Treatment.

- Dab Spot Treatment or Blemish Blend on individual blemishes several times a day, as needed, to clear them quickly.

- At least twice a week, massage Grainy Scrub into your skin to discourage blackheads and blemishes.

- Once a week, apply Clearing Mask to remove impurities and to regulate oiliness. Adding enzymes to the Clearing Mask formula will help the mask to remove dead skin cells that can block pores and contribute to blemishes.

- Once a week, steam your face with Acne-Clearing Facial Steam to loosen sebum and bacteria that clog pores. Follow with Green Clay Cleanser, Grainy Scrub, or Clearing Mask.

- Men can use Blemish-Banishing After-Shave to prevent blemishes and infected ingrown hairs.

AROMATHERAPY BLENDS

The aromatherapy blends below are essential oil formulas you can prepare at home. For a more detailed explanation of how to put together and use these blends, see Taking Care of Your Skin on page 184 and/or FACIAL STEAM BATHS in Part Four. For a quick review of general guidelines for using essential oils, see page 91.

❧ Green Clay Cleanser

1 teaspoon French green clay powder
1 teaspoon honey or water

1 drop geranium oil
1 drop lavender oil
1 drop tea tree oil

Mix all the ingredients into a paste in your palm. Massage the paste into your skin until it feels clean. Rinse. Repeat if necessary.

❧ Skin-Clearing Toner

8 ounces distilled water
2 drops lavender oil
1 drop palmarosa oil
1 drop rosewood oil

Place the water in a clean bottle, add the essential oils, and shake it to blend. Saturate a cotton ball with toner and apply it to your skin after cleansing. Blend the mixture again before each use.

❧ Oily Skin Treatment

1 ounce jojoba oil
3 drops lavender oil
2 drops lemon oil
2 drops tea tree oil
2 drops ylang ylang oil
1 drop geranium oil
1 drop orange oil
1 drop rosewood oil

Place the jojoba oil in a clean container, add the essential oils, and turn the container upside down several times or roll it between your hands for a few minutes to blend. Apply one or two drops to your skin as a moisturizer. Jojoba oil is very similar in composition to your skin's own natural oils, and helps to balance oil production. It does not aggravate acne.

🐦 Spot Treatment

⅛ ounce jojoba oil
20 drops lavender oil
20 drops tea tree oil

Place the jojoba oil in a clean container and add the essential oils. Turn the container upside down a few times or roll it between your hands for a few minutes to blend. Apply a dab of Spot Treatment directly to each blemish several times daily.

🐦 Blemish Blend

⅛ ounce jojoba oil
8 drops lavender oil
8 drops rosewood oil
8 drops tea tree oil
4 drops chamomile oil
4 drops geranium oil
4 drops helichrysum oil
4 drops lemon oil

Place the jojoba oil in a clean container, add the essential oils, and turn the container upside down a few times or roll it between your hands to blend. Dab a bit of the mixture on each blemish several times daily.

🐦 Grainy Scrub

½ teaspoon oat flour
½ teaspoon blue cornmeal
1 drop lemon oil
1 drop ylang ylang oil
½ teaspoon (approximately) honey or water

Combine the oat flour, blue cornmeal, lemon oil, and ylang ylang oil in your palm. Add enough honey or water to form a paste. Massage the paste into clean skin for one minute. Rinse.

🐦 Clearing Mask

1 teaspoon French green clay or bentonite
1 teaspoon honey
1 drop helichrysum oil
1 drop orange oil
1 drop rosemary oil
¼ teaspoon enzyme powder (optional)

Mix all the ingredients together well in your palm. Apply the mask to clean skin and leave it on for ten minutes. Rinse thoroughly.

🐦 Acne-Clearing Facial Steam

1 quart steaming water
2 drops tea tree oil
1 drop clary sage oil
1 drop lemon oil
1 drop palmarosa oil
1 drop ylang ylang oil

Pour the water into a two-quart glass bowl. Drop the oils into the water and gently disperse them. Lean your clean face over the bowl and drape a towel over both your head and the bowl to capture the steam. Steam your face for five minutes. Cleanse your skin afterwards with Green Clay Cleanser or your favorite cleanser.

🐦 Blemish-Banishing After-Shave

8 ounces distilled water
2 drops sandalwood oil
1 drop cedarwood oil
1 drop tea tree oil
1 drop vetiver oil

Add the water to a clean bottle, drop in the essential oils, and shake to combine. Splash the mixture on your skin after shaving. Shake again before each use.

Anxiety

Everyone fears or worries about something sometime. But when your fears or apprehensions begin to dominate or interfere with your life, you have anxiety. The most extreme manifestation of anxiety is an anxiety attack. Your heart pounds rapidly in your chest. Breathing becomes difficult. An awful gnawing sensation in your stomach nauseates you. Your head pounds. Panic sets in.

Anxiety can become the focal point of your life and, paradoxically, prevent you from dealing with the very problems that are causing it. Anxiety shows up in your health, on your skin, and in your attitude. Chronic anxiety can weaken your immune system, making you more susceptible to disease of every kind.

Many different factors can contribute to or aggravate anxiety. Some of the most common are the consumption of caffeine and other stimulants, chemical sensitivities, childhood trauma, emotional difficulties, environmental pollutants, heredity, lifestyle factors such as problems at work or in relationships, nutritional deficiencies, physical illness, poor diet, and stress, especially chronic stress.

Cigarette smoking, the use of alcohol or other drugs (whether legal or illegal, prescription or over-the-counter), the consumption of too much salt or sugar, and exposure to pesticides, household or industrial chemicals, or synthetic fragrances contribute to anxiety attacks in many people. Monosodium glutamate (MSG), an additive that is found in many processed food products and is often added to Chinese and fast food, can also trigger anxietylike symptoms in susceptible people.

HELPFUL TREATMENTS

If you cannot change the situation that is the focus of your anxiety, try to determine what you can do to change your way of handling or responding to problems. Remember, chronic anxiety takes its toll on both physical and emotional health. If you find you simply cannot manage your anxiety, consulting a qualified counsellor may help. If your anxiety has led to health problems, consult your health care professional.

If you suffer from anxiety, you should eliminate or reduce your intake of caffeine, which is present not only in coffee and tea but often also in candy, chocolate, cocoa, medications, and soft drinks. Read product labels carefully. Avoid additive-laden processed foods. Keep track of the foods you eat and your reactions to them, and then avoid any foods that seem to trigger your anxiety. Do the same with other substances you may be exposed to. Sometimes taking supplements of nutrients, especially the B-complex vitamins, calcium, magnesium, and potassium, all of which are vital for nerve health, can help reduce anxiety.

Relaxation and stress reduction are important parts of any program to overcome anxiety. Aromatherapy can relax you and strengthen your emotional stamina, allowing you to deal better with anxiety-provoking situations. Essential oils such as benzoin, bergamot, cedarwood, chamomile, clary sage, coriander, frankincense, geranium, jasmine, juniper, marjoram, neroli, orange, patchouli, rose, rosewood, vetiver, and ylang ylang help reduce anxiety. During trying times, disperse Anxiety Diffuser Blend throughout your home or office. Bathe in Anxiety Bath Blend once or twice daily to keep anxiety under control. Carry Quick-Fix Anxiety Inhalant with you and inhale it directly from the bottle as often as necessary to remain calm.

AROMATHERAPY BLENDS

The aromatherapy blends below are essential oil formulas you can prepare at home. For a more detailed explanation of how to put together and use these blends, see BATHS; DIFFUSERS AND LAMPS and/or INHALANTS in Part Four. For a quick review of general guidelines for using essential oils, see page 91.

Anxiety Diffuser Blend

15 drops clary sage oil
10 drops bergamot oil
10 drops geranium oil
8 drops chamomile oil
8 drops marjoram oil
5 drops ylang ylang oil

Drop the essential oils into a small glass bottle and gently turn the bottle upside down a few times or roll it between your hands to blend. Add some of the mixture to your diffuser or lamp bowl. Run your diffuser or lamp as necessary to prevent or reduce anxiety.

Anxiety Bath Blend

2 drops frankincense oil
2 drops geranium oil
2 drops neroli oil
2 drops patchouli oil

Disperse the essential oils in a bathtub filled with warm water. Enjoy a calming soak for twenty to thirty minutes.

Quick-Fix Anxiety Inhalant

3 drops neroli oil
2 drops benzoin resin
2 drops geranium oil
2 drops rosewood oil
2 drops ylang ylang oil

1 drop frankincense oil
1 drop rose oil

Drop the essential oils into a small glass bottle with an airtight cover and blend. Inhale directly from the bottle to prevent or alleviate an anxiety attack. Repeat as often as needed.

Appetite Disturbances

Some people experience a loss of appetite; others have difficulty controlling theirs. When considering disturbances of appetite, it is important to remember that while hunger is a physical sensation, appetite is a psychological one. The hypothalamus area of the brain, which controls appetite, is closely connected with the emotions.

Alcohol, cigarettes, drugs, allergies, depression, emotional upset, illness, nutritional deficiencies, stress, and weather—among other things—can affect appetite. Sometimes simply seeing or talking about a favorite food can stimulate your appetite, even if you've just eaten. Conversely, the sight of an unappealing or disliked food can decrease your appetite, even when you're hungry. In times of stress, anxiety, tension, or emotional upset, some people tend to react by overindulging in food, while others stop eating completely.

HELPFUL TREATMENTS

If you experience a notable change in appetite—whether a loss of appetite or excessive appetite—you should first consult a health practitioner or nutritionist to rule out any underlying physical illness or nutritional deficiencies. Whether you wish to stimulate or to curb your appetite, changing the way you eat may help. If you want to increase your appetite, more frequent small meals of healthy and nutritious foods may be more appetizing than two or three larger ones. Avoid fast food and processed foods, which offer little appeal and poor nutritional value. Instead, concentrate on eating a diet that contains a lot of fresh vegetables, fruits, and whole grains, which look and smell more tempting, are nutritionally safer choices, and are more likely to satisfy hunger.

If you want to suppress your appetite, you should also change your diet to one that focuses on fresh, healthy foods. Eating fresh vegetables and whole grains as your primary foods will help you to feel full while furnishing your body with necessary nutrients. When your nutritional needs are met, you won't get as hungry between meals.

Aromatherapy can help regulate appetite. Essential oils that come from culinary herbs, including basil, black pepper, clary sage, coriander, ginger, marjoram, peppermint, rosemary, and thyme, are particularly good for stimulating appetite. Several other oils—bergamot, chamomile, juniper, myrrh, palmarosa, and orange—also arouse the appetite. Aromatherapy can help if loss of appetite is linked to stress or depression, because it can work directly on those problems. Aromatherapy may also help some people with eating disorders such as anorexia nervosa. Used in conjunction with medical and psychological attention, essential oils may help an anorexic regain her appetite and feel better about herself. If you want to increase your appetite, breathing in Appetite-Stimulating Inhalation, beginning thirty minutes to one hour before mealtime, can help. You can repeat this as necessary. Massage Appetite-Stimulating Stomach Rub over your entire abdominal area several times a day.

Some people wish to suppress their appetites, usually for the purpose of losing weight. Bergamot, fennel, and patchouli can decrease or regulate the desire for food, according to the body's needs. If you want to tame your appetite, breathe in Appetite-Suppressing Inhalation whenever you get the urge to eat between meals. Massage Appetite-Suppressing Stomach Rub over your entire abdominal area as many times a day as necessary to curb your appetite.

AROMATHERAPY BLENDS TO STIMULATE APPETITE

The aromatherapy blends below are essential oil formulas you can prepare at home. For a more detailed explanation of how to put together and use these blends, see INHALANTS and/or MASSAGE in Part Four. For a quick review of general guidelines for using essential oils, see page 91.

Appetite-Stimulating Inhalant

8 drops clary sage oil
6 drops coriander oil
4 drops black pepper oil
3 drops ginger oil
1 drop peppermint oil

Drop the essential oils into a small glass bottle with an airtight cover, and gently turn the bottle upside down a few times or roll it between your hands to blend. Inhale directly from the container as necessary.

Appetite-Stimulating Stomach Rub

½ ounce carrier oil
4 drops basil oil
4 drops orange oil
4 drops thyme oil
3 drops coriander oil
3 drops rosemary oil

Place the carrier oil in a clean container, add the essential oils, and blend well. Massage the mixture over your stomach and abdominal area as needed.

AROMATHERAPY BLENDS TO SUPPRESS APPETITE

The aromatherapy blends below are essential oil formulas you can prepare at home. For a more detailed explanation of how to put together and use these blends, see INHALANTS and/or MASSAGE in Part Four. For a quick review of general guidelines for using essential oils, see page 91.

❧ Appetite-Suppressing Inhalant

15 drops bergamot oil
10 drops fennel oil

Drop the bergamot and fennel oils into a small glass bottle with an airtight cover. Gently turn the bottle over a few times or roll it between your hands to blend. Inhale directly from the container as necessary.

❧ Appetite-Suppressing Stomach Rub

½ ounce carrier oil
10 drops fennel oil
5 drops bergamot oil
3 drops patchouli oil

Place the carrier oil in a clean container, add the essential oils, and blend. Massage the mixture over your stomach and abdominal area several times daily, as needed.

Note: Bergamot oil increases sensitivity to the sun. Omit it from the formula if your skin will be exposed to sunlight.

Arthritis

Arthritis (which literally means "joint inflammation"), may appear in the joints of the elbows, fingers, hips, knees, neck, shoulders, toes, or wrists, or along the spine. Medically, arthritis is a general category that includes over 100 different joint disorders with symptoms ranging from mild aches and pains, stiffness, and swelling to severe, crippling pain and deformities. Osteoarthritis and rheumatoid arthritis are the most common forms of arthritis.

Osteoarthritis, or degenerative joint disease, involves wear and tear on the joints due to use and aging. The cartilage at the end of the bones becomes rough and the ligaments, muscles, and tendons weaken. Bones begin to grind against each other during movement. Symptoms of osteoarthritis include stiffness, soreness, and pain in the joints of the feet, toes, thumbs, and weight-bearing bones. A number of different factors, including heredity, physical stress, and injuries affect a person's chances of developing osteoarthritis.

Rheumatoid arthritis affects both the bones and the surrounding tissue. It is an autoimmune disease, which means that the immune system begins attacking the body's own tissues. Rheumatoid arthritis often destroys the bone surface, the cartilage, and the tissues surrounding the joint. Fluids accumulate and inflame the joints. The small joints of the ankles, feet, hands, knees, and wrists are most often affected, although rheumatoid arthritis can attack any joint in the body. It causes pain, stiffness, swelling, and sometimes disabling deformities.

The exact cause or causes of most cases of rheumatoid arthritis are unknown, but abnormal bowel function, food allergies, heredity, infections, nutritional deficiencies, and weakened immunity have been implicated. Another possibility is increased intestinal permeability, which allows bacterial toxins or tiny particles of undigested food to leak from the intestines into the bloodstream, where they can initiate an immune response. Foods that can trigger or aggravate arthritis in susceptible people include alcohol, corn, dairy products, sugar, and wheat. Members of the nightshade family—which includes potatoes, eggplant, peppers, tomatoes, and tobacco—may also promote joint inflammation and interfere with joint repair in some people.

HELPFUL TREATMENTS

In many cases, good nutrition can play a big role in controlling arthritis. Consult your nutritionist or health care professional to check for and help you correct any nutritional deficiencies. A low-fat, low-sugar diet centered on fresh vegetables and whole grains may bring relief. Some people find that avoiding citrus fruits, dairy products, processed and refined foods, red meat, salt, and sugar, as well as vegetables in the nightshade family, diminishes inflammation. Iron supplements can exacerbate arthritis, while supplemental flaxseed oil, essential fatty acids, and garlic may bring relief. Physical therapy and exercise may help to maintain and restore muscle strength and, in some cases, can decrease symptoms.

Aromatherapy complements other treatments for arthritis. Essential oils that benefit arthritis include basil, benzoin, black pepper, cedarwood, chamomile, coriander, elemi, eucalyptus, fennel, ginger, helichrysum, juniper, lemon, marjoram, myrrh, pine, rosemary, thyme, and vetiver. These oils can ease pain and discomfort, reduce swelling, and relieve sore muscles.

Soak in Arthritis Bath Blend daily to relieve pain and discomfort. Apply Arthritis Massage Blend

over your entire body for a detoxifying and pain-relieving effect. Massage Deep Relief Arthritis Oil into your joints and muscles as often as necessary to relieve pain and reduce swelling.

AROMATHERAPY BLENDS

The aromatherapy blends below are essential oil formulas you can prepare at home. For a more detailed explanation of how to put together and use these blends, see BATHS and/or MASSAGE in Part Four. For a quick review of general guidelines for using essential oils, see page 91.

🐦 Arthritis Bath Blend

> 3 drops lemon oil
> 2 drops coriander oil
> 2 drops helichrysum oil
> 2 drops marjoram oil

Drop the oils into a bathtub filled with warm water and gently disperse them. Enjoy a leisurely soak for twenty to thirty minutes. Repeat as necessary.

🐦 Arthritis Massage Blend

> 1½ ounces carrier oil
> ½ ounce flaxseed oil
> 6 drops chamomile oil
> 4 drops marjoram oil
> 3 drops coriander oil
> 3 drops rosemary oil
> 2 drops benzoin resin
> 1 drop black pepper oil
> 1 drop ginger oil

Place the carrier oil in a clean container, add the essential oils, and gently turn the container upside down several times or roll it between your hands to blend. Massage the mixture over your joints and muscles as necessary.

❧ Deep Relief Arthritis Oil

1½ ounces carrier oil
½ ounce flaxseed oil
4 drops chamomile oil
4 drops helichrysum oil
4 drops lemon oil
3 drops fennel oil
3 drops juniper oil
3 drops marjoram oil
2 drops ginger oil

Mix the carrier oil and the flaxseed oil together in a clean container. Add the essential oils and blend. Apply the mixture to your joints and muscles as needed.

Asthma and Bronchitis

An asthma attack occurs when the muscles around the bronchi, the two main breathing tubes that lead from the windpipe to the lungs, go into spasms. The bronchi narrow and breathing becomes difficult. Sometimes inflammation also swells the lining of these air tubes, preventing proper breathing. Mucous secretions may increase and block the bronchi. As a result, air cannot pass into or out of the lungs as easily as it normally does. Carbon dioxide becomes trapped in the lungs and cannot be exhaled; fresh oxygen cannot be inhaled. Coughing and wheezing result from a desperate attempt to breathe.

A wide variety of factors can trigger or contribute to an asthma attack, including airborne and food allergies, especially allergies to dairy products, wheat, and yeast- or mold-containing foods; chemical sensitivities; exposure to cigarette smoke; changes in climate, humidity, and/or temperature; a diet high in dairy products, fried foods, and sugar; subnormal functioning of the adrenal glands; hypoglycemia; infections; poor circulation; reactions to food additives and preservatives; and stress. Aspirin, chemical irritants, emotional upset, sinusitis, exercise, and exposure to food colorings, monosodium glutamate, newsprint, sulfites, or synthetic fragrances may also trigger asthma attacks or aggravate symptoms.

Bronchitis is a condition in which the bronchial walls become inflamed, and thick, sticky mucus accumulates in the bronchi. In some cases, this is accompanied by bronchial spasms. The swelling and mucus block the exchange of oxygen and carbon dioxide in the lungs. Breathing becomes difficult, and coughing results as the body attempts to expel the mucus. The cough is at first a "dry" cough, but it usually becomes productive after several days.

Bronchitis most often occurs as part of an upper respiratory infection such as a cold. Exposure to cigarette smoke (whether by smoking or inhaling secondhand smoke) and other irritants, such as environmental pollutants and noxious chemicals, may contribute to or predispose a person to developing bronchitis. Poor nutrition and fatigue are also believed to play a role.

HELPFUL TREATMENTS

If you have asthma or are prone to developing bronchitis, you should avoid exposure to cigarette smoke. If you smoke, quit. Practice deep breathing exercises, engage in mild aerobic exercise such as walking or swimming, do yoga, and eat a healthy diet. Avoid contact with noxious chemicals. Try to determine which foods or food ingredients seem to be connected with acute attacks, and eliminate those items from your diet.

If you have bronchitis, rest is important. It is not usually advisable to suppress the cough; it is necessary to clear mucus from the lungs and restore breathing. Instead, drink plenty of fluids, which thin secretions and make them easier to cough out.

Whether you are suffering from asthma or bronchitis, aromatherapy can help you breathe more easily by clearing congestion, reducing inflammation, and releasing excess mucus. Essential oils that can calm or prevent asthma attacks include benzoin, clary sage, cypress, eucalyptus, frankincense, helichrysum, lavender, lemon, marjoram, peppermint, myrrh, pine, rose, rosemary, and tea tree. Essential oils useful for treating bronchitis include benzoin, cedarwood, cypress, elemi, eucalyptus, frankincense, helichrysum, lavender, lemon, marjoram, peppermint, myrrh, orange, pine, rosemary, sandalwood, and tea tree. There are also essential oils that can soothe coughs, such as basil, benzoin, black pepper, cedarwood, clary sage, elemi, eucalyptus, ginger, lavender, marjoram, myrrh, pine, rose, rosemary, tea tree, and thyme.

To relieve respiratory congestion or improve your breathing, breathe in Respiratory Relief Steam Inhalation as necessary. Apply Respiratory Rub or Breathe Easier Blend to your chest, back, and throat. Use your diffuser or lamp to circulate All-Purpose Diffuser Breathing Blend through your room, home, or office. To ward off an asthma attack, breathe in Asthma Inhalant directly from the bottle as needed. Ease the pain of coughing by massaging Chest Rub for Coughs over your chest, back, and throat.

AROMATHERAPY BLENDS

The aromatherapy blends below are essential oil formulas you can prepare at home. For a more detailed explanation of how to put together and use these blends, see ATOMIZERS; DIFFUSERS AND LAMPS; INHALANTS; MASSAGE; and/or STEAM INHALATIONS in Part Four. For a quick review of general guidelines for using essential oils, see page 91.

Respiratory Relief Steam Inhalation

    1 quart steaming water
    3 drops frankincense oil
    2 drops myrrh oil
    1 drop peppermint oil

Pour the water into a two-quart glass bowl and add the essential oils. Lean your face over the bowl and drape a towel over both your head and the bowl to capture the steam. Inhale the steam for five minutes. Repeat as necessary.

Respiratory Rub

    1 ounce jojoba oil
    3 drops eucalyptus oil
    3 drops pine oil
    3 drops tea tree oil
    2 drops frankincense oil
    2 drops myrrh oil
    2 drops thyme oil

Place the jojoba oil in a clean container, add the essential oils, and gently turn the container upside down a few times or roll it between your hands to blend. Massage the mixture over your chest and back as needed to aid breathing and to clear excess mucus.

Breathe Easier Blend

    1 ounce carrier oil
    3 drops eucalyptus oil
    3 drops tea tree oil
    2 drops helichrysum oil
    2 drops lavender oil
    1 drop rosemary oil

In a clean container, add the essential oils to the carrier oil and blend. Apply the mixture to your chest, throat, and back. Repeat as necessary.

☙ All-Purpose Diffuser Breathing Blend

12 drops eucalyptus oil
10 drops lemon oil
8 drops clary sage oil
8 drops thyme oil
6 drops cypress oil
6 drops marjoram oil
4 drops frankincense oil
4 drops rosemary oil

Drop the essential oils into a small glass bottle. Gently turn the bottle upside down a few times or roll it between your hands to blend. Add some of the mixture to your diffuser, lamp bowl, or atomizer. Run your diffuser, lamp, or atomizer as necessary to ease breathing.

☙ Asthma Inhalant

10 drops eucalyptus oil
10 drops rosemary oil
8 drops lavender oil
6 drops pine oil
4 drops cypress oil
4 drops myrrh oil

Add all the ingredients to a small glass bottle with an airtight cover and blend well. Inhale directly from the bottle as necessary to prevent asthma attacks.

☙ Chest Rub for Coughs

1 ounce carrier oil
4 drops cedarwood oil
3 drops elemi oil
2 drops pine oil

2 drops thyme oil
1 drop tea tree oil

Place the carrier oil in a clean container, add the essential oils, and blend. Massage the oil over your chest, neck, and throat as necessary.

CAUTIONS

People with asthma should exercise caution when using essential oils. Certain oils may trigger an asthma attack in susceptible individuals. If you have asthma, consult with your medical practitioner before using any essential oils.

Athlete's Foot

Over 30 percent of all Americans suffer from athlete's foot, or *tinea pedis,* at some time in their lives. This is a contagious fungal infection that most commonly occurs between the toes and on the soles of the feet.

Fungi thrive in dark and damp areas with little light or air. The warm, moist area between the toes, enclosed in nylons or socks and shoes most of the time, is a perfect breeding ground for these microbes. The dead skin cells that accumulate between your toes sustain them. Athlete's foot causes the skin to itch, flake, and burn, and it becomes irritated and inflamed.

HELPFUL TREATMENTS

Good hygiene is vital. Keeping your feet clean and dry is crucial for eliminating athlete's foot. Whenever possible, go barefoot or wear open sandals to allow air to circulate between your toes. Change socks and shoes several times a day. Freshen your shoes, particularly athletic shoes, by wiping them out with a clean cloth sprinkled with three drops of tea tree oil. Fungi hide in public showers and locker rooms, so you should always wear shoes in public showers, gyms, and locker rooms.

Essential oils such as elemi, eucalyptus, lavender, myrrh, patchouli, tea tree, and thyme fight athlete's foot by destroying fungi. These oils also relieve the uncomfortable burning, flaking, inflammation, and itching. Twice a day, give your feet a soak in Tea Tree Oil Foot Bath or Athlete's Foot Bath. Afterwards, apply Athlete's Foot Relief Oil. Once your athlete's foot is under control, weekly treatments should prevent its return.

AROMATHERAPY BLENDS

The aromatherapy blends below are essential oil formulas you can prepare at home. For a more detailed explanation of how to put together and use these blends, see FOOT BATHS and/or MASSAGE in Part Four. For a quick review of general guidelines for using essential oils, see page 91.

❧ Tea Tree Oil Foot Bath

Add 10 drops of tea tree oil to a small tub or foot bath filled with warm water. Soak your feet for ten to twenty minutes. Dry thoroughly, especially between the toes, and apply Athlete's Foot Relief Oil.

❧ Athlete's Foot Bath

5 drops tea tree oil
4 drops patchouli oil
2 drops myrrh oil

Add the oils to a small tub or foot bath filled with warm water. Soak your feet for ten to twenty minutes. Dry your feet well and apply Athlete's Foot Relief Oil.

❧ Athlete's Foot Relief Oil

2 ounces carrier oil
10 drops tea tree oil
8 drops eucalyptus oil
6 drops myrrh oil
6 drops thyme oil

Place the carrier oil in a clean container, add the essential oils, and turn the container upside down a few times or roll it between your hands to blend. Apply a few drops of the mixture directly to the affected areas, making sure your feet are clean and dry first. Use this blend before putting on your shoes.

Blood Pressure Problems

See HIGH BLOOD PRESSURE; LOW BLOOD PRESSURE.

Bronchitis

See ASTHMA AND BRONCHITIS.

Bruises

See CUTS AND BRUISES.

Candidiasis

Candida albicans is a single-celled fungus that is one of a number of microorganisms normally found in the intestines, the colon, and the genitourinary tract. In most people, the body is able to maintain a healthy balance between all of these microorganisms, but if this balance is disrupted, candida (also often called yeast) may thrive and even spread to other parts of the body, causing the infection known as candidiasis.

Antibiotics are one major contributing factor in candidiasis; they kill not only the bacteria that cause infections but also the beneficial bacteria, which are the body's natural defenses that keep candida under control. Other factors that can upset the body's natural balance include birth control pills, anti-inflammatory drugs, immunosuppressant drugs, and cortisone; a diet high in sugar, refined carbohydrates, and yeast-laden foods; food allergies; pregnancy; stress; and hormonal imbalances. Sugar is a major culprit, because yeast thrive on sugar. This includes not only refined white sugar but also brown sugar, corn syrup, fructose, honey, maple syrup, and sucrose. Other foods and food ingredients that can contribute to or aggravate candidiasis are alcohol; dairy products; fresh or dried fruits and fruit juices; grains such as barley, oats, rye, and wheat; and certain yeast-containing foods, such as breads and nutritional yeast.

Two of the most common manifestations of candida infection occur in the mouth, where it is called oral thrush, and in the vagina, where it is called vaginitis or a yeast infection (see VAGINITIS). However, candidiasis is often hard to pin down, because it can cause or contribute to a host of different physical symptoms, including acne, arthritis, asthma, athlete's foot, blurred vision, chemical sensitivity, chronic fatigue, clumsiness, constipation, cystitis, diabetes, diaper rash, diarrhea, dizziness, eczema, endometriosis, headaches, hyperactivity, hypoglycemia, hypothyroidism, indigestion, lethargy, loss of libido, menstrual difficulties or irregularity, muscular aches and pains, premenstrual syndrome, respiratory ailments, sinusitis, skin disorders, sore throat, and even cravings for sugar. In addition, many mental or emotional symptoms may appear, among them anxiety, depression, difficulty coping, impaired memory, irritability, lack of confidence, low self-esteem, mood swings, and poor concentration.

A candida infection may surface on the skin around the mouth, on the throat, and in the corners of the ears, eyes, mouth and nose. It appears as a dry, scaly, weeping rash or tiny cuts or cracks in the skin. It itches and burns and it may be painful and become inflamed.

HELPFUL TREATMENTS

Many alternative health care practitioners have designed programs to combat or control candida. All treatment for candidiasis is long-term and involves making changes in lifestyle and diet to minimize symptoms and eliminate, or at least control, the cause. Successful treatment includes reestablishing the proper balance of intestinal bacteria, usually by taking acidophilus and digestive enzymes; avoiding foods that trigger symptoms; and strengthening the immune system. All types of sugar should be eliminated from the diet, as should the other foods mentioned above that can contribute to candidiasis. A diet to control candida centers around fresh vegetables, fresh fish, brown rice, millet, and quinoa, plus at least eight to ten glasses of water daily to help flush out wastes.

Australian physicians treat candida with therapeutic-grade tea tree oil, taken internally. However, only a medical professional trained in medical aromatherapy is qualified to recommend the internal use of any essential oil. Many health care professionals suggest using tea tree oil suppositories as an adjunct therapy.

Aromatherapy alone cannot eliminate candida, but in conjunction with a good medical program, it can speed your recovery. The essential oils of chamomile, eucalyptus, geranium, lavender, marjoram, myrrh, patchouli, rosemary, tea tree, and thyme are helpful in treating candidiasis.

Regular use of Candida Bath Treatment and Candida Immune-Boosting Body Oil will help to fight candida, strengthen immunity, and soothe stress. You can bathe in Candida Bath Treatment once or twice daily, and apply Candida Immune-Boosting Body Oil to your entire body once or twice daily, as necessary. If a candida infection appears on your face, keep your skin clean and avoid wearing makeup. Apply Candida Facial Oil to the affected areas several times daily, as needed.

AROMATHERAPY BLENDS

The aromatherapy blends below are essential oil formulas you can prepare at home. For a more detailed explanation of how to put together and use these blends, see BATHS and/or MASSAGE in Part Four. For a quick review of general guidelines for using essential oils, see page 91.

ᘒᗏ Candida Bath Treatment

6 drops tea tree oil
3 drops eucalyptus oil
2 drops patchouli oil

Once or twice daily, add these oils to a bathtub filled with warm water. Soak for twenty minutes.

ᘒᗏ Candida Immune-Boosting Body Oil

4 ounces carrier oil
10 drops rosemary oil
10 drops tea tree oil
8 drops geranium oil
8 drops lavender oil
6 drops elemi oil
6 drops thyme oil
4 drops patchouli oil

Place the carrier oil in a clean container, add the essential oils, and gently turn the container upside down a few times or roll it between your hands to blend. Massage the mixture onto your skin daily until symptoms cease.

Note: Geranium oil can lower your blood sugar level. Use it with caution (or omit it) if you have hypoglycemia (low blood sugar).

ᘒᗏ Candida Facial Oil

¼ ounce jojoba oil
4 drops tea tree oil
3 drops geranium oil
2 drops myrrh oil
2 drops patchouli oil

Place the jojoba oil in a clean container, add the essential oils, and blend. Apply several drops of the mixture to soothe skin and relieve irritation. Apply to the affected areas as needed, until symptoms subside.

Capillaries, Broken

Broken capillaries usually appear on dry, delicate, or mature skin that is thin and fragile. Sometimes called thread veins, spider veins, or couperose skin, the condition occurs when cells in the capillary walls become weak, causing the capillaries to lose their elasticity. Normally, capillaries—like all blood vessels—expand and contract in a more or less rhythmic fashion; this is what moves the blood through the circulatory system. But when capillaries lose their elasticity, they are unable to return to their normal size after dilation. They then collapse and the skin appears red.

Broken capillaries most commonly appear on the face, but they can occur elsewhere on the body as well. A number of factors may cause or contribute to the development of broken capillaries, including the use of abrasive cleansers and facial scrubs; the consumption of alcohol, caffeine, and/or certain drugs; exposure to cold weather, harsh winds, or extreme changes in temperature; the use of certain cosmetics; forceful massage; overexposure to the sun; rough handling of the skin; and the consumption of spicy food and stimulants.

HELPFUL TREATMENTS

If you have broken capillaries, you should avoid alcohol, caffeine, drugs, extremes of temperature, facial steaming, saunas, harsh or irritating cosmetics, spicy food, and stimulants. Always protect your skin in cold or windy weather, and always touch your skin gently. Bioflavonoid supplements may reduce redness and strengthen capillaries.

Aromatherapy treatment can achieve good results but it requires time. Certain essential oils, including cypress, geranium, lemon, neroli, palmarosa, and rose, help restore elasticity to blood vessels and diminish the redness on the surface of the skin. Some carrier oils, such as borage oil, evening primrose oil, and rose hip seed oil, enhance the effectiveness of aromatherapy blends in reducing broken capillaries.

Apply Facial Oil for Broken Capillaries or Floral Facial Oil for Broken Capillaries to the affected area every day. It may take several months to see results, and treatment should be continued thereafter in order to maintain results. If you have broken capillaries on your body, use Capillary-Conditioning Body Oil daily.

AROMATHERAPY BLENDS

The aromatherapy blends below are essential oil formulas you can prepare at home. For a more detailed explanation of how to put together and use these blends, see Taking Care of Your Skin on page 184 and/or MASSAGE in Part Four. For a quick review of general guidelines for using essential oils, see page 91.

❧ Facial Oil for Broken Capillaries

½ ounce jojoba oil
¼ ounce rose hip seed oil
10 drops borage oil
10 drops evening primrose oil
4 drops cypress oil
3 drops lemon oil
2 drops palmarosa oil

Mix the jojoba and rose hip seed oils together in a clean container, add the essential oils, and gently turn the container upside down a few times or roll it between your hands to blend. Apply the mixture to the affected area once or twice a day.

❧ Floral Facial Oil for Broken Capillaries

½ ounce jojoba oil
¼ ounce rose hip seed oil
10 drops borage oil
10 drops evening primrose oil
3 drops neroli oil
3 drops rose oil
2 drops geranium oil

Mix the jojoba and rose hip seed oils together in a clean container, add the essential oils, and blend well. Apply the oil to the affected areas daily.

❧ Capillary-Conditioning Body Oil

1½ ounces sunflower oil
¼ ounce rose hip seed oil
20 drops borage oil
20 drops evening primrose oil
10 drops geranium oil
8 drops lemon oil
6 drops cypress oil
6 drops palmarosa oil
2 drops neroli oil
2 drops rose oil

Mix the sunflower and rose hip seed oils together in a clean container, add the essential oils, and gently turn the container upside down a few times to blend. Massage the oil over the affected areas daily.

Note: Geranium oil can lower your blood sugar level. Use it with caution (or omit it) if you have hypoglycemia (low blood sugar).

Cellulite

Approximately 90 percent of all females over the age of eighteen have cellulite, those unsightly fatty deposits also known as "orange-peel skin." Cellulite is more than ordinary fat; it is a combination of fat, cellular wastes, and water. It forms a gellike mass that is trapped in the connective tissue below the skin's surface, causing visible ripples, bumps, and bulges. Cellulite usually appears on the hips and thighs, but can also show up on the arms, abdomen, and upper back.

Such factors as bad diet, constipation, poor posture, a sedentary lifestyle, and sluggish blood and lymphatic circulation allow cellular wastes to accumulate. Hormonal imbalances may also contribute to cellulite; these can occur as a result of an internal metabolic problem or some external factor, such as the use of oral contraceptives, which completely disrupt hormonal balance. Stress can also be involved, because it taxes the body, impairing circulation and obstructing elimination. Possible dietary culprits include alcohol, caffeine, carbonated sodas, dairy products, fatty and fried foods, meats and animal products, pesticide residues, preservatives, processed foods, salt, and sugar. Inadequate water intake also contributes to sluggish circulation and inhibits the elimination of wastes.

HELPFUL TREATMENTS

To conquer cellulite, first identify the factors that may be causing your cellulite and take steps to minimize or eliminate them. This will probably mean drinking more water, exercising regularly, improving your posture, modifying your diet, practicing deep breathing, and reducing stress. A diet that focuses on fresh vegetables and fruits, whole grains, and lots of water will help cleanse your body. Plenty of exercise—walking, swimming, bicycling, or anything else that gets circulation pumping to your extremities—will benefit you and help your body eliminate cellulite wastes. Reprogramming your posture to eliminate exaggerated lower back or lumbar curves will boost circulation to your lower body. Breathing deeply will improve circulation, delivering more oxygen and nutrients to your cells and promptly removing wastes.

Eliminating cellulite takes time, but after all, it usually takes several years or even decades for it to accumulate in the first place. Essential oils that help combat cellulite include basil, cedarwood, clary sage, cypress, fennel, juniper, lemon, orange, patchouli, rosemary, and thyme. Aromatherapy baths and body oils help counteract cellulite by improving circulation, encouraging the elimination of wastes, and restoring hormonal balance. Seaweed or algae powder, added to the bath, is especially effective for eliminating toxins.

Skin brushing boosts circulation to the surface of the skin. Apply Skin-Brushing Blend and brush your body before taking the Cellulite Bath. Afterwards, apply Cellulite Skin Oil to all affected areas. Repeat this regimen daily for the best results. Once you achieve the desired effect, continue brushing daily, and use a Cellulite Bath and Cellulite Skin Oil at least once or twice weekly to maintain results.

AROMATHERAPY BLENDS

The aromatherapy blends below are essential oil formulas you can prepare at home. For a more detailed explanation of how to put together and use these blends, see BATHS; MASSAGE; and/or SKIN BRUSHING in Part Four. For a quick review of general guidelines for using essential oils, see page 91.

❧ Skin-Brushing Blend

2 ounces carrier oil
10 drops lemon oil
5 drops cypress oil
5 drops juniper oil
5 drops orange oil
2 drops fennel oil

Place the carrier oil in a clean container and add the essential oils. Gently turn the container upside down a few times or roll it between your hands to blend. Massage a few drops of the mixture onto the areas with cellulite. Then dry-brush your skin.

❧ Cellulite Bath

¼ cup algae or seaweed powder

4 drops lemon oil
2 drops cypress oil
2 drops fennel oil
2 drops rosemary oil

Add the algae or seaweed powder to a bathtub filled with warm water. Drop the essential oils into the tub and disperse well. Soak in the bath for twenty to thirty minutes.

❧ Cellulite Skin Oil

4 ounces carrier oil
10 drops cypress oil
10 drops lemon oil
10 drops orange oil
5 drops rosemary oil
4 drops cedarwood oil
4 drops coriander oil
3 drops fennel oil
3 drops clary sage oil
2 drops patchouli oil

Place the carrier oil in a clean container, add the essential oils, and blend. Apply the mixture to the affected areas after bathing or showering.

Chronic Fatigue Syndrome

Chronic fatigue syndrome (CFS) is a chronic, debilitating illness, usually lasting several years or longer. It is believed to be a result of infection with the Epstein-Barr virus, which is a member of the herpes family of viruses and the same virus that causes infectious mononucleosis. Other herpes viruses include herpes simplex viruses (which cause cold sores and genital herpes) and varicella-zoster (which causes herpes zoster, or shingles, and chickenpox).

The physical symptoms of CFS are highly variable. They include lethargy or incapacitating fatigue, fever, sore throat, swollen glands, cough, diarrhea, digestive and intestinal problems, dizziness, fever, headaches, outbreaks of herpes or fever blisters, hot flashes (unrelated to menopause), insomnia, joint pain, menstrual problems, muscular aches and pains, nausea, recurrent sore throat, respiratory ailments, ringing in the ears, skin rashes, sweating or flushing (unrelated to physical exertion), swelling or dark circles around the eyes, tingling or numbness in different parts of the body, and weight loss. There may also be mental and emotional symptoms, including anxiety, confusion, depression, difficulty concentrating, emotional stress, lack of interest in pleasurable activities, low self-esteem, temporary memory loss, mood swings, panic attacks, unexplained feelings of sadness or guilt, and thoughts of suicide.

The Epstein-Barr virus can be spread by kissing, sharing food, and other forms of intimate contact, including sexual contact. Once infected with the virus, a person remains infected for life, although symptoms may diminish or disappear if the virus goes dormant. However, any weakening of the immune system can then reactivate the latent virus.

Most people who suffer from CFS have weakened immune systems and many have a history of mononucleosis. Other factors have also been implicated in CFS, including anemia; emotional imbalances; exposure to environmental pollutants and cigarette smoke; hypoglycemia; hypothyroidism; various types of infection; long-term antibiotic, cortisone, or steroid drug therapy; mental or physical stress; mercury poisoning from amalgam dental fillings; overuse of prescription, over-the-counter, or recreational drugs; intestinal parasites; and reactions to vaccinations.

HELPFUL TREATMENTS

Treatment for CFS usually includes a detoxifying program, elimination of contributing factors, stress reduction, measures to strengthen the immune system, and a healthy diet supplemented with vitamins and herbs. Many medical specialists consider stress reduction as important as nutritional therapy in fighting this syndrome.

There are a number of different essential oils that can can help with CFS by reducing stress, boosting immunity, and eliminating toxins. These include basil, bergamot, chamomile, clary sage, coriander, geranium, lavender, lemon, marjoram, orange, peppermint, rosemary, thyme, and tea tree. If you are suffering from CFS, bathe in Energizing Bath Blend daily. Apply Therapeutic Body Oil for CFS over your entire body once or twice daily, and inhale Stimulating Inhalant for CFS as needed to energize you.

AROMATHERAPY BLENDS

The aromatherapy blends below are essential oil formulas you can prepare at home. For a more detailed explanation of how to put together and use these blends, see BATHS; INHALANTS; and/or MASSAGE in Part Four. For a quick review of general guidelines for using essential oils, see page 91.

૨ Energizing Bath Blend

> 3 drops rosemary oil
> 2 drops thyme oil
> 2 drops tea tree oil
> 1 drop peppermint oil

Drop the essential oils into a bathtub filled with warm water. Soak in the bath for fifteen to twenty minutes.

🐝 Therapeutic Body Oil for CFS

2 ounces carrier oil
6 drops geranium oil
6 drops lavender oil
3 drops marjoram oil
2 drops coriander oil
2 drops thyme oil

Place the carrier oil in a clean container and add the essential oils. Gently turn the container upside down several times or roll it between your hands for a few minutes to blend. Massage the mixture onto your skin daily.

🐝 Stimulating Inhalant for CFS

8 drops geranium oil
6 drops basil oil
6 drops coriander oil
4 drops bergamot oil
4 drops rosemary oil
2 drops peppermint oil

Drop the essential oils into a small glass bottle with an airtight cover and blend. Inhale directly from the bottle as needed.

Note: Geranium oil can lower your blood sugar level. Use it with caution (or omit it from the above blends) if you have hypoglycemia (low blood sugar).

Circulation, Poor

The circulation of blood throughout the body provides all of the cells in the body with nutrients and oxygen, laying the foundation for good health.

Poor or sluggish circulation detracts from health and can contribute to many illnesses and diseases.

Sluggish circulation can result from clogged arteries, constipation, excess weight, illness, incorrect posture, lack of exercise, low blood pressure, poor diet, a sedentary lifestyle, or failure to eliminate toxins properly. Symptoms may include cold feet and hands, dizziness, difficulty concentrating, dull-looking skin, fatigue, a high cholesterol level, poor memory, shortness of breath, and varicose veins.

HELPFUL TREATMENTS

Daily exercise, such as doing aerobics, taking a brisk walk, or doing yoga will stimulate circulation. If you are overweight, losing the excess weight will probably help. Eat a healthy diet centered around fresh vegetables and fruits, whole grains, and legumes. Drink eight to ten glasses of water daily. Massaging and brushing your skin will encourage circulation to extremities and to the surface of the skin.

There are many essential oils that stimulate circulation, including basil, benzoin, black pepper, cedarwood, coriander, cypress, fennel, geranium, ginger, juniper, lavender, lemon, marjoram, myrrh, neroli, orange, palmarosa, peppermint, pine, rose, rosemary, thyme, vetiver, and ylang ylang. Apply a few drops of Circulation-Boosting Body-Brushing Oil to your body and brush your skin every morning to invigorate your circulation. Then take a Circulation-Boosting Bath. Apply Circulation-Boosting Body Oil once or twice daily to your entire body, especially to your extremities.

As your circulation improves, your blood cells will bring more nutrients into the tissues and take away wastes more efficiently. Your health will begin to improve at the cellular level, and your entire body will function better.

AROMATHERAPY BLENDS

The aromatherapy blends below are essential oil formulas you can prepare at home. For a more detailed explanation of how to put together and use these blends, see BATHS; MASSAGE; and/or SKIN BRUSHING in Part Four. For a quick review of general guidelines for using essential oils, see page 91.

❧ Circulation-Boosting Body-Brushing Oil

2 ounces carrier oil
6 drops rosemary oil
4 drops lemon oil
4 drops palmarosa oil
4 drops thyme oil
2 drops basil oil
2 drops fennel oil
1 drop black pepper oil
1 drop ginger oil

Blend all the ingredients together well in a clean container. Apply a few drops to your skin and brush.

❧ Circulation-Boosting Bath

2 drops cypress oil
2 drops juniper oil
2 drops peppermint oil
2 drops pine oil
2 drops rosemary oil

Add the essential oils to a bathtub filled with warm water. Soak in the bath for twenty to thirty minutes.

❧ Circulation-Boosting Body Oil

2 ounces carrier oil
8 drops rosemary oil
6 drops lemon oil

4 drops orange oil
3 drops geranium oil
2 drops benzoin resin
2 drops myrrh oil
1 drop ginger oil
1 drop vetiver oil

Add the essential oils to the carrier oil and blend. Apply the oil to your skin as needed to stimulate circulation.

Note: Rosemary and peppermint oils are extremely stimulating. If you plan to use any of the above blends before going to bed at night, you may wish to omit these two oils from the formula so that they do not interfere with your sleep.

Cold Sores

See HERPES VIRUS.

Colds and Flu

Congestion, coughs, fatigue, fever, chills, grogginess, headache, runny nose, sore throat, swollen glands, and watery or burning eyes can signal an approaching cold. Many different viruses cause colds. Colds are the most common communicable diseases and they spread easily from person to person.

Symptoms of the flu are similar to those of a cold, but usually include a higher temperature and an all-over feeling of achiness. The runny nose, sore throat, and watery eyes that are charactaristic of a cold may or may not be present with the flu.

Like colds, the flu is a highly contagious viral illness that spreads rapidly from one person to another. Because the structure of the flu virus changes every two or three years or so, the disease normally occurs in epidemics, as the population is exposed to a new type of flu virus.

Colds and flu are most likely to strike when a person's immunity is low as a result of inadequate rest, overwork, poor nutrition, or stress. You are more susceptible at these times because your defenses are too weak to fight off invading viruses.

HELPFUL TREATMENTS

Since there is no cure for the common cold, or for the flu, assisting the body in fighting the infection is the best course of action. Sleeping and resting, drinking lots of liquids, and avoiding sugar and sweets will help your immune system to recuperate. Taking supplements of vitamin C, beta-carotene, and zinc can help. The herbs echinacea, goldenseal, and licorice root are helpful as well, because they fight viruses and strengthen immunity.

Essential oils can help fight colds and flu in two ways. First, they can ward off illness or hasten recovery by boosting immunity. Second, they can ease many of the discomforts of colds and the flu when used in baths, chest rubs, compresses, and inhalants, as well as in the diffuser. Essential oils that can help are basil, benzoin, bergamot, black pepper, clary sage, elemi, eucalyptus, fennel, frankincense, ginger, helichrysum, juniper, lemon, marjoram, myrrh, orange, palmarosa, pine, rosemary, rosewood, tea tree, and thyme.

At the first sign of a cold or the flu, take a Cold- and Flu-Fighting Bath. Then prepare an Inhalant for Cold and Flu and use it in a steam inhalation or inhale it directly from the bottle. Massage Cold and Flu Chest Rub onto your chest, throat, and back. Then get in bed! If you have a fever or chills, you can apply a Compress for Chills or Fever (choose cool water for fever, hot water for chills). Drink lots of liquids. Disperse Cold-Combatting Diffuser Blend throughout your room. Repeat this entire treatment once or twice daily for several days or until symptoms subside.

AROMATHERAPY BLENDS

The aromatherapy blends below are essential oil formulas you can prepare at home. For a more detailed explanation of how to put together and use these blends, see BATHS; COMPRESSES; DIFFUSERS AND LAMPS; INHALANTS; and/or MASSAGE in Part Four. For a quick review of general guidelines for using essential oils, see page 91.

❧ Cold- and Flu-Fighting Bath

> 3 drops lemon oil
> 3 drops tea tree oil
> 2 drops elemi oil
> 1 drop marjoram oil
> 1 drop myrrh oil

Disperse the essential oils in a bathtub filled with warm water. Soak in the bath for twenty to thirty minutes, taking care not to become chilled. Repeat as necessary.

❧ Inhalant for Colds and Flu

> 8 drops bergamot oil
> 4 drops rosewood oil
> 3 drops ginger oil
> 3 drops helichrysum oil
> 2 drops basil oil
> 2 drops black pepper oil
> 2 drops eucalyptus oil

Add all the oils to a small glass bottle with an airtight cover and blend well. You can inhale the mixture directly from the bottle, apply two drops to a tissue, or add three drops to a bowl of steaming water and lean your face over the bowl for five minutes while inhaling the steam.

ᘓ Cold and Flu Chest Rub

> 1 ounce carrier oil
> 4 drops pine oil
> 3 drops eucalyptus oil
> 2 drops frankincense oil
> 2 drops rosemary oil
> 2 drops thyme oil
> 1 drop ginger oil

Place the carrier oil in a clean container, add the essential oils, and blend. Massage the oil over your chest and back several times daily until your symptoms subside.

ᘓ Compress for Fevers or Chills

> 1 quart hot or cool water
> 2 drops orange oil
> 2 drops pine oil
> 1 drop black pepper oil
> 1 drop ginger oil

Pour the water into a two-quart glass bowl (use cool water for fever, hot water for chills) and add the essential oils to the water. Soak a clean cloth in the water and apply it to your chest or forehead as needed.

ᘓ Cold-Combatting Diffuser Blend

> 20 drops orange oil
> 10 drops eucalyptus oil
> 10 drops juniper oil
> 10 drops pine oil
> 6 drops basil oil
> 6 drops rosewood oil
> 4 drops ginger oil

One by one, drop the essential oils into a small glass bottle with an airtight cover. Turn the bottle upside down several times or roll it between your hands for a few minutes to blend the oils, and add some of the mixture to your diffuser. Run the diffuser as necessary.

Constipation

Constipation, a condition in which bowel movements decrease in frequency, is a common digestive complaint. Dehydration, poor diet, a sedentary lifestyle, and stress can all contribute to constipation.

The average American diet lacks sufficient amounts of fiber, the indigestible portion of plant foods that binds with wastes in the intestines so that the wastes can be eliminated. Instead, most Americans eat a diet loaded with chemical additives, fats, pesticide residues, preservatives, salt, and sugar, which are difficult to digest, difficult to assimilate, and difficult to eliminate. Such a diet burdens the digestive tract with wastes that are not eliminated. Particles of waste can become impacted on the intestinal walls, making complete elimination difficult or impossible.

A sedentary lifestyle can contribute to constipation because it does not give the body enough stimulation to keep everything moving properly. Stress overloads the body, preventing it from functioning normally. Insufficient water intake keeps the body from eliminating wastes as it should.

HELPFUL TREATMENTS

Eating a diet that focuses on fresh vegetables, fruits, and whole grains will provide necessary dietary fiber; drinking lots of water (at least eight 8-ounce glasses a day is recommended) will help flush out wastes. Regular exercise, such as walking, swimming, or doing yoga, is useful for stimulating circulation, digestion, and elimination. Finding ways to manage stress is also important (see STRESS).

Essential oils can help by improving digestion, increasing peristalsis (the rhythmic contractions of intestinal muscles that push wastes out of the body), and encouraging the elimination of wastes. Essential oils can also reduce stress. Basil, chamomile, coriander, fennel, ginger, lavender, lemon, marjoram, orange, rose, and rosemary are essential oils that can help overcome constipation. If you suffer from constipation, massage Constipation Abdominal Rub over your abdomen every morning and every evening to encourage regular bowel movements.

AROMATHERAPY BLENDS

The aromatherapy blend below is an essential oil formula you can prepare at home. For a more detailed explanation of how to put together and use this blend, see MASSAGE in Part Four. For a quick review of general guidelines for using essential oils, see page 91.

❧ Constipation Abdominal Rub

    4 ounces carrier oil
    12 drops fennel oil
    10 drops marjoram oil
    8 drops Roman chamomile oil
    8 drops coriander oil
    8 drops lemon oil
    6 drops lavender oil
    6 drops rosemary oil

Place the carrier oil in a clean container, add the essential oils, and gently turn the container upside down a few times or roll it between your hands to blend. Twice a day, massage the oil over your abdominal area, moving clockwise from right to left.

Cuts and Bruises

Cuts and bruises usually result from injuries to or incisions into the skin. Most superficial cuts and wounds require little treatment and will heal naturally. Immediately after the skin is broken, the blood begins clotting to stop the bleeding. A scab forms, protecting the underlying tissue and allowing the skin to regenerate and repair itself.

Because skin acts as a barrier to prevent foreign matter and microorganisms from invading the body, any break in the skin increases the possibility of infection. Cuts and wounds also can result in scarring if they are extensive or if they are not cleansed and treated properly. Seek medical attention for any wound that is caused by a rusty metal object or a deep puncture, or that bleeds heavily.

Bruising occurs when an injury damages tiny blood vessels under the skin. Black, blue, and purple discoloration occurs as blood leaks from the damaged blood vessels into the surrounding tissues. As the blood is absorbed, the bruise will fade and heal naturally. Anemic or obese people, and people with nutritional deficiencies, may bruise more easily than others. A variety of medications, including anti-inflammatory drugs, anticoagulants, painkillers, steroids, and some antibiotics, can also increase susceptibility to bruising.

HELPFUL TREATMENTS

Thoroughly cleanse and treat cuts and wounds immediately to reduce pain, speed healing, and minimize scarring. Essential oils that can help prevent infection and speed healing of cuts and wounds are benzoin, bergamot, clary sage, cypress, elemi, eucalyptus, frankincense, helichrysum, juniper, lavender, lemon, myrrh, palmarosa, patchouli, pine, rose, rosemary, rosewood, sandalwood, tea tree, thyme, and vetiver. Essential oils that help diminish scarring include benzoin, frankincense, geranium, palmarosa, patchouli, and rosewood. Neroli oil reputedly will prevent scarring if applied to the cut or wound regularly. The properties of certain carrier oils make them particularly suitable for use in aromatherapy blends for injuries that break the skin. Both rose hip seed oil and vitamin E oil reduce scarring, while camellia oil prevents the formation of keloids, an unsightly thickening of scar tissue.

To speed the healing of an injury that breaks the skin, apply Cut- and Wound-Healing Oil to the injured area several times daily. To prevent or lessen scarring, once the wound has healed, massage Scar Massage Oil onto the affected area once or twice daily, until the scar fades.

Everyone gets bruises from time to time. If you bruise easily or frequently, however, you may wish to consult a nutritionist to check for a vitamin C or vitamin K deficiency. If you think you are bruising much more easily than you used to, it may be wise to consult a medical professional to check for the possibility of an underlying health problem. Essential oils to use on bruises include geranium, ginger, helichrysum, juniper, lavender, marjoram, and thyme. Immediately after an injury, apply ice or a cold Muscle Strain Compress to the area. Rub Bruise-Diminishing Blend over the bruised area two or more times daily to speed healing and stimulate blood flow through the bruised area.

AROMATHERAPY BLENDS

The aromatherapy blends below are essential oil formulas you can prepare at home. For a more detailed explanation of how to put together and use these blends, see COMPRESSES and/or MASSAGE in Part Four. For a quick review of general guidelines for using essential oils, see page 91.

❧ Cut- and Wound-Healing Oil

1 ounce carrier oil
10 drops tea tree oil
6 drops lavender oil
4 drops cypress oil
3 drops helichrysum oil
2 drops lemon oil
1 drop myrrh oil

Place the carrier oil in a clean container, add the essential oils, and blend. After thoroughly cleansing a cut or wound, apply this mixture to the affected area. Repeat the application several times daily, as needed.

❧ Scar Massage Oil

1 ounce camellia oil
½ ounce flaxseed oil
10 drops vitamin E oil
4 drops geranium oil
4 drops neroli oil
3 drops palmarosa oil
3 drops rosewood oil
2 drops benzoin resin
2 drops frankincense oil
2 drops patchouli oil

Mix the camellia, flaxseed, and vitamin E oils together in a clean container. Add the essential oils and gently turn the container upside down a few times to blend all the ingredients together. Once the wound has closed and healed over, apply the oil to your skin once or twice daily to prevent or minimize the appearance of scars.

‹❧ Muscle Strain Compress

1 quart cold water
2 drops chamomile oil
2 drops marjoram oil
1 drop rosemary oil

Pour the water into a two-quart glass bowl and add the essential oils. Saturate a clean cloth in the water and apply it to the affected area for at least ten minutes. Do this immediately after an injury and repeat the treatment often for the first twenty-four hours thereafter.

‹❧ Bruise-Diminishing Blend

2 ounces carrier oil
4 drops marjoram oil
3 drops geranium oil
3 drops helichrysum oil
3 drops lavender oil
2 drops ginger oil
2 drops juniper oil
2 drops thyme oil

In a clean container, add the essential oils to the carrier oil and blend. Apply the mixture to the bruised area several times daily.

Cystitis

Cystitis is an infection or inflammation of the bladder. It is usually caused by bacteria from outside that invade the urethra, the passageway that carries urine from the bladder for elimination. Common symptoms of cystitis are frequent or painful urination, a burning sensation when urinating, and a nearly constant urge to urinate.

These are occasionally accompanied by back pain, blood or mucus in the urine, fever, nausea, or vomiting. Failure to treat cystitis promptly can allow the infection to spread to the kidneys and cause permanent damage.

Bladder infections affect women more often than men, because the female urethra is shorter and located very near the anus; bacteria often migrate from the anal area to the urethra. Women who are pregnant and persons of either sex who have weakened immune systems are more likely than others to get cystitis. A number of external factors can contribute to an attack of cystitis, including poor personal hygiene and the use of such products as scented toilet tissue, deodorant tampons or sanitary pads, diaphragms, spermicidal creams, feminine hygiene sprays, perfumed bath oils, bubble baths, and soaps. Holding onto urine, engaging in sexual intercourse (especially if a diaphragm is used), and wearing tight-fitting clothing or underwear that doesn't "breathe" may also be involved.

HELPFUL TREATMENTS

To discourage cystitis, it is best to eliminate any possible contributing causes. Drink eight to ten glasses of water daily. Avoid wearing tight-fitting clothes like pantyhose, girdles, and jeans, and choose underwear made of natural fibers. Cranberries contain a substance that prevents bacteria from clinging to the interior surface of the bladder and the urinary tract. Drinking several glasses of unsweetened cranberry juice daily can speed recovery and prevent future infections.

Hygiene is important for both preventing and treating cystitis. Women should keep the vaginal area clean by wiping from front to back after bowel movements. Urinating after bathing and before and after intercourse also reduces the risk of bacterial infection.

Aromatherapy can be used to minimize the discomfort of cystitis and speed recovery. Aromatherapy may also prevent recurring bouts of cystitis. Essential oils such as benzoin, bergamot, cedarwood, cypress, elemi, eucalyptus, frankincense, juniper, pine, sandalwood, tea tree, and thyme help cystitis. Benzoin, eucalyptus, sandalwood, tea tree, and thyme oils are especially effective against bacterial infection. In addition, benzoin, cedarwood, cypress, eucalyptus, juniper, pine, sandalwood, and thyme oils are diuretics and increase urination, which cleanses the bladder. This is helpful if cystitis makes urination difficult.

If you develop cystitis, immerse yourself in Sitz Bath for Cystitis once or twice a day until your symptoms subside. Apply Cystitis Massage Oil to your abdomen, lower back, pubic area, and pelvic region several times daily.

AROMATHERAPY BLENDS

The aromatherapy blends below are essential oil formulas you can prepare at home. For a more detailed explanation of how to put together and use these blends, see MASSAGE and/or SITZ BATHS in Part Four. For a quick review of general guidelines for using essential oils, see page 91.

❧ Sitz Bath for Cystitis

> 3 drops tea tree oil
> 2 drops bergamot oil
> 2 drops cypress oil
> 2 drops thyme oil
> 1 drop eucalyptus oil

Add the oils to a shallow tub filled with warm water. Sit hip-deep in the tub for fifteen minutes. Repeat once or twice each day until your symptoms subside.

❧ Cystitis Massage Oil

> 1 ounce carrier oil
> 3 drops sandalwood oil
> 2 drops cedarwood oil
> 2 drops cypress oil
> 1 drop benzoin resin
> 1 drop frankincense oil

Add all the ingredients to a clean container and blend. Massage the mixture over your abdomen, lower back, and pelvic area. Repeat several times daily until symptoms cease.

Depression

Although many people use the word "depression" to describe passing feelings of sadness, true depression is actually an illness classified as a mood disorder. The many faces of depression may show up as anger, anxiety, feelings of worthlessness, confusion, diminished sex drive, fatigue, hyperactivity, insomnia, irritability, lethargy, loss of interest in usual activities, loss of appetite (or overeating), mood swings, poor concentration, thoughts of suicide, and weight loss or weight gain.

The cause or causes of depression are not well understood. Life events and circumstances—such as loss of a loved one, a job, or reputation—may be related to the onset of depression, but such events are likely to cause the condition only in susceptible people. Many cases of depression occur without any traumatic incident.

There are a multitude of physical conditions that can lead to or exacerbate symptoms of depression. These include allergies, overconsumption of caffeine or alcohol, candidiasis, chemical sensitivities, chronic fatigue syndrome, cigarette smoking, digestive disorders, endometriosis, exposure to environmental pollutants, high sugar intake, hormonal imbalances, hypoglycemia, nutritional deficiencies, chronic illness, poor diet, certain drugs, stress, and thyroid disorders.

HELPFUL TREATMENTS

If you are experiencing symptoms of depression, you should consider seeking psychological counselling. It may also be helpful to consult your health care professional to rule out any physical problems or nutritional deficiencies.

Changing your diet and correcting nutritional deficiencies can often have a positive impact on the way you feel. Eliminate all junk food, refined foods, and sugar, as well as most fats, from your diet. Focus on eating whole grains, fresh vegetables, and other complex carbohydrates. Regular physical exercise has also been shown to diminish depression. Keep as involved and active as possible. Reducing stress often helps to decrease depression.

Aromatherapy can help to alter your moods. The aroma of certain essential oils can stimulate the production of neurotransmitters within your brain that regulate your behavior and moods. If you want to be more calm and relaxed, use benzoin, chamomile, clary sage, jasmine, lavender, neroli, patchouli, rose, rosewood, sandalwood, vetiver, and ylang ylang oils. If you're feeling lethargic or sluggish, stimulate your stamina with basil, bergamot, geranium, helichrysum, jasmine, lavender, lemon, neroli, orange, patchouli, peppermint, rose, and rosemary oils. For the quickest relief, simply open a bottle of one of the above oils and sniff it.

Depending on how your depression manifests itself, you should take either a Sedating Anti-Depression Bath or a Stimulating Anti-Depression Bath every day. Follow this by applying either Calming Anti-Depression Massage Oil or Energizing Anti-Depression Massage Oil, again depending

on your needs. Several times a day, apply either Relaxing Personal Fragrance or Uplifting Personal Perfume—or inhale it directly from the bottle. You can also disperse Anti-Depression Diffuser Blend throughout your home or office during the day as needed.

AROMATHERAPY BLENDS

The aromatherapy blends below are essential oil formulas you can prepare at home. For a more detailed explanation of how to put together and use these blends, see BATHS; DIFFUSERS AND LAMPS; MASSAGE; and/or PERSONAL FRAGRANCES AND PERFUMES in Part Four. For a quick review of general guidelines for using essential oils, see page 91.

❧ Sedating Anti-Depression Bath

2 drops chamomile oil
2 drops clary sage oil
2 drops lavender oil
1 drop ylang ylang oil

Add the oils to a bathtub filled with warm water. Soak in the bath for twenty minutes before bedtime. Follow with Calming Anti-Depression Massage Oil.

❧ Stimulating Anti-Depression Bath

4 drops lavender oil
3 drops rosemary oil
2 drops geranium oil
2 drops lemon oil

Add the oils to a bathtub filled with warm water and soak for twenty minutes. Follow with an application of Energizing Anti-Depression Massage Oil.

❧ Calming Anti-Depression Massage Oil

1 ounce carrier oil
4 drops sandalwood oil

3 drops German chamomile oil

3 drops rosewood oil

2 drops benzoin resin

2 drops ylang ylang oil

1 drop jasmine absolute or enfleurage

Place the carrier oil in a clean container and add the essential oils. Gently turn the container upside down several times or roll it between your hands for a few minutes to blend. Massage the oil into your body daily, as necessary.

❧ Energizing Anti-Depression Massage Oil

1 ounce carrier oil

3 drops orange oil

2 drops helichrysum oil

2 drops rosemary oil

1 drop basil oil

1 drop peppermint oil

Place the carrier oil in a clean container, add the essential oils, and blend. Massage the mixture into your skin daily.

❧ Relaxing Personal Fragrance

⅛ ounce jojoba oil

4 drops sandalwood oil

3 drops clary sage oil

2 drops jasmine absolute or enfleurage

2 drops ylang ylang oil

1 drop benzoin resin

1 drop vetiver oil

In a clean container, add the essential oils to the jojoba oil and gently turn the container over several times or roll it between your hands to blend. Dab the mixture on your pulse points or inhale the fragrance directly from the bottle, as needed.

❧ Uplifting Personal Perfume

⅛ ounce jojoba oil

4 drops neroli oil

3 drops geranium oil

3 drops lavender oil

2 drops bergamot oil

2 drops rose oil

Place the jojoba oil in a clean container and add the essential oils. Gently turn the container upside down several times or roll it between your hands to blend the oils. Apply the blend to your pulse points as a perfume. You can also inhale it directly from the bottle. Use it as needed.

❧ Anti-Depression Diffuser Blend

20 drops lavender oil

15 drops geranium oil

8 drops bergamot oil

6 drops lemon oil

6 drops ylang ylang oil

4 drops rosewood oil

3 drops patchouli oil

2 drops helichrysum oil

Drop the essential oils into a small glass bottle with an airtight cover and blend. Add some of the mixture to your diffuser as necessary.

Dermatitis

Dermatitis is a broad category of skin disorders characterized by inflammation and, usually, itching. Many cases of dermatitis occur when the skin comes into contact with a substance that causes an allergic reaction. There are also forms of dermatitis that can result from a deficiency of essential fatty acids, a high-acid diet, overuse of drugs, stress, or the presence of too many refined foods or saturated fats in the diet.

Of the many kinds of dermatitis, the most common is contact dermatitis. Contact dermatitis occurs as a reaction to one or more of a variety of chemicals or other environmental elements to which an individual is sensitive. Skin that comes into contact with an offending substance becomes irritated and inflamed, with itching and redness. It may be dry and flaky. Some of the things that most commonly cause contact dermatitis are antiperspirants and deodorants, cleaning products, fabric dyes, cosmetics, detergents, fragrances, hair coloring and permanent solutions, leather-processing chemicals, plants, rubber compounds, solvents, and certain metals, especially nickel, which may be present in jewelry, bra closures, wristwatches, and zippers. Eczema is a type of dermatitis that causes patches of skin to become dry and red, frequently with cracking, crusting, and weeping or watery blistered areas (see ECZEMA).

HELPFUL TREATMENTS

If you suffer from dermatitis, pinpointing the cause or causes of the problem—and then eliminating or minimizing your exposure to them—is the first step toward alleviating the symptoms. Aromatherapy can help ease or eliminate symptoms as well. Essential oils such as benzoin, cedarwood, chamomile, elemi, geranium, helichrysum, jasmine, juniper, lavender, neroli, orange, patchouli, peppermint, rose, rosemary, rosewood, sandalwood, tea tree, thyme, and ylang ylang soothe irritated skin, reduce inflammation, prevent dryness and itching, and subdue stress.

To ease irritation and inflammation and to combat dryness, bathe in Dermatitis-Soothing Bath once a day or several times a week, depending on the severity of your condition. Apply a Cool Compress for Dermatitis to the affected areas to soothe hot, inflamed skin. Massage Dermatitis Skin Oil into your skin several times daily as needed.

Many cases of dermatitis improve after bathing the skin in Dead Sea salts or seaweed or algae powder. The addition of essential oils will make the bath even more effective.

AROMATHERAPY BLENDS

The aromatherapy blends below are essential oil formulas you can prepare at home. For a more detailed explanation of how to put together and use these blends, see BATHS; COMPRESSES; and/or MASSAGE in Part Four. For a quick review of general guidelines for using essential oils, see page 91.

❧ Dermatitis-Soothing Bath

    3 drops chamomile oil
    3 drops lavender oil
    2 drops rosewood oil
    1 drop helichrysum oil
    1 drop ylang ylang oil
    1 cup Dead Sea salts (optional)
    ¼ cup seaweed or algae powder (optional)

Add all the essential oils to a bathtub filled with warm water, together with the Dead Sea salts and seaweed or algae powder, if desired. Soak in the bath for twenty minutes.

❧ Cool Compress for Dermatitis

    1 quart cool water
    1 drop benzoin resin
    1 drop cedarwood oil
    1 drop patchouli oil
    1 drop sandalwood oil

Pour the water into a two-quart glass bowl and

add the essential oils. Soak a clean cloth in the water and apply it to the affected areas as needed.

❧ Dermatitis Skin Oil

    1 ounce jojoba or hazelnut oil
    2 drops chamomile oil
    2 drops lavender oil
    2 drops neroli oil
    2 drops rose oil
    1 drop benzoin resin

Place the jojoba or hazelnut oil in a clean container, add the essential oils, and gently turn the container upside down a few times or roll it between your hands to blend. Apply the oil to your skin as needed.

Diarrhea

Frequent, watery bowel movements accompanied by abdominal pain and cramping are characteristic of diarrhea. Diarrhea is one way in which the body can rapidly rid itself of toxins and foreign substances. It may result from a bacterial or viral infection, food allergies, food poisoning, the consumption of caffeine or impure water, emotional upset, poor or inadequate digestion of food, reactions to drugs, a condition known as spastic colon, or stress.

HELPFUL TREATMENTS

Diarrhea is usually a sign that the body is attempting to cleanse itself. When you experience a bout of diarrhea, it is better not to eat anything, but you should drink plenty of pure water to prevent dehydration and to help your body flush out toxins. If you are travelling in a foreign country and are unsure about the water, drink only bottled water and avoid any "hidden" sources of the local water, such as raw fruits and vegetables washed in local water.

Aromatherapy can relieve some of the discomforts of diarrhea. Black pepper, chamomile, coriander, ginger, lavender, and peppermint oils relieve stomach spasms; myrrh, patchouli, tea tree, and thyme oils fight infection caused by bacteria and other microbial infections. Cypress oil helps to restore balance when the body is excreting excessive amounts of fluids. Calming oils such as chamomile, geranium, orange, neroli, and sandalwood are soothing, both physically and emotionally, and are useful when stress or nerves are factors.

If you are suffering a bout of diarrhea, massage All-Purpose Diarrhea Diminisher over your abdomen and lower back several times daily until symptoms subside.

AROMATHERAPY BLENDS

The aromatherapy blend below is an essential oil formula you can prepare at home. For a more detailed explanation of how to put together and use this blend, see MASSAGE in Part Four. For a quick review of general guidelines for using essential oils, see page 91.

❧ All-Purpose Diarrhea Diminisher

    2 ounces carrier oil
    8 drops cypress oil
    8 drops lemon oil
    6 drops tea tree oil
    4 drops chamomile oil
    4 drops peppermint oil
    3 drops lavender oil
    2 drops coriander oil

Place the carrier oil in a clean container, add the essential oils, and gently turn the container upside down a few times or roll it between your hands to blend. Massage the mixture over your abdominal area and lower back as necessary.

Digestive Disorders

See CONSTIPATION; DIARRHEA; INDIGESTION.

Earache

An earache can produce a dull ache, sharp stabbing pains, ringing, or throbbing in the ear. Earaches that result from bacterial infection often occur when fluid builds up in the eustachian tube, which connects the middle ear with the nasal cavity and throat and equalizes pressure on both sides of the eardrum. The eustachian tube also permits excess secretions to drain away from the ear. If the eustachian tube is not draining properly, these secretions build up in the middle ear, pressure in the ear rises, and you may experience pain in the ear. In addition, microorganisms may migrate from the nose and throat to the ear by means of the eustachian tube, causing infection.

Respiratory allergies, respiratory infections, food allergies, and middle ear infections are the most common causes of earaches. Sometimes an earache can be prompted by a rapid change in air pressure (such as occurs with changes in altitude or decompression of an airplane's cabin), or exposure to cold climates. Infants and young children are more often affected by earaches than older children and adults are.

HELPFUL TREATMENTS

If you have an earache, you should see a medical practitioner as soon as possible, as it may signal a problem requiring a doctor's treatment.

A weakened immune system, chronic respiratory infections, and food allergies are all factors that can contribute to frequent earaches. If you suffer from recurring earaches, use an elimination diet or food diary to determine whether food allergies may be involved and, if so, which foods are causing your allergies. Start by eliminating the most common offenders: dairy products, eggs, wheat, corn, citrus fruits, peanuts, and peanut butter.

Aromatherapy can help by decreasing discomfort until you see your medical professional. Aromatherapy can also strengthen your immune system to fight respiratory ailments. Basil, chamomile, lavender, rosemary, sandalwood, and tea tree oils are essential oils that can ease the discomfort of earaches.

Massage Earache Oil Blend on and around your ears. Then apply an Earache Compress. Or put one drop of any of the oils listed above on a cotton ball, place it in your ear, and apply the Earache Compress on top of it.

AROMATHERAPY BLENDS

The aromatherapy blends below are essential oil formulas you can prepare at home. For a more detailed explanation of how to put together and use these blends, see COMPRESSES and/or MASSAGE in Part Four. For a quick review of general guidelines for using essential oils, see page 91.

❧ Earache Oil Blend

    1 ounce carrier oil
    4 drops chamomile oil
    3 drops lavender oil
    2 drops sandalwood oil
    1 drop basil oil

Place the carrier oil in a clean container, add the essential oils, and gently turn the container upside down several times or roll it between your hands for a few minutes to blend. Massage the mixture over your ears as needed.

❧ Earache Compress

    1 quart hot water
    2 drops chamomile oil
    1 drop basil oil
    1 drop lavender oil
    1 drop sandalwood oil

Pour the water into a two-quart glass bowl and disperse the essential oils in the water. Soak a clean cloth in the water and apply it to your ear for fifteen minutes. Repeat as necessary.

Eczema

Eczema is a type of dermatitis that appears as dry patches of skin with cracking, crusting, redness, and swelling, often with weeping sores or watery blisters. The skin becomes hot and inflamed and it itches.

Many different factors can cause or contribute to eczema in susceptible individuals. Stress can cause or aggravate eczema, as can exposure to cleaning compounds, colognes, cosmetics, detergents, household chemicals, soaps, and synthetic perfumes.

Food allergies can often trigger an outbreak of eczema. Corn, dairy products, tomatoes, vinegar, and wheat are among the foods that most commonly cause the allergies that show up as skin problems. Acidic, hot, or spicy foods can also activate skin rashes in some people. Deficiencies of nutrients, such as essential fatty acids, can contribute to eczema as well.

HELPFUL TREATMENTS

The best approach for clearing or controlling eczema—and most other skin disorders—is to follow a healthy diet, minimize stress, and avoid synthetically fragranced cosmetics, perfumes, and other products, as well as all harsh chemicals. Keep track of your outbreaks to find out what may be triggering your skin sensitivities; then avoid those things.

Flaxseed oil, applied externally or taken internally, often eases symptoms of eczema.

Aromatherapy can help relieve eczema by decreasing stress, calming inflammation, and helping the skin to heal. Bathing the skin in Dead Sea salts and seaweed or algae powder has soothed many people's symptoms. Essential oils boost the effectiveness of the salts. Essential oils that help eczema are benzoin, bergamot, chamomile, clary sage, elemi, geranium, helichrysum, jasmine, lavender, lemon, myrrh, neroli, orange, patchouli, peppermint, pine, rose, rosemary, rosewood, sandalwood, tea tree, thyme, and ylang ylang.

To help control eczema, bathe in Eczema-Calming Bath daily. Apply a Skin-Cooling Compress to the affected areas for additional relief. Several times each day, apply Eczema Body Oil or Eczema Facial Oil to the affected areas to reduce inflammation and irritation and to promote healing.

AROMATHERAPY BLENDS

The aromatherapy blends below are essential oil

formulas you can prepare at home. For a more detailed explanation of how to put together and use these blends, see BATHS; COMPRESSES; and/or MASSAGE in Part Four. For a quick review of general guidelines for using essential oils, see page 91.

❧ Eczema-Calming Bath

3 drops chamomile oil
3 drops geranium oil
3 drops lemon oil
2 drops elemi oil
2 drops sandalwood oil
1 cup Dead Sea salts (optional)
¼ cup seaweed or algae powder (optional)

Disperse all the ingredients in a bathtub filled with warm water. Enjoy a leisurely thirty-minute soak.

❧ Skin-Cooling Compress

1 quart cool water
2 drops chamomile oil
2 drops lavender oil
1 drop helichrysum oil

Pour the water into a two-quart glass bowl, add the essential oils, and blend. Soak a clean cotton cloth in the water. Apply the cloth to the affected area as needed.

❧ Eczema Body Oil

1½ ounces carrier oil
½ ounce flaxseed oil
6 drops geranium oil
4 drops elemi oil
4 drops tea tree oil
3 drops lemon oil
3 drops ylang ylang oil
2 drops benzoin resin

Mix the carrier oil and the flaxseed oil together in a clean container and add the essential oils. Gently turn the container upside down several times or roll it between your hands for a few minutes to blend all the ingredients together. Apply the oil to the affected areas as necessary.

Note: Geranium oil can lower your blood sugar level. Use it with caution (or omit it) if you have hypoglycemia (low blood sugar).

❧ Eczema Facial Oil

¼ ounce jojoba oil
2 drops clary sage oil
2 drops neroli oil
1 drop helichrysum oil
1 drop myrrh oil

Place the jojoba oil in a clean container, add the essential oils, and blend well. Apply the mixture to your face as necessary.

Emotional Issues

Everyone experiences emotional challenges from time to time. Emotions may manifest themselves in many ways and have a multitude of causes. Some emotions, like grief and sadness, may be a normal response to unavoidable circumstances. Others may be more within your control. Emotions like anger and impatience are often destructive and usually serve little or no purpose, except perhaps to signal the need to change some aspect of your life, such as your work, your relationships, or your manner of relating to others. On the other hand, desirable feelings such as love, joy, and confidence have a positive impact and help to improve the quality of your life.

Expressing emotions is natural and healthy. Yet many people deal with their emotions, especially negative ones, by repressing them. They prefer to become engrossed with such things as work, food, alcohol, or drugs—often to the point of obsession—in an attempt not to feel any unpleasant feelings. Other people withdraw into themselves, denying their feelings entirely. Unexpressed feelings and repressed emotions can often contribute to poor health, weakened immunity, and physical illness.

Chemical sensitivities, environmental pollutants, food additives and preservatives, nutritional deficiencies, and a poor diet can activate or aggravate certain emotional problems. Heredity and past experience can also be a factor. Emotional upsets are often related to physical problems as well. Physical illness or disease can lead to emotional and psychological problems; conversely, emotional and psychological issues can lead to physical illness.

HELPFUL TREATMENTS

If you find yourself facing constant challenges with your emotions, or if you are having trouble handling them, it is best to seek counselling. A good counsellor can help you understand your feelings and discover new ways of dealing with your problems. It may take work, but you can change your emotional state and responses.

Among aromatherapy's greatest strengths are its abilities to soothe emotional upsets, to help you get through trying times, and to speed recovery from emotional distress. Aromatherapy can help you work on releasing undesirable emotions as well as on developing or increasing desirable ones. Many European physicians, psychologists, and psychiatrists regularly prescribe essential oils as part of the treatment for their patients. Aromatherapy works well with other therapies.

Essential oils can calm and soothe emotional upset, help you create a positive emotional environment, and help you manage your emotions, change the way you feel, and improve the quality of your life. Throughout history, people in many different cultures have used essential oils for emotional and psychological purposes.

Aromatherapy can help you cope with challenging circumstances in your life by providing support during difficult times, by lifting your spirits, and by helping you improve or maintain an optimistic outlook. Take an emotional inventory. Which emotions and feelings would you like to subdue or eliminate? Which ones would you like to develop or enhance? Look at the Aromatherapy Blends for Undesirable Emotions and the Aromatherapy Blends for Enhancing Positive Emotions in this section for blends that can be used in the method or methods that work best for you and suit your lifestyle. Included are recommendations for personal blends, baths, and diffusers or lamps. Use the following general instructions for preparing and using these aromatherapy treatments:

- **Personal blends.** In a clean container, add a total of 8 to 12 drops of any single oil or combination of oils of your choice to $1/8$ ounce of jojoba oil, or mix one of the recommended blends. Mix the oils by gently turning the container upside down several times or by rolling it between your hands for a few minutes. Do not shake the mixture forcefully. Apply the blend as a fragrance or simply inhale it directly from the bottle, as needed.

- **Baths.** Add a total of 3 to 10 drops of any single oil or combination of oils you choose, or one of the blends suggested in this section, to a bathtub filled with warm water. Soak in the bath for twenty minutes. Repeat as needed.

- **Diffuser or lamp blends.** Choose any of the single oils mentioned, a combination of two or more of those oils, or one of the recommended blends. Drop the essential oils into a small glass bottle with an airtight cover and combine. Add the blend to your diffuser or lamp. For a diffuser, follow the manufacturer's directions. For a lamp, place 10 to 20 drops of a single oil or blend in the lamp bowl. Run the diffuser or lamp as needed.

AROMATHERAPY BLENDS FOR UNDESIRABLE EMOTIONS

Essential oils can help you overcome or rise above emotions that are no longer benefitting you. For any undesirable emotions you wish to change, use the oils suggested, either individually or in any combination you choose, or make one of the recommended blends.

AGGRESSION

Essential oils that combat aggression include bergamot, chamomile, juniper, lemon, marjoram, rosemary, and ylang ylang. For instructions on using these essential oils, see page 126. Or use one or more of the aromatherapy blends that follow.

❧ Anti-Aggression Personal Blend

⅛ ounce jojoba oil
4 drops lemon oil
3 drops ylang ylang oil
2 drops bergamot oil
2 drops chamomile oil

Add the essential oils to the jojoba oil and blend. Wear as a fragrance or inhale directly from the bottle, as needed.

Note: Bergamot and lemon oils increase sensitivity to the sun. Omit them from your formula if your skin will be exposed to sunlight.

❧ Nighttime Bath for Easing Aggression

3 drops chamomile oil
3 drops marjoram oil
2 drops juniper oil
2 drops ylang ylang oil

Disperse the essential oils in a bathtubful of warm water. Soak in the bath for twenty minutes before going to bed.

❧ Aggression Diffuser Blend

20 drops lemon oil
15 drops chamomile oil
15 drops ylang ylang oil
5 drops juniper oil
5 drops rosemary oil

Drop the essential oils into a small glass container with an airtight cover and combine. Add some of the blend to your diffuser or lamp as necessary.

ANGER

Essential oils recommended for fighting feelings of anger are chamomile, jasmine, marjoram, rose, rosemary, and ylang ylang. For instructions on using these essential oils, see page 126. Or use one or more of the aromatherapy blends that follow.

❧ Calming Personal Blend

⅛ ounce jojoba oil
3 drops chamomile oil
3 drops ylang ylang oil
1 drop jasmine absolute or enfleurage
1 drop rose oil

Add the essential oils to the jojoba oil and blend. Wear as a fragrance or inhale directly from the bottle, as needed.

๏ Bath Blend for Releasing Anger

3 drops chamomile oil
3 drops ylang ylang oil
2 drops marjoram oil

Disperse the essential oils in a bathtubful of warm water. Soak in the bath for twenty minutes. Repeat as needed.

๏ Diffuser Blend for Diminishing Anger

20 drops chamomile oil
18 drops rosemary oil
10 drops ylang ylang oil

Drop the essential oils into a small glass container with an airtight cover and combine. Add some of the blend to your diffuser or lamp as necessary.

DISAPPOINTMENT

Essential oils recommended for easing disappointment are jasmine and rose. For instructions on using these essential oils, see page 126. Or use one or more of the aromatherapy blends that follow.

๏ Personal Blend for Decreasing Disappointment

⅛ ounce jojoba oil
4 drops jasmine absolute or enfleurage
4 drops rose oil

Add the essential oils to the jojoba oil and blend. Wear as a fragrance or inhale directly from the bottle, as needed.

๏ Bath Blend for Dealing with Disappointment

2 drops jasmine absolute or enfleurage
2 drops rose oil

Disperse the essential oils in a bathtubful of warm water. Soak in the bath for twenty minutes. Repeat as needed.

FEAR

Essential oils recommended for easing feelings of fear are cedarwood, fennel, ginger, patchouli, sandalwood, and thyme. For instructions on using these essential oils, see page 126. Or use one or more of the aromatherapy blends that follow.

๏ Fear-Less Personal Blend

⅛ ounce jojoba oil
8 drops sandalwood oil
2 drops cedarwood oil
1 drop ginger oil
1 drop patchouli oil

Add the essential oils to the jojoba oil and blend. Wear as a fragrance or inhale directly from the bottle, as needed.

๏ Fear-Free Bath Blend

3 drops fennel oil
3 drops sandalwood oil
2 drops cedarwood oil
1 drop thyme oil

Disperse the essential oils in a bathtubful of warm water. Soak in the bath for twenty minutes. Repeat as needed.

๏ Diffuser Blend for Combatting Fear

20 drops cedarwood oil
20 drops sandalwood oil
5 drops fennel oil
5 drops ginger oil
5 drops lemon thyme oil

Drop the essential oils into a small glass container with an airtight cover and combine. Add some of the blend to your diffuser or lamp as necessary.

GRIEF

Essential oils recommended for dealing with grief are bergamot, chamomile, jasmine, marjoram, neroli, and rose. For instructions on using these essential oils, see page 126. Or use one or more of the aromatherapy blends that follow.

Be aware that bergamot oil increases sensitivity to the sun. Omit it from your formula if your skin will be exposed to sunlight.

❧ Grief Relief Personal Blend

⅛ ounce jojoba oil
4 drops neroli oil
2 drops chamomile oil
2 drops jasmine absolute or enfleurage
1 drop rose oil

Add the essential oils to the jojoba oil and blend. Wear as a fragrance or inhale directly from the bottle, as needed.

❧ Bath Blend for Getting Through Grief

4 drops chamomile oil
3 drops bergamot oil
3 drops marjoram oil

Disperse the essential oils in a bathtubful of warm water. Soak in the bath for twenty minutes. Repeat as needed.

❧ Grief Release Diffuser Blend

25 drops bergamot oil
15 drops chamomile oil
5 drops marjoram oil

Drop the essential oils into a small glass container with an airtight cover and combine. Add some of the blend to your diffuser or lamp as necessary.

HYSTERIA

Essential oils recommended for combatting hysteria are chamomile, lavender, neroli, orange, and tea tree. For instructions on using these essential oils, see page 126. Or use one or more of the aromatherapy blends that follow.

❧ Tranquil Personal Blend

⅛ ounce jojoba oil
4 drops chamomile oil
4 drops lavender oil
1 drop neroli oil
1 drop orange oil

Add the essential oils to the jojoba oil and blend. Wear as a fragrance or inhale directly from the bottle, as needed.

❧ Hysteria-Calming Bath Blend

4 drops chamomile oil
4 drops lavender oil
2 drops orange oil
1 drop tea tree oil

Disperse the essential oils in a bathtubful of warm water. Soak in the bath for twenty minutes. Repeat as needed.

IMPATIENCE/IRRITABILITY

Essential oils recommended for reducing impatience or irritability are chamomile, clary sage, frankincense, and lavender. For instructions on using these essential oils, see page 126. Or use the following aromatherapy blend.

☙ Impatience/Irritability Eliminator Personal Blend

1/8 ounce jojoba oil
4 drops lavender oil
3 drops chamomile oil
2 drops clary sage oil
1 drop frankincense oil

Add the essential oils to the jojoba oil and blend. Wear as a fragrance or inhale directly from the bottle, as needed.

INDECISION/INDIFFERENCE

Essential oils recommended for overcoming indecision or indifference are basil, clary sage, cypress, jasmine, patchouli, and peppermint. For instructions on using these essential oils, see page 126. Or use one or more of the aromatherapy blends that follow.

☙ Personal Decisiveness Blend

1/8 ounce jojoba oil
6 drops clary sage oil
2 drops jasmine absolute or enfleurage
1 drop patchouli oil

Add the essential oils to the jojoba oil and blend. Wear as a fragrance or inhale directly from the bottle, as needed.

☙ Bath Blend for Overcoming Indifference

4 drops clary sage oil
3 drops cypress oil
1 drop peppermint oil

Disperse the essential oils in a bathtubful of warm water. Soak in the bath for twenty minutes. Repeat as needed.

☙ Decision-Making Diffuser Blend

20 drops clary sage oil
15 drops basil oil
8 drops cypress oil
5 drops peppermint oil

Drop the essential oils into a small glass container with an airtight cover and combine. Add some of the blend to your diffuser or lamp as necessary.

JEALOUSY/RESENTMENT

Essential oils recommended for dealing with feelings of jealousy and resentment are jasmine and rose. For instructions on using these essential oils, see page 126. Or use the following aromatherapy blend.

☙ Personal Blend for Overcoming Jealousy

1/8 ounce jojoba oil
5 drops jasmine absolute or enfleurage
4 drops rose oil

Add the essential oils to the jojoba oil and blend. Wear as a fragrance or inhale directly from the bottle, as needed.

LONELINESS

Essential oils recommended for comforting loneliness are benzoin and marjoram. For instructions on using these essential oils, see page 126. Or use the following aromatherapy blend.

☙ Loneliness-Easing Bath

8 drops marjoram oil
2 drops benzoin resin

Disperse the essential oils in a bathtubful of

warm water. Soak in the bath for twenty minutes. Repeat as needed.

MENTAL/EMOTIONAL FATIGUE

Essential oils recommended for combatting mental or emotional fatigue include basil, clary sage, coriander, ginger, helichrysum, jasmine, juniper, orange, palmarosa, peppermint, rosemary, thyme, vetiver, and ylang ylang. For instructions on using these essential oils, see page 126. Or use one or more of the aromatherapy blends that follow.

❧ Stimulating Personal Blend

⅛ ounce jojoba oil
3 drops orange oil
2 drops clary sage oil
2 drops coriander oil
1 drop helichrysum oil
1 drop jasmine absolute or enfleurage
1 drop palmarosa oil
1 drop vetiver oil

Add the essential oils to the jojoba oil and blend. Wear as a fragrance or inhale directly from the bottle, as needed.

❧ Stimulating Morning Bath

3 drops rosemary oil
2 drops basil oil
1 drop juniper oil
1 drop peppermint oil

Disperse the essential oils in a bathtubful of warm water. Soak in the bath for twenty minutes. Repeat as needed.

❧ Mind-Activating Diffuser Blend

10 drops basil oil
8 drops coriander oil
8 drops rosemary oil
5 drops ginger oil
5 drops peppermint oil
3 drops ylang ylang oil

Drop the essential oils into a small glass container with an airtight cover and combine. Add some of the blend to your diffuser or lamp as necessary.

NERVOUSNESS

Essential oils recommended for reducing nervousness are chamomile, clary sage, coriander, frankincense, neroli, orange, and vetiver. Essential oils that act as nervous system tonics, which can be used for toning and strengthening the nervous system as a preventative measure, are bergamot, black pepper, cedarwood, chamomile, clary sage, coriander, lemon, peppermint, pine, orange, neroli, rosemary, and thyme. For instructions on using these essential oils, see page 126. Or use one or more of the aromatherapy blends that follow.

❧ Nerve-Settling Personal Blend

⅛ ounce jojoba oil
4 drops clary sage oil
3 drops orange oil
2 drops chamomile oil
1 drop frankincense oil
1 drop neroli oil

Add the essential oils to the jojoba oil and blend. Wear as a fragrance or inhale directly from the bottle, as needed.

❧ Nerve-Calming Bath

4 drops chamomile oil
3 drops clary sage oil
2 drops orange oil
1 drop vetiver oil

Disperse the essential oils in a bathtubful of warm water. Soak in the bath for twenty minutes. Repeat as needed.

❧ Nerve Tonic Personal Blend

⅛ ounce jojoba oil
4 drops lavender oil
3 drops clary sage oil
3 drops sandalwood oil
2 drops neroli oil
1 drop coriander oil
1 drop vetiver oil

Add the essential oils to the jojoba oil and blend. Wear as a fragrance or inhale directly from the bottle, as needed.

❧ Nighttime Nerve Tonic Bath

3 drops chamomile oil
2 drops thyme oil
2 drops pine oil
1 drop cedarwood oil
1 drop orange oil

Disperse the essential oils in a bathtubful of warm water. Soak in the bath for twenty minutes. Repeat as needed.

❧ Tangy Nerve Tonic Diffuser Blend

25 drops bergamot oil
20 drops lemon oil
15 drops orange oil
8 drops ylang ylang oil
2 drops black pepper oil
1 drop peppermint oil

Drop the essential oils into a small glass container with an airtight cover and combine. Add some of the blend to your diffuser or lamp as necessary.

Note: Bergamot and lemon oils increase sensitivity to the sun. Omit them from your formula if your skin will be exposed to sunlight.

PANIC

Essential oils recommended for alleviating panic are chamomile, clary sage, geranium, jasmine, juniper, lavender, neroli, and ylang ylang. For instructions on using these essential oils, see page 126. Or use one or more of the aromatherapy blends that follow.

❧ Floral Panic-Preventing Personal Blend

⅛ ounce jojoba oil
4 drops geranium oil
2 drops chamomile oil
2 drops lavender oil
1 drop jasmine absolute or enfleurage
1 drop neroli oil
1 drop ylang ylang oil

Add the essential oils to the jojoba oil and blend. Wear as a fragrance or inhale directly from the bottle, as needed.

❧ Panic-Soothing Bath Blend

4 drops clary sage oil
3 drops geranium oil
2 drops juniper oil
1 drop ylang ylang oil

Disperse the essential oils in a bathtubful of warm water. Soak in the bath for twenty minutes. Repeat as needed.

❧ Panic-Stopping Diffuser Blend

20 drops chamomile oil
15 drops lavender oil

10 drops clary sage oil
10 drops geranium oil
5 drops ylang ylang oil

Drop the essential oils into a small glass container with an airtight cover and combine. Add some of the blend to your diffuser or lamp as necessary.

SADNESS

Essential oils recommended to help lift feelings of sadness are benzoin, jasmine, rose, and rosewood. For instructions on using these essential oils, see page 126. Or use the following aromatherapy blend.

❧ So Long Sadness Personal Blend

⅛ ounce jojoba oil
6 drops rosewood oil
2 drops benzoin resin
2 drops jasmine absolute or enfleurage
1 drop rose oil

Add the essential oils to the jojoba oil and blend. Wear as a fragrance or inhale directly from the bottle, as needed.

SHOCK

Essential oils recommended for easing feelings of shock are lavender, neroli, rose, and tea tree. For instructions on using these essential oils, see page 126. Or use one or more of the aromatherapy blends that follow.

❧ Shock-Soothing Personal Blend

⅛ ounce jojoba oil
6 drops lavender oil
2 drops neroli oil
1 drop rose oil

Add the essential oils to the jojoba oil and blend. Wear as a fragrance or inhale directly from the bottle, as needed.

❧ Shock Bath Therapy

8 drops lavender oil
2 drops tea tree oil

Disperse the essential oils in a bathtubful of warm water. Soak in the bath for twenty minutes. Repeat as needed.

SHYNESS

The best essential oil for overcoming shyness is jasmine. For instructions on using it in a bath, diffuser, or lamp, see page 126. Or use the following aromatherapy blend.

❧ Shyness Personal Blend

⅛ ounce jojoba oil
8 drops jasmine absolute or enfleurage

Add the jasmine to the jojoba oil and blend. Wear as a fragrance or inhale directly from the bottle, as needed.

SUSPICION

Essential oils recommended for releasing feelings of suspicion are jasmine and lavender. For instructions on using these essential oils, see page 126. Or use the following aromatherapy blend.

❧ Suspicion-Soothing Personal Blend

⅛ ounce jojoba oil
6 drops lavender oil
2 drops jasmine absolute or enfleurage

Add the essential oils to the jojoba oil and

blend. Wear as a fragrance or inhale directly from the bottle, as needed.

TENSION

Essential oils recommended for easing tension are chamomile, clary sage, cypress, frankincense, geranium, jasmine, lavender, lemon, marjoram, neroli, orange, rose, rosewood, sandalwood, and ylang ylang. For instructions on using these essential oils, see page 126. Or use one or more of the aromatherapy blends that follow.

❧ Tension-Tamer Personal Blend

⅛ ounce jojoba oil
3 drops sandalwood oil
2 drops rosewood oil
2 drops neroli oil
1 drop frankincense oil
1 drop jasmine absolute or enfleurage
1 drop ylang ylang oil

Add the essential oils to the jojoba oil and blend. Wear as a fragrance or inhale directly from the bottle, as needed.

❧ Tension-Easing Bath Blend

4 drops lavender oil
3 drops marjoram oil
2 drops chamomile oil
2 drops cypress oil

Disperse the essential oils in a bathtubful of warm water. Soak in the bath for twenty minutes. Repeat as needed.

❧ Tension-Release Diffuser Blend

15 drops lavender oil
10 drops clary sage oil
10 drops lemon oil

8 drops rosewood oil
6 drops marjoram oil
4 drops geranium oil
2 drops ylang ylang oil

Drop the essential oils into a small glass container with an airtight cover and combine. Add some of the blend to your diffuser or lamp as necessary.

AROMATHERAPY BLENDS FOR POSITIVE EMOTIONS

Essential oils can have a positive influence on your mental state by helping to restore equilibrium and balance in your life. For any positive feelings, emotions, or mental conditions you wish to develop or deepen, use the suggested essential oils, either singly or in any combination you choose, or use the recommended aromatherapy blends.

DEALING WITH CHANGE

Essential oils recommended for emotions connected with facing and handling change are black pepper, clary sage, cypress, frankincense, and myrrh. For instructions on using these essential oils, see page 126. Or use the following aromatherapy blend.

❧ Transition Tonic Personal Blend

⅛ ounce jojoba oil
3 drops clary sage oil
2 drops frankincense oil
2 drops myrrh oil
1 drop black pepper oil
1 drop cypress oil

Add the essential oils to the jojoba oil and blend. Wear as a fragrance or inhale directly from the bottle, as needed.

CONCENTRATION

Essential oils recommended for increasing concentration are basil, ginger, peppermint, and rosemary. For instructions on using these essential oils, see page 126. Or use one or more of the aromatherapy blends that follow.

❧ Concentration Bath Blend

3 drops basil oil
2 drops rosemary oil
1 drop ginger oil
1 drop peppermint oil

Disperse the essential oils in a bathtubful of warm water. Soak in the bath for twenty minutes. Repeat as needed.

❧ Concentration Diffuser Blend

20 drops rosemary oil
10 drops peppermint oil
8 drops basil oil
5 drops ginger oil

Drop the essential oils into a small glass container with an airtight cover and combine. Add some of the blend to your diffuser or lamp as necessary.

CONFIDENCE

Essential oils recommended for boosting confidence are jasmine, marjoram, neroli, patchouli, peppermint, rose, rosemary, and ylang ylang. For instructions on using these essential oils, see page 126. Or use one or more of the aromatherapy blends that follow.

❧ Confidence-Building Personal Blend

⅛ ounce jojoba oil
3 drops geranium oil

3 drops neroli oil
2 drops jasmine absolute or enfleurage
2 drops rose oil
2 drops ylang ylang oil
1 drop chamomile oil

Add the essential oils to the jojoba oil and blend. Wear as a fragrance or inhale directly from the bottle, as needed.

❧ Self-Confidence Bath

3 drops ylang ylang oil
2 drops marjoram oil
1 drop jasmine absolute or enfleurage

Disperse the essential oils in a bathtubful of warm water. Soak in the bath for twenty minutes. Repeat as needed.

COURAGE

Essential oils recommended to heighten courage are black pepper, fennel, ginger, and thyme. For instructions on using these essential oils, see page 126. Or use the following aromatherapy blend.

❧ Courage-Boosting Bath Blend

4 drops thyme oil
3 drops fennel oil
1 drop ginger oil
1 drop black pepper oil

Disperse the essential oils in a bathtubful of warm water. Soak in the bath for twenty minutes. Repeat as needed.

CREATIVITY

Essential oils recommended for enhancing creativity are clary sage, helichrysum, neroli, rose, and rosewood. For instructions on using these essential oils, see page 126. Or use one or more of the aromatherapy blends that follow.

❧ Creativity Perfume Blend

⅛ ounce jojoba oil
5 drops rosewood oil
4 drops helichrysum oil
2 drops clary sage oil
2 drops neroli oil
2 drops rose oil

Add the essential oils to the jojoba oil and blend. Wear as a fragrance or inhale directly from the bottle, as needed.

❧ Creative Diffuser Blend

15 drops rosewood oil
12 drops clary sage oil
8 drops helichrysum oil
3 drops neroli oil

Drop the essential oils into a small glass container with an airtight cover and combine. Add some of the blend to your diffuser or lamp as necessary.

HAPPINESS/JOY

Essential oils recommended for promoting feelings of happiness and joy are basil, bergamot, neroli, orange, and rose. For instructions on using these essential oils, see page 126. Or use one or more of the aromatherapy blends that follow.

Be aware that bergamot and orange oils increase sensitivity to the sun. Omit them from your formulas if your skin will be exposed to sunlight.

❧ Joyous Personal Blend

⅛ ounce jojoba oil
4 drops bergamot oil
4 drops neroli oil
3 drops rose oil
1 drop orange oil

Add the essential oils to the jojoba oil and blend. Wear as a fragrance or inhale directly from the bottle, as needed.

❧ Happy Bath Blend

4 drops bergamot oil
3 drops orange oil
1 drop basil oil

Disperse the essential oils in a bathtubful of warm water. Soak in the bath for twenty minutes. Repeat as needed.

❧ Joyous Diffuser Blend

20 drops bergamot oil
20 drops orange oil
5 drops basil oil

Drop the essential oils into a small glass container with an airtight cover and combine. Add some of the blend to your diffuser or lamp as necessary.

HARMONY/BALANCE

Essential oils recommended for deepening feelings of harmony and balance are cedarwood, elemi, geranium, lavender, and vetiver. For instructions on using these essential oils, see page 126. Or use one or more of the aromatherapy blends that follow.

❧ Harmony Personal Blend

⅛ ounce jojoba oil
6 drops lavender oil
4 drops geranium oil
2 drops ylang ylang oil
1 drop vetiver oil

Add the essential oils to the jojoba oil and blend. Wear as a fragrance or inhale directly from the bottle, as needed.

❧ Balancing Bath Blend

4 drops geranium oil
4 drops lavender oil
1 drop cedarwood oil
1 drop vetiver oil

Disperse the essential oils in a bathtubful of warm water. Soak in the bath for twenty minutes. Repeat as needed.

❧ Equilibrium Diffuser Blend

20 drops lavender oil
15 drops elemi oil
15 drops geranium oil
10 drops cedarwood oil
5 drops vetiver oil

Drop the essential oils into a small glass container with an airtight cover and combine. Add some of the blend to your diffuser or lamp as necessary.

INTUITION

Essential oils recommended for enhancing intuition are helichrysum, rose, and rosewood. For instructions on using these essential oils, see page 126. Or use the following aromatherapy blend.

❧ Intuition Personal Blend

1/8 ounce jojoba oil
4 drops helichrysum oil
4 drops rosewood oil
1 drop rose oil

Add the essential oils to the jojoba oil and blend. Wear as a fragrance or inhale directly from the bottle, as needed.

LOVE

Essential oils recommended for deepening feelings of love are benzoin, coriander, ginger, jasmine, lavender, neroli, palmarosa, rose, rosemary, and ylang ylang. For instructions on using these essential oils, see page 126. Or use one or more of the aromatherapy blends that follow.

❧ Love Potion Personal Blend

1/8 ounce jojoba oil
2 drops jasmine absolute or enfleurage
2 drops neroli oil
2 drops ylang ylang oil
1 drop benzoin resin
1 drop coriander oil
1 drop ginger oil
1 drop rose oil

Add the essential oils to the jojoba oil and blend. Wear as a fragrance or inhale directly from the bottle, as needed.

❧ Loving Bath Blend

3 drops lavender oil
3 drops ylang ylang oil
2 drops coriander oil
1 drop neroli oil

Disperse the essential oils in a bathtubful of warm water. Soak in the bath for twenty minutes. Repeat as needed.

❧ Love Diffuser Blend

10 drops lavender oil
10 drops ylang ylang
8 drops coriander oil
6 drops benzoin resin
6 drops palmarosa oil
4 drops ginger oil

Drop the essential oils into a small glass container with an airtight cover and combine. Add some of the blend to your diffuser or lamp as necessary.

MEDITATION

Essential oils recommended for heightening meditation include benzoin, black pepper, cedarwood, chamomile, clary sage, elemi, frankincense, helichrysum, jasmine, juniper, myrrh, rosewood, sandalwood, and vetiver. For instructions on using these essential oils, see page 126. Or use the following aromatherapy blend.

❧ Meditation Diffuser Blend

20 drops sandalwood oil
12 drops rosewood oil
10 drops elemi oil
5 drops cedarwood oil
5 drops frankincense oil
5 drops myrrh oil
5 drops vetiver oil

Drop the essential oils into a small glass container with an airtight cover and combine. Add some of the blend to your diffuser or lamp as necessary.

MEMORY

Essential oils recommended for improving memory are basil, clary sage, coriander, fennel, ginger, peppermint, and rosemary. For instructions on using these essential oils, see page 126. Or use one or more of the aromatherapy blends that follow.

❧ Brain Tonic Bath Blend

3 drops rosemary oil
2 drops clary sage oil
2 drops coriander oil
1 drop fennel oil
1 drop basil oil

Disperse the essential oils in a bathtubful of warm water. Soak in the bath for twenty minutes. Repeat as needed.

❧ Memory-Jogger Diffuser Blend

25 drops clary sage oil
10 drops coriander oil
10 drops ginger oil
8 drops rosemary oil
3 drops peppermint oil

Drop the essential oils into a small glass container with an airtight cover and combine. Add some of the blend to your diffuser or lamp as necessary.

PEACE/SERENITY/CALMNESS

Essential oils recommended for deepening feelings of peace, serenity, and calmness are benzoin, bergamot, chamomile, clary sage, elemi, geranium, ginger, helichrysum, jasmine, lavender, marjoram, neroli, rose, rosewood, sandalwood, and ylang ylang. For instructions on using these essential oils, see page 126. Or use one or more of the aromatherapy blends that follow.

❧ Serenity Personal Blend

⅛ ounce jojoba oil
4 drops sandalwood oil
2 drops clary sage oil
2 drops jasmine absolute or enfleurage
2 drops lavender oil
2 drops rosewood oil
1 drop chamomile oil
1 drop neroli oil

Add the essential oils to the jojoba oil and blend. Wear as a fragrance or inhale directly from the bottle, as needed.

🐦 Composure Bath Blend

3 drops rosewood oil
2 drops clary sage oil
2 drops sandalwood oil
1 drop chamomile oil
1 drop elemi oil
1 drop marjoram oil

Disperse the essential oils in a bathtubful of warm water. Soak in the bath for twenty minutes. Repeat as needed.

🐦 Calming Diffuser Blend

18 drops lavender oil
15 drops rosewood oil
12 drops chamomile oil
12 drops geranium oil
10 drops clary sage oil
10 drops ylang ylang oil
8 drops marjoram oil

Drop the essential oils into a small glass container with an airtight cover and combine. Add some of the blend to your diffuser or lamp as necessary.

RELEASING THE PAST

Essential oils recommended to help you let go of the past are black pepper, cypress, frankincense, myrrh, and rose. For instructions on using these essential oils, see page 126. Or use the following aromatherapy blend.

🐦 Letting Go Personal Blend

1/8 ounce jojoba oil
3 drops frankincense oil
2 drops myrrh oil
2 drops rose oil
1 drop black pepper oil

Add the essential oils to the jojoba oil and blend. Wear as a fragrance or inhale directly from the bottle, as needed.

SELF-ESTEEM

Essential oils recommended for boosting self-esteem are marjoram, patchouli, peppermint, rosemary, and ylang ylang. For instructions on using these essential oils, see page 126. Or use one or more of the aromatherapy blends that follow.

🐦 Self-Esteem Personal Blend

1/8 ounce jojoba oil
6 drops ylang ylang oil
4 drops marjoram oil
1 drop patchouli oil

Add the essential oils to the jojoba oil and blend. Wear as a fragrance or inhale directly from the bottle, as needed.

🐦 Esteem-Boosting Bath

3 drops rosemary oil
2 drops ylang ylang oil
1 drop patchouli oil
1 drop peppermint oil

Disperse the essential oils in a bathtubful of warm water. Soak in the bath for twenty minutes. Repeat as needed.

SEXUAL DESIRE

Essential oils recommended for their aphrodisiac properties include benzoin, clary sage, coriander, ginger, jasmine, lavender, neroli, patchouli, rose, rosewood, sandalwood, vetiver, and ylang ylang. For instructions on using these essential oils, see page 126. Or use one or more of the aromatherapy blends that follow.

🐦 All-Purpose Aphrodisiac Personal Blend

⅛ ounce jojoba oil
4 drops neroli oil
4 drops sandalwood oil
2 drops benzoin resin
2 drops jasmine absolute or enfleurage
1 drop rose oil
1 drop vetiver oil

Add the essential oils to the jojoba oil and blend. Wear as a fragrance or inhale directly from the bottle, as needed.

🐦 Sensuality Bath

3 drops sandalwood oil
2 drops rosewood oil
2 drops ylang ylang oil
1 drop patchouli oil

Disperse the essential oils in a bathtubful of warm water. Soak in the bath for twenty minutes. Repeat as needed.

🐦 Sensual Diffuser Blend

15 drops lavender oil
10 drops clary sage oil
6 drops ylang ylang oil
4 drops coriander oil
3 drops ginger oil
2 drops vetiver oil

Drop the essential oils into a small glass container with an airtight cover and combine. Add some of the blend to your diffuser or lamp as necessary.

SPIRITUAL PURITY

Essential oils recommended for spiritual purifica-
tion and cleansing are eucalyptus, ginger, juniper, lemon, neroli, orange, pine, and rosemary. For instructions on using these essential oils, see page 126. Or use the following aromatherapy blend.

🐦 Purifying Bath Blend

3 drops juniper oil
3 drops lemon oil
2 drops pine oil
2 drops rosemary oil
1 drop eucalyptus oil

Disperse the essential oils in a bathtubful of warm water. Soak in the bath for twenty minutes. Repeat as needed.

Fatigue

Fatigue is the condition of not having enough energy to function, so much so that you need to stop and rest or sleep. Other symptoms may include dizziness, headaches, nausea, or nervousness. Mental weariness can also accompany physical fatigue.

Fatigue is a signal that your body needs to conserve its energy or strength. It can mean simply that you are expending more energy than your body produces. Fatigue can also be a symptom of an underlying health problem. Adrenal malfunction, allergies, anemia, candidiasis, depression, diabetes, hormonal imbalances, hypoglycemia, low blood pressure, poor absorption of nutrients, nutritional deficiencies, poor diet, stress, and thyroid disorders can all produce fatigue, as can virtually any infectious illness. In some cases, fatigue can be the first sign of a developing physical or emotional problem.

HELPFUL TREATMENTS

If you are bothered by fatigue, you should see a health care professional to check for low blood pressure and to rule out physical illness as the cause of your sluggishness. If illness is the cause of your fatigue, your doctor can recommend appropriate treatment and you should begin a program to improve your immunity (see WEAKENED IMMUNE SYSTEM).

If no underlying illness or other cause for your fatigue is found, begin a regimen including regular exercise, a healthy diet, nutritional supplementation, relaxation, and regular, restful sleep. This alone may be sufficient to restore your energy. You should also avoid such energy-depleting habits as smoking, drinking, overworking, and taking drugs. Learn how to manage stress and balance your emotions. Avoid taking on too many responsibilities. If you do all of these things and your fatigue continues for more than several months, chronic fatigue syndrome may be a possibility (see CHRONIC FATIGUE SYNDROME).

Aromatherapy can help you to increase your energy, improve your body's immune response, and reduce stress. Stimulating essential oils such as basil, coriander, elemi, geranium, ginger, lavender, lemon, orange, patchouli, peppermint, pine, rosemary, and thyme can boost your energy level.

Take a Fatigue-Fighting Bath every morning. Apply Energizing Body Oil over your body once or twice daily and breathe in Energy Inhalant Oil during the day, as needed. You can also disperse Energy-Boosting Diffuser Blend in your home or office.

AROMATHERAPY BLENDS

The aromatherapy blends below are essential oil formulas you can prepare at home. For a more detailed explanation of how to put together and use these blends, see BATHS; DIFFUSERS AND LAMPS; INHALANTS; and/or MASSAGE in Part Four. For a quick review of general guidelines for using essential oils, see page 91.

࿏ Fatigue-Fighting Bath

3 drops rosemary oil
2 drops orange oil
1 drop peppermint oil
1 drop thyme oil

Disperse all the ingredients in a bathtub filled with warm water and soak in the tub for twenty to thirty minutes. Repeat as necessary.

࿏ Energizing Body Oil

2 ounces carrier oil
6 drops lavender oil
4 drops rosemary oil
3 drops geranium oil
3 drops lemon oil
2 drops coriander oil
2 drops patchouli oil

Place the carrier oil in a clean container, add the essential oils, and gently turn the container over several times or roll it between your hands to blend. Massage the oil into your skin once a day, as needed.

࿏ Energy Inhalant Oil

8 drops rosemary oil
6 drops elemi oil
4 drops peppermint oil
3 drops basil oil
1 drop ginger oil

Add the oils to a small glass bottle with an airtight cover and blend well. Inhale directly from the bottle any time you need a boost of energy.

🐚 Energy-Boosting Diffuser Blend

15 drops rosemary oil
12 drops pine oil
10 drops lavender oil
10 drops lemon oil
2 drops peppermint oil

Combine all the ingredients in a small glass bottle with an airtight cover. Add some of the mixture to your diffuser or lamp bowl as desired.

Gas, Intestinal

See INDIGESTION.

Gum Disease

When the gums or the tissues supporting the teeth become damaged or inflamed, gum disease (periodontal disease) can threaten oral health. Most cases of periodontal disease are related to poor oral hygiene. Plaque, a sticky bacterial substance, adheres to the teeth, especially along the gum line. When minerals present in saliva combine with plaque, it hardens into tartar, which pushes the gums back; the bacteria in the tartar can then cause infection of the gum tissue. Periodontal disease may also arise from or be aggravated by faulty dental work, the presence of mercury amalgam fillings, mouth-breathing, the use of cigarettes or chewing tobacco, and grinding one's teeth. Systemic disorders such as anemia, collagen diseases, diabetes, impaired immunity, leukemia, and vitamin deficiencies can cause periodontal disease as well.

Gingivitis, or inflammation of the gums, is the most common form of periodontal disease. The gums swell and become sensitive and bleed easily. The breath may smell offensive. If gingivitis is not treated, periodontitis may develop. In periodontitis, the tissue surrounding the teeth becomes inflamed, and the bones supporting the teeth gradually deteriorate. Finally, the gums recede and weaken; teeth become loose and may fall out. Periodontitis is the major cause of tooth loss in adults.

HELPFUL TREATMENTS

Good oral hygiene is the best way to prevent gum problems (see Oral Hygiene, page 143). If you already have gum problems, good oral hygiene may reverse some of the damage and prevent the problem from progressing further. You should also see your dentist for proper treatment.

Essential oils can be used along with your dentist's treatment to minimize the pain and discomfort of periodontal disease. Lemon, myrrh, orange, rose, and tea tree oils are recommended for gingivitis; cypress, myrrh, and tea tree are the best essential oils for the more advanced problems associated with periodontitis. Cypress, lemon, and tea tree oils help prevent bleeding gums; basil, fennel, and thyme oils can help fight gum infections; and basil, bergamot, lemon, myrrh, orange, and tea tree oils help heal mouth ulcers. All of these essential oils help to restore gum health and prevent additional problems.

Once or twice daily, after brushing your teeth, rub Gingivitis Gum Massage Oil into your gums to promote circulation and encourage gum health. Alternate this treatment with the use of Gum-Strengthening Mouthwash or Infection-Fighting Mouthwash.

Oral Hygiene

Good oral hygiene combines proper home care with the professional care of your dentist and oral hygienist to keep your teeth and gums healthy. Proper brushing after eating removes plaque, a soft and sticky colorless film comprised of bacteria and mucus. Plaque coats your teeth, attacks tooth enamel, and contributes to cavities. Take your time when brushing, and make sure you brush your tongue as well as your teeth. It is better to give your mouth one complete brushing each day than to brush several times quickly and miss certain areas again and again. Use a soft-bristle toothbrush, and replace it frequently (approximately every three months). Daily flossing also removes plaque and discourages the formation of tartar, the hardened deposit that forms on the teeth when calcium from your saliva combines with plaque. If you have any doubts about proper brushing or flossing technique, ask your dentist or dental hygienist.

When combined with good home care, regular dental checkups and professional cleanings can prevent cavities and most dental problems. Most dentists recommend a cleaning and a checkup every six months. You should also consult your dentist between scheduled visits if you suspect you may be developing any tooth or gum problems.

Aromatherapy can be a valuable addition to your oral hygiene program. Lemon, myrrh, orange, peppermint, and tea tree oils fight the bacteria that cause plaque. Myrrh oil also helps preserve or restore gum health, while peppermint, orange, and lemon oils freshen breath. Many manufacturers fortify toothpastes, mouthwashes, dental flosses, and toothpicks with essential oils.

You can use the aromatherapy blends below to help you maintain good dental health. Therapeutic Breath-Freshening Mouthwash will freshen your breath as it contributes to gum health. Gum Therapy Oil will help maintain or improve the condition of your gums.

❧ Therapeutic Breath-Freshening Mouthwash

    8 ounces distilled water
    2 drops myrrh oil
    2 drops tea tree oil
    1 drop peppermint oil

Mix all the ingredients together in a clean bottle. Swish about $\frac{1}{2}$ ounce around in your mouth after brushing your teeth or after meals, as needed. Shake well before using.

❧ Gum Therapy Oil

    $\frac{1}{8}$ ounce carrier oil
    10 drops tea tree oil
    6 drops myrrh oil
    3 drops lemon oil
    1 drop peppermint oil

Place the carrier oil in a clean container, add the essential oils, and blend. Massage the mixture into your gums once a day, after brushing your teeth and rinsing your mouth with mouthwash.

AROMATHERAPY BLENDS

The aromatherapy blends below are essential oil formulas you can prepare at home. For a more detailed explanation of how to put together and use these blends, see MOUTHWASHES, GARGLES, AND GUM TREATMENTS in Part Four. For a quick review of general guidelines for using essential oils, see page 91.

❧ Gingivitis Gum Massage Oil

1/8 ounce carrier oil
8 drops tea tree oil
4 drops myrrh oil
3 drops lemon oil
1 drop orange oil

Place the carrier oil in a clean container, add the essential oils, and turn the container over a few times or gently roll it between your hands to blend. Once or twice daily, after brushing your teeth, massage a couple of drops onto your gums.

❧ Gum-Strengthening Mouthwash

8 ounces distilled water
2 drops myrrh oil
2 drops fennel oil
2 drops tea tree oil
1 drop bergamot oil
1 drop peppermint oil

Pour the water into a bottle and add the essential oils to the water. Shake to blend. After brushing your teeth, rinse your mouth thoroughly with about 1/2 ounce of the mixture. Shake well before each use.

❧ Infection-Fighting Mouthwash

8 ounces distilled water
2 drops basil oil

2 drops fennel oil
2 drops thyme oil

Pour the water into a bottle, add the essential oils, and shake well. After brushing your teeth, rinse your mouth thoroughly, using about 1/2 ounce of the mouthwash. Shake the bottle before each use.

Hair and Scalp Problems

A healthy head of hair begins with a healthy scalp. Normal hair is shiny, silky, and full of body. It is neither too dry nor too oily. Hair and scalp problems often result from imbalances in the body. These may be caused by nutritional deficiencies, poor diet, or stress. Sometimes heredity and environmental factors, such as the chemicals found in hair dyes and perm solutions or heat from electric styling appliances, play a role as well. The most common hair- and scalp-related problems include dry hair, oily hair, dandruff, and hair loss.

Most hair and scalp problems respond to a healthier diet and to the use of appropriate hair care products. When nutritional deficiencies are corrected, hair and scalp conditions usually improve. No matter what type of problem you have with your hair, it is beneficial to eliminate all fatty and fried foods from your diet, and to keep your hair and scalp clean.

Aromatherapy hair care products help improve the condition of your hair and scalp by stimulating circulation to your scalp and adding luster and shine to your hair. They can also help balance your scalp's oil secretions.

NORMAL HAIR

If your hair is normal, you already have a proper balance of oil secretions. You can maintain this balance and keep your hair looking healthy and shiny with chamomile, lavender, thyme, and ylang ylang oils. Use Normal Hair Shampoo as needed.

❧ Normal Hair Shampoo

4 ounces unscented shampoo
8 drops lavender oil
6 drops chamomile oil
3 drops thyme oil
3 drops ylang ylang oil

Add all the oils to the unscented shampoo. Turn the bottle upside down several times or roll it between between your hands for a few minutes to blend. Use the mixture to shampoo your hair as necessary.

DRY HAIR

Dry hair appears dull and lifeless. The sebaceous, or oil, glands in the scalp secrete too little oil to sufficiently lubricate the hair. Little or no oil in the diet can contribute to dry hair, as can a poor diet or nutritional deficiencies.

Many external factors can dry out your hair. The overuse of curling irons, electric curlers, hair dryers, hair dyes, hair styling products, and perms can all dry out and even damage your hair. If you have dry hair, give your hair a rest from electric appliances, hair dyes, and perms.

Essential oils that help improve the condition of dry hair are cedarwood, chamomile, clary sage, lavender, and rosemary. Several times a week, apply Dry Hair Conditioning Treatment to your hair and scalp. Shampoo with Dry Hair Shampoo as needed.

❧ Dry Hair Conditioning Treatment

2 ounces jojoba oil
8 drops cedarwood oil
8 drops clary sage oil
4 drops lavender oil

Place the jojoba oil in a clean container and add the essential oils. Turn the container upside down several times or roll it between your hands for a few minutes to blend. At least once a week (more if needed), massage some of the treatment into your scalp and hair and leave it on for thirty to forty-five minutes or overnight. Then shampoo your hair with Dry Hair Shampoo.

❧ Dry Hair Shampoo

4 ounces unscented shampoo for dry hair
8 drops chamomile oil
8 drops lavender oil
4 drops rosemary oil

Add the chamomile, lavender, and rosemary oils to the unscented shampoo and blend well. Use the mixture to shampoo as necessary.

OILY HAIR

Oily hair can appear greasy and may cling to the scalp. Just as underactive sebaceous glands in the scalp lead to dry hair, oil glands that secrete too much oil cause oily hair. Other contributing factors may include a diet high in fats, refined carbohydrates, and sugar; the use of hair conditioners or hair styling gels; hormonal imbalances; and too-infrequent washing.

Oily hair often responds to dietary changes. If you have oily hair, reduce your fat intake and eliminate all fried foods, refined carbohydrates, and sugar from your diet. Essential oils such as bergamot, cedarwood, clary sage, cypress, juniper, lavender, lemon, patchouli, pine, rosemary, tea tree, thyme, and ylang ylang can help reduce oiliness. Wash your hair every day with Oily Hair Shampoo.

❧ Oily Hair Shampoo

> 4 ounces unscented shampoo for oily hair
> 6 drops lemon oil
> 4 drops bergamot oil
> 4 drops cedarwood oil
> 4 drops rosemary oil
> 2 drops ylang ylang oil

Add the essential oils to the unscented shampoo. Turn the bottle of shampoo upside down a few times or roll it between your hands for a few minutes to blend. Use this shampoo daily.

DANDRUFF

Dandruff can appear on both dry and oily scalps. It results from abnormal activity of the sebaceous, or oil-secreting, glands in the scalp. This causes fine white scales to form. These flakes of dead skin accumulate on the scalp and then fall off onto clothing.

People who have dandruff often eat diets high in saturated fats and fried foods. Infrequent shampooing can contribute to the condition as well. Most commercial dandruff shampoos contain harsh chemicals and coal tar. These ingredients may control dandruff but usually do not eliminate the underlying problem.

Essential oils that fight dandruff include cedarwood, clary sage, cypress, lemon, patchouli, pine, rosemary, and tea tree. Dandruff Scalp Treatment is useful because it helps to regulate the secretions of the sebaceous glands, thereby minimizing scalp problems. Use Dandruff-Diminishing Shampoo daily.

❧ Dandruff Scalp Treatment

> 2 ounces jojoba oil
> 8 drops tea tree oil
> 6 drops rosemary oil
> 4 drops cedarwood oil
> 3 drops pine oil

Place the jojoba oil in a clean container, add the essential oils, and blend. Massage some of the mixture into your clean scalp and leave it on for thirty minutes or overnight, then shampoo with Dandruff-Diminishing Shampoo. Repeat the treatment several times a week, as needed.

❧ Dandruff-Diminishing Shampoo

> 8 ounces unscented shampoo
> 10 drops tea tree oil
> 8 drops cedarwood oil
> 6 drops pine oil
> 6 drops rosemary oil
> 4 drops clary sage oil
> 4 drops lemon oil

Add the oils to the unscented shampoo and blend thoroughly. Use this shampoo daily.

HAIR LOSS

Many people—both men and women—worry about hair loss. A daily loss of about 150 to 200 strands of hair is normal. If you lose more hair than that, you probably will not grow enough new hair to replace it and the loss will become noticeable.

Hair loss can occur in patches or over the entire scalp or body. Most cases of hair loss, or *alopecia*, are probably related to aging, heredity, and hormones. In addition, sebum, or oil secretions, can build up on the scalp, plug the hair follicles, and interfere with new hair growth. Other causes of hair loss include chemotherapy or radiation treatments, diabetes, certain drugs, hypothyroidism, impaired circulation, poor diet, nutritional deficiencies, pregnancy, skin disorders such as psoriasis and seborrhea, and stress.

Hair loss is a problem that may not be reversible, but you can often prevent further loss of hair by reducing some of the contributing factors. Avoid stress as much as possible. Avoid using hair styling products on your hair. These can clog hair follicles and that can discourage new hair growth. Massage Scalp-Stimulating Hair-Growth Formula into your scalp daily. Keep your hair and scalp clean by shampooing with Hair-Growth Shampoo every day.

❧ Scalp-Stimulating Hair-Growth Formula

1 ounce jojoba oil
4 drops clary sage oil
4 drops rosemary oil
2 drops cedarwood oil
2 drops ylang ylang oil

Place the jojoba oil in a clean container and add the essential oils. Gently turn the container upside down several times or roll it between your hands for a few minutes to blend. Massage some of the mixture into your scalp daily. Leave it on for thirty minutes or overnight, then shampoo with Hair-Growth Shampoo.

❧ Hair-Growth Shampoo

8 ounces unscented shampoo
12 drops rosemary oil
10 drops clary sage oil
8 drops cedarwood oil
6 drops ylang ylang oil

Add the rosemary, clary sage, cedarwood, and ylang ylang oils to the unscented shampoo and blend. Use this shampoo daily.

Headache

Headaches can take the form of dull throbbing or sharp, stabbing pain, on one or both sides of the head. Sometimes the pain localizes in the temple area or behind the eyes. Blurred vision, pressure in the sinus cavities, and sensitivity to light can accompany headaches.

Most headaches result from tension. Tension produces muscle spasms in the head, neck, scalp, and shoulders that can interfere with circulation to the head. Feelings such as aggression, anxiety, anger, depression, fear, guilt, humiliation, rage, and rejection can cause or contribute to tension headaches, especially when these feelings are repressed. Headaches often increase irritability and can lead to insomnia.

Headaches may be related to any of a number of other health problems, including anemia, arthritis, brain disorders, candidiasis, constipation, digestive difficulties, eyestrain, fatigue, high blood pressure, head injury, low blood pressure, low blood sugar, nutritional imbalances, premenstrual syndrome (PMS), poor circulation, poor posture, sinusitis, spinal misalignment, stress, sun exposure, or throat, nose, or eye disorders. They can also be triggered by certain foods and food additives, especially alcohol, caffeine, chocolate, dairy products, monosodium glutamate (MSG), refined and processed foods, sugar, and yeast, as well as by certain drugs or by exposure to cigarette smoke, certain smells, synthetic fragrances, chemicals, or environmental pollutants. Even just being in a poorly ventilated room for a period of time may cause a headache in some people.

Migraine is a type of headache that occurs when the arteries leading to the head bulge with excess blood, exerting pressure against the brain and the surrounding tissue. An abnormal flow of blood to the brain results, alternately constricting and dilating blood vessels, first restricting the brain's blood supply and then flooding the brain with blood. Pressure within the blood vessels can irritate nerve endings and contribute to the pain. The pain of a migraine may last for several hours or several days. While tension headaches are often relieved by a night's sleep, this is not necessarily the case with migraines.

Migraines cause severe pain, sometimes beginning with a throbbing pain on one or both sides of the head. Some migraine sufferers experience visual auras—flashes of lights, hallucinatory-type effects, or holes in the field of vision—prior to the onset of a migraine. Nausea and vomiting, as well as stiffness and aches in the neck, often accompany migraines. Migraines can cause painful sensitivity to bright lights or sunlight.

Migraines are frequently related to food and environmental allergies. Foods that may trigger migraines include chicken, chocolate, corn, dairy products, fried foods, fruits, grains, red meat, nuts, potatoes, soy products, sugar, tomatoes, and yeast. Alcohol (especially red wines), caffeine, salt, monosodium glutamate (MSG), preservatives, and other food additives are common culprits as well. Migraines may also be brought on by changes in humidity, chemical sensitivities, poor circulation, constipation, a disturbance in one's sleep pattern, emotional upset, hormonal fluctuations (many women say that their migraines are related to menopause or certain phases of the menstrual cycle), liver malfunction, nutritional imbalances, poor diet, sun exposure, temporomandibular joint (TMJ) dysfunction, and stress. Self-inflicted stress, like that which comes from striving to be perfect, or feelings of anger, anxiety, depression, fear, frustration, or hatred can lead to migraines.

HELPFUL TREATMENTS

Because headaches can be a symptom of an underlying illness, if you get frequent or unusually severe headaches, you should consult with your health care practitioner to rule out this possibility. In most cases, however, a headache—whether a tension headache or a migraine—indicates that your body needs to slow down and rest, or stop whatever you're doing at the moment. Painkillers may relieve the pain, but they do nothing to eliminate the cause of a headache; they may even mask symptoms that are your body's cry for changes in your behavior or lifestyle.

Because low blood sugar can provoke headaches, make sure that you eat regular, nutritious meals. You may wish to consult a nutritionist for advice about your diet and possible vitamin deficiencies. Focus on eating complex carbohydrates such as fresh vegetables and whole grains, and eliminate the most common dietary culprits—alcohol, artificial sweeteners, caffeine, dairy products (especially cheese), chicken, chocolate, fruits, processed meats, sugar, vinegar, and yeast products—as well as any other foods you suspect. After several weeks, if you find that your headaches have diminished, you can—slowly, and one at a time—reintroduce the banished foods back into your diet. If your headaches return, you will then know which food or foods are causing the problem. If your headaches or migraines occur when you are hungry, or when you haven't eaten for a while, have your doctor check for hypoglycemia. You may need to eat small meals throughout the day to stabilize your blood sugar.

If you suspect that your spine may be misaligned and contributing to your headaches, visit a chiropractor for an evaluation. Biofeedback, deep breathing techniques, meditation, relaxation, visualization, and yoga are other methods that are effective for many people, especially migraine sufferers. Avoid exposure to cigarette smoke, cleaning compounds, paints, and other chemicals, as well as anything with a synthetic fragrance or perfume.

Aromatherapy can help you beat—and avoid—headaches by relaxing you physically and emotionally and by reducing stress (see STRESS). It can also help with some of the underlying conditions that can lead to headaches, such as arthritis, candidiasis, constipation, digestive problems, fatigue, high or low blood pressure, premenstrual syndrome, poor circulation, and sinusitis (see ARTHRITIS; CANDIDIASIS; CIRCULATION, POOR; CONSTIPATION; FATIGUE; HIGH BLOOD PRESSURE; INDIGESTION; LOW BLOOD PRESSURE; PREMENSTRUAL SYNDROME; and/or SINUSITIS).

Essential oils such as basil, chamomile, clary sage, coriander, eucalyptus, ginger, helichrysum, lavender, lemon, marjoram, peppermint, rose, rosemary, rosewood, and thyme are helpful in preventing or easing headache pain. Apply Peppermint Pain Reliever to your forehead, neck, and shoulders whenever you feel a tension headache or a migraine coming on; it will help to reduce or eliminate the pain. Bathe in Headache Relief Bath to relax your muscles and reduce muscular tension. Then apply an Icy Migraine Compress to your head to prevent a headache from progressing. You can repeat this regimen as necessary. To relieve muscular tension, rub Tension-Easing Massage Oil into your shoulders and neck. Apply a Warm Compress for Muscular Pain to your neck and shoulders. If at all possible, rest in bed until your symptoms subside.

AROMATHERAPY BLENDS

The aromatherapy blends below are essential oil formulas you can prepare at home. For a more detailed explanation of how to put together and use these blends, see BATHS; COMPRESSES; and/or MASSAGE in Part Four. For a quick review of general guidelines for using essential oils, see page 91.

❧ Peppermint Pain Reliever

½ ounce carrier oil
12 drops peppermint oil

In a clean container, add the peppermint oil to the carrier oil and blend. At the first sign of a headache, apply the blend to the painful site, avoiding the eye area. Repeat the treatment as necessary.

❧ Headache Relief Bath

3 drops chamomile oil
3 drops lavender oil
2 drops marjoram oil
2 drops thyme oil
1 drop coriander oil

Disperse the oils in a bathtub filled with warm water. Soak in the bath for twenty to thirty minutes. Repeat as necessary.

❧ Icy Migraine Compress

1 quart ice-cold water
2 drops peppermint oil
1 drop ginger oil
1 drop marjoram oil

Pour the water into a two-quart glass bowl and add the essential oils. Soak a clean cloth in the water and apply it to your head, forehead, or neck at the first sign of a developing migraine. Avoid letting the compress come into contact with your eyes. You can apply an ice pack over the compress to keep it from getting warm.

🐦 Tension-Easing Massage Oil

1 ounce carrier oil
4 drops marjoram oil
3 drops chamomile oil
3 drops lavender oil
2 drops coriander oil
2 drops helichrysum oil
1 drop basil oil
1 drop ginger oil

Place the carrier oil in a clean container and add the essential oils. Gently turn the container upside down several times or roll it between your hands for a few minutes to blend all the ingredients together. Massage the mixture over your neck and shoulders to relieve muscular tension. Repeat as necessary.

🐦 Warm Compress for Muscular Pain

1 quart hot water
2 drops marjoram oil
1 drop ginger oil
1 drop peppermint oil
1 drop rosemary oil

Pour the water into a two-quart glass bowl and disperse the oils in the water. Soak a clean cloth in the water and apply it to your neck and shoulders as needed.

Heartburn

See INDIGESTION.

Hemorrhoids

One quarter of all adults suffer from hemorrhoids at some time in their lives. Hemorrhoids are dilated, stretched, or swollen veins that appear in or around the rectal opening. There may be blood clots within the veins, and sometimes hemorrhoids protrude out of the rectum. They may itch, tear, bleed, and cause extreme pain. In some cases, blood may be visible on the surface of the stools or on toilet paper.

Poor circulation and weakness of the blood vessels contribute to hemorrhoids. Straining during bowel movements can aggravate hemorrhoids or lead to their development. Other contributing factors include allergies, recurrent constipation, lack of exercise, lifting heavy objects, obesity, poor nutrition, and standing or sitting for long periods of time. Pregnant women often get hemorrhoids as a result of the added pressure and weight on their pelvic veins.

HELPFUL TREATMENTS

A high-fiber diet reduces constipation and therefore straining during elimination. Eating more fresh vegetables, whole grains, fruits, and legumes will promote normal bowel movements. Make sure to drink plenty of pure water as well. Regular exercise also helps; begin an exercise program to improve your circulation. As much as possible, avoid standing or sitting in one position for prolonged periods of time.

Aromatherapy can help ease the discomfort of hemorrhoids by improving circulation, soothing the pain, and promoting the regeneration and healing of tissue. Essential oils that are effective in treating hemorrhoids include coriander, cypress, juniper, myrrh, and tea tree. Tea tree oil, applied topically or used in suppositories, offers relief in many instances.

A daily Hemorrhoid Sitz Bath can decrease discomfort, stimulate circulation, and promote healing. Apply Hemorrhoid Massage Oil throughout the day, as needed.

AROMATHERAPY BLENDS

The aromatherapy blends below are essential oil formulas you can prepare at home. For a more detailed explanation of how to put together and use these blends, see MASSAGE and/or SITZ BATHS in Part Four. For a quick review of general guidelines for using essential oils, see page 91.

❧ Hemorrhoid Sitz Bath

2 drops cypress oil
2 drops juniper oil

Add the cypress and juniper oils to a shallow tub filled with warm water. Sit hip-deep in the bath for twenty minutes.

❧ Hemorrhoid Massage Oil

1 ounce jojoba oil
4 drops cypress oil
4 drops tea tree oil
3 drops coriander oil
3 drops myrrh oil

Place the jojoba oil in a clean container, add the essential oils, and gently turn the container upside down several times or roll it between your hands to blend. Apply the oil externally, as needed.

Herpes Virus

The herpes viruses are a group of viruses that cause skin eruptions or blisters. Herpes simplex virus 1 (HSV1) causes cold sores. It is spread by direct contact with the fluids of a cold sore, fever blister, or skin eruption of someone who carries the virus. Herpes simplex 2 (HSV2) affects the genitals and is usually transmitted sexually. Other herpes viruses are responsible for chickenpox, shingles, and mononucleosis, among other illnesses. This section addresses oral and genital herpes, the problems caused by HSV1 and HSV2.

Once an individual is infected with herpes, the virus remains in the body, usually lying dormant until some other factor—emotional upset, exposure to the sun, an infection, poor diet, stress, or weakened immunity—triggers an outbreak. When this happens, small, painful, fluid-filled blisters form on and around the mouth or in the genital area within a few hours. Several days later, the blisters break, pus seeps out, and ulcers remain. It can take two to three weeks for them to heal completely. Certain foods, such as alcohol, citrus fruits and juices, caffeine, coffee, processed food, refined carbohydrates, and sugar, can aggravate symptoms.

HELPFUL TREATMENTS

Although there is no cure for herpes, you can take precautions to prevent outbreaks. Herpes viruses thrive on low levels of the amino acid lysine and high levels of the amino acid arginine. If you have herpes, you should therefore limit your consumption of foods with a high arginine content. These include chicken, chocolate, corn (including popcorn), rice, carob, oats, dairy products, nuts, seeds, and whole-wheat products. When lysine levels exceed those of arginine, lysine suppresses the herpes virus. Foods high in lysine include eggs, fish, lima beans, potatoes, red meat, soy products, and yeast. Lysine is also available in supplement form. The B-complex vitamins, vitamins C and E, beta-carotene, and zinc supplements may also help control herpes. Boosting immunity will discourage the recurrence of herpes outbreaks.

Aromatherapy helps with herpes by improving immunity, relieving stress, and easing the pain and discomfort. Immediate treatment with essential oils such as bergamot, clary sage, eucalyptus, geranium, lavender, lemon, myrrh, rose, and tea tree will often reduce the severity and the length of an outbreak. At first signs of an oral herpes outbreak, apply a Cold Sore Compress frequently. Follow this with an application of Healing Oil for Herpes. Repeat these treatments regularly during the outbreak. For genital herpes, take a Herpes Sitz Bath two or three times a day as soon as symptoms first appear. Follow with a Cold Sore Compress and Healing Oil for Herpes. Repeat this regimen as often as necessary.

AROMATHERAPY BLENDS

The aromatherapy blends below are essential oil formulas you can prepare at home. For a more detailed explanation of how to put together and use these blends, see COMPRESSES; MASSAGE; and/or SITZ BATHS in Part Four. For a quick review of general guidelines for using essential oils, see page 91.

❧ Cold Sore Compress

1 pint (16 ounces) cold or ice water
2 drops lemon oil
2 drops tea tree oil
1 drop bergamot oil

Pour the water into a one-quart glass bowl, add the essential oils, and blend. Soak a clean cloth in the water to make a compress; apply the compress to the affected area. Repeat frequently.

❧ Healing Oil for Herpes

1 ounce jojoba oil
6 drops bergamot oil
4 drops myrrh oil
3 drops tea tree oil
2 drops clary sage oil

Mix all the ingredients togther in a clean container. Apply the oil to the affected area after treatment with the Cold Sore Compress.

Note: Bergamot oil increases sensitivity to the sun, increasing the possibility of sunburn and uneven darkening of the skin. Omit it from the formula if your skin will be exposed to sunlight.

❧ Herpes Sitz Bath

3 drops bergamot oil
3 drops tea tree oil
2 drops eucalyptus oil
2 drops geranium oil

Disperse the oils in a shallow tub filled with warm water. Sit hip-deep in the water for twenty minutes. Repeat as necessary.

High Blood Pressure

As blood courses through the arteries, it exerts pressure against the walls of the blood vessels. When the blood encounters greater than normal difficulty flowing through the arteries, the pressure of the blood against the walls of the blood vessels rises. This condition is called high blood pressure, or hypertension. It commonly results when fatty deposits, called plaque, form inside the walls of blood vessels, thickening the arterial walls and making them relatively rigid. While it is normal for blood pressure to rise in response to stress or physical exertion and then fall again when the stressful situation is over or exercise ends, a person with hypertension will consistently show an elevated blood pressure (usually 140/90 or higher), even when at rest.

Alcohol, drugs, obesity, a lack of exercise, too much sodium in the diet, oral contraceptives, smoking, stress, and the regular consumption of stimulants such as coffee and tea can cause or contribute to high blood pressure. Heredity may also be a factor.

High blood pressure puts extra strain on the heart, forcing it to work harder to pump blood throughout the body. Over time, it can damage other internal organs, notably the kidneys and blood vessels. It can lead to heart attacks, kidney problems, and strokes.

HELPFUL TREATMENTS

In many cases, a low- or no-sodium, low-fat, caffeine-free, and alcohol-free diet can reduce blood pressure. Losing weight is often helpful as well. A diet that focuses on fresh fruits and vegetables and whole grains, which are high in nutrients and fiber, is recommended. Exercise and stress-reduction techniques can further reduce blood pressure. Many people with high blood pressure have difficulty relaxing. Because of the serious dangers associated with high blood pressure, if your blood pressure does not respond to dietary and lifestyle changes, you should consult a medical professional for treatment.

Aromatherapy massages and baths can help by calming and relaxing you. Certain essential oils—clary sage, lavender, lemon, marjoram, and ylang ylang—may actually lower blood pressure. Studies in England indicate that a massage with these oils can lower blood pressure for several days following the massage. Take a Blood-Pressure-Reducing Bath every evening for its relaxing and calming benefits. Rub Hypertension Massage Oil over your body once or twice a day or have your massage therapist use it for massages. Disperse Diffuser Blend for Hypertension in your home or office or inhale it directly from the bottle during stressful situations.

AROMATHERAPY BLENDS

The aromatherapy blends below are essential oil formulas you can prepare at home. For a more detailed explanation of how to put together and use these blends, see BATHS; DIFFUSERS AND LAMPS; and/or MASSAGE in Part Four. For a quick review of general guidelines for using essential oils, see page 91.

❧ Blood-Pressure-Reducing Bath

4 drops ylang ylang oil
3 drops clary sage oil
2 drops marjoram oil

Add the oils to a bathtub filled with warm water and soak in the bath for twenty minutes.

❧ Hypertension Massage Oil

1 ounce carrier oil
4 drops lavender oil
4 drops ylang ylang oil
2 drops clary sage oil
2 drops marjoram oil
1 drop neroli oil

Place the carrier oil in a clean container and add the essential oils. Gently turn the container upside down several times or roll it between your hands for a few minutes to blend. Massage the oil onto your skin daily.

🐚 Diffuser Blend for Hypertension

10 drops clary sage oil
10 drops lavender oil
10 drops lemon oil
8 drops ylang ylang oil
4 drops marjoram oil

Drop the oils into a small glass bottle with an airtight cover and combine. Add some of the mixture to your diffuser or lamp bowl as necessary.

CAUTIONS

Certain essential oils can elevate blood pressure. These include hyssop, peppermint, pine, rosemary, sage, and thyme oils. If you suffer from high blood pressure, you should avoid using these essential oils.

Hyperactivity

Hyperactivity usually affects children, although adults may be hyperactive as well. Some signs of hyperactivity include persistent impatience, impulsiveness, an inability to sit still, a short attention span, aggressiveness, anger, clumsiness, emotional instability, failure to listen or follow directions, frequent frustration, headaches, lack of motor coordination, learning disabilities, lying, poor concentration, self-destructive behavior, sleep disturbances, stomach pains, and tantrums.

The exact cause or causes of hyperactivity are unknown, but many cases appear to be related to one or more of the following: reactions to food additives, especially sugar, salicylates, caffeine, artificial colors and flavorings, artificial sweeteners, nitrates, and preservatives, particularly BHA and BHT; exposure to environmental pollutants; food allergies and sensitivities, especially to foods with phosphates or with high phosphorous contents, such as meats, fats, and carbonated beverages; heavy metal poisoning from cadmium, copper, lead, manganese, or mercury; hyperthyroidism; hypoglycemia; a poor diet, especially one that is deficient in protein; nutritional deficiencies; and vision or hearing loss. Heredity may play a role as well. A child may become hyperactive if his or her mother smoked or used alcohol or drugs during pregnancy, if there was prenatal trauma, or if the child was deprived of oxygen at birth.

HELPFUL TREATMENTS

Diet can often successfully treat hyperactivity; dietary changes frequently bring about an immediate improvement. A person who is hyperactive should avoid all of the foods listed above that trigger hyperactivity. Other products to avoid include antacids, bacon, candy, catsup, chocolate, cough drops and throat lozenges, ham, hot dogs, ice cream, luncheon meats, milk, margarine, perfume, processed foods, salt, soft drinks, soy sauce, cider vinegar, and *anything* with artificial coloring, flavoring, or sweeteners. Read labels carefully. Some butter, cheeses, teas, and toothpastes, among other things, may contain these additives. Eliminating salicylates is a bit more difficult because these occur naturally in certain foods. Natural sources of salicylates include almonds, apples, apricots, berries, cherries, cucumbers, currants, oranges, peaches, plums, prunes, and tomatoes.

Aromatherapy can help calm and relax hyperactive individuals with such essential oils as basil, benzoin, cedarwood, chamomile, coriander, fennel, frankincense, lavender, marjoram, myrrh, neroli, rose, rosewood, sandalwood, vetiver, and ylang ylang. Disperse Diffuser Blend for Hyperactivity throughout the house or in the hyperactive individual's room or office. A daily bath in Relaxing Bath Blend can quickly calm down a hyperactive person, as will applying Calming Skin Oil. Use Children's Bath Blend and Children's Skin Blend for an infant or small child who is hyperactive.

AROMATHERAPY BLENDS

The aromatherapy blends below are essential oil formulas you can prepare at home. For a more detailed explanation of how to put together and use these blends, see BATHS; DIFFUSERS; and/or MASSAGE in Part Four. For a quick review of general guidelines for using essential oils, see page 91.

❧ Diffuser Blend for Hyperactivity

    25 drops lavender oil
    20 drops chamomile oil
    10 drops rosewood oil
    10 drops sandalwood oil
    8 drops cedarwood oil
    6 drops ylang ylang oil
    4 drops coriander oil

Blend all the oils together in a clean glass container. Use the mixture in your diffuser or lamp as necessary.

❧ Relaxing Bath Blend

    3 drops lavender oil
    2 drops basil oil
    2 drops marjoram oil
    1 drop fennel oil
    1 drop vetiver oil

Disperse the oils in a bathtub filled with warm water. Soak in the bath for ten to twenty minutes, or as long as possible. Repeat as necessary.

❧ Calming Skin Oil

    2 ounces carrier oil
    6 drops lavender oil
    4 drops chamomile oil
    4 drops rosewood oil
    2 drops benzoin resin
    2 drops neroli oil
    1 drop rose oil
    1 drop ylang ylang oil

Place the carrier oil in a clean container and add the essential oils. Gently turn the container upside down several times or roll it between your hands for a few minutes to blend. Massage the oil into your skin once or more daily, as needed.

❧ Children's Bath Blend

    1 drop chamomile oil
    1 drop lavender oil

Add the chamomile and lavender oils to a bathtub filled with warm water. Have the child soak in the bath for five to fifteen minutes (or for as long as you can persuade him or her to stay in the tub). Repeat as necessary.

❧ Children's Skin Blend

    1 ounce carrier oil
    2 drops chamomile oil
    2 drops lavender oil

In a clean container, add the chamomile and lavender oils to the carrier oil and blend. Massage the mixture onto the child's skin once or more daily as needed.

Immune System Disorders

See WEAKENED IMMUNE SYSTEM.

Impotence

A man who cannot achieve or keep an erection, or who cannot complete the sexual act, is said to be impotent. Impotence may be an occasional, frequent, or permanent problem. Physical causes can include overall poor health, anatomical defects, diabetes, drug abuse, lower back problems, liver or kidney disorders, nervous system injury or disorders, and the use of alcohol, tobacco, and certain drugs, especially heart and blood pressure medications, antihistamines, and decongestants. However, most cases of impotence are related to psychological or emotional factors such as anxiety, depression, and relationship problems.

HELPFUL TREATMENTS

If you suffer from recurring impotence, you should visit your health care provider to rule out any underlying medical problems or illness. If you suspect that stress is at the root of the problem, begin a stress management program (see STRESS). If emotional or relationship problems are part of the problem, it may be helpful to seek individual or joint counselling.

Aromatherapy can help you overcome impotence by reducing stress and creating a sensual atmosphere for lovemaking. Certain essential oils have aphrodisiac properties and can stir sexual desire (see the recommendations for enhancing sexual desire on pages 139–140). Benzoin, clary sage, coriander, ginger, jasmine, rose, rosemary, rosewood, sandalwood, and ylang ylang all have reportedly helped many men overcome impotence. In addition, benzoin may help prevent premature ejaculation.

Bathe in Sexuality Bath—with your partner if possible. Afterwards, massage each other with Sexuality Massage Oil. Disperse Sexuality Diffuser Blend throughout your bedroom or home.

AROMATHERAPY BLENDS

The aromatherapy blends below are essential oil formulas you can prepare at home. For a more detailed explanation of how to put together and use these blends, see BATHS; DIFFUSERS AND LAMPS; and/or MASSAGE in Part Four. For a quick review of general guidelines for using essential oils, see page 91.

❧ Sexuality Bath

4 drops sandalwood oil
3 drops clary sage oil
2 drops coriander oil
2 drops ylang ylang oil

Add the essential oils to a bathtub filled with warm water. Soak in the bath (preferably with your partner) for fifteen to twenty minutes.

❧ Sexuality Massage Oil

2 ounces carrier oil
10 drops sandalwood oil
6 drops clary sage oil

4 drops ylang ylang oil

3 drops coriander oil

3 drops rosewood oil

2 drops benzoin resin

1 drop ginger oil

1 drop jasmine absolute or enfleurage

1 drop rose oil

Place the carrier oil in a clean container and add the essential oils. Gently turn the container upside down several times or roll it between your hands for a few minutes to blend. Use the mixture to massage your partner's body; then have your partner massage you.

❧ Sexuality Diffuser Blend

20 drops sandalwood oil

12 drops clary sage oil

8 drops ylang ylang oil

6 drops coriander oil

4 drops ginger oil

Combine all the ingredients in a small glass bottle with an airtight cover. Add some of the blend to your diffuser or lamp bowl as desired.

Indigestion

Indigestion can take the form of bloating, constipation, diarrhea, gas, heartburn, queasiness, or nausea. Poor digestion may be a result of the aging process, anxiety, eating too quickly, emotional upset or stress, improper food combinations, food allergies, lack of digestive enzymes, low fiber intake, nutritional deficiencies, poor diet, failure to chew food thoroughly, overeating, overweight, pregnancy, eating spicy or hot foods, or stress. When the body's ability to digest food decreases, tiny particles of partially digested food can enter the bloodstream through the intestinal mucosa. This can cause autoimmune disorders, food allergies, joint problems, and abdominal aches and pains.

Gas, or flatulence, usually results from digestive enzyme deficiencies, poor diet, or poor eating habits such as eating too quickly, overeating, or swallowing foods without chewing them thoroughly. In addition, certain foods—notably legumes and carbonated beverages—and certain combinations of foods commonly cause gas.

Gastritis is an inflammation of the stomach or stomach lining that typically causes a burning sensation in the stomach, nausea, or vomiting. It is usually related to the consumption of a specific irritant such as alcohol, caffeine, tobacco, or certain drugs.

Heartburn is a tight, burning feeling in the middle of chest or the upper abdominal area that extends upward through the esophagus and causes unpleasant belching, bloating, or gas. Heartburn can be a result of anxiety, bacterial infection, eating too rapidly, gastritis, an imbalance of stomach acids, improper food combinations, nervousness, poor diet, stress, or ulcers. Heartburn can also result if the lining of the stomach becomes unable to produce the mucus that normally protects it from attack by stomach acid.

Nausea is a queasy, uneasy feeling and may result in vomiting. It often occurs after eating spoiled foods or foods that disagree with you. Anxiety, morning sickness, motion sickness, nervousness, and stress can also cause nausea.

HELPFUL TREATMENTS

Use a food diary to keep track of what you eat and how you feel afterwards. This can help you see if certain foods, or combinations of foods, are causing your digestive distress. Always chew your food thoroughly. Certain food combinations can cause digestive difficulties. Avoid eating proteins with carbohydrates, fruits, sugars, or starches. Eat sweet fruits, such as bananas, dates, raisins, and dried fruits, either by themselves or in combination with the sub-acid fruits—grapes, papayas, mangoes, and fruits with cores or pits, such as apples, peaches, and pears. Eat acid fruits, including pineapples, citrus fruits, tomatoes, and most berries, either by themselves or in combination with sub-acid fruits; never combine them with sweet fruits. Melons should always be eaten by themselves. You may wish to check with a nutritionist to determine whether you have any nutritional deficiencies and ask for suggestions to improve your diet.

Digestive enzymes, available in health food stores, may be helpful. If feelings of anxiety, nervousness, or stress are interfering with your digestion, find ways to reduce them. Many culinary herbs, such as basil, black pepper, cardamom, coriander, cumin, fennel, ginger, marjoram, parsley, rosemary, sage, tarragon, and thyme, promote better digestion. You can often enhance both your dining pleasure and your digestion by seasoning your favorite dishes with these herbs.

Essential oils can help by aiding the digestive process, relieving gas, easing heartburn, and soothing nausea. Essential oils that improve digestion include basil, bergamot, black pepper, chamomile, clary sage, coriander, fennel, frankincense, ginger, helichrysum, lemon, marjoram, neroli, palmarosa, peppermint, and thyme. Oils that relieve gas include basil, benzoin, black pepper, clary sage, coriander, fennel, ginger, marjoram, myrrh, peppermint, rosemary, and thyme. For heartburn, use black pepper, chamomile, coriander, fennel, ginger, lemon, marjoram, and/or peppermint oils. Sandalwood and thyme oils are specifics for gastritis; basil, black pepper, coriander, fennel, ginger, peppermint, rose, rosewood, and sandalwood oils soothe nausea.

For any digestive difficulty, use All-Purpose Digest-Aid Oil to massage your abdomen twice a day.

AROMATHERAPY BLENDS

The aromatherapy blend below is an essential oil formula you can prepare at home. For a more detailed explanation of how to put together and use this blend, see MASSAGE in Part Four. For a quick review of general guidelines for using essential oils, see page 91.

❧ All-Purpose Digest-Aid Oil

    1 ounce carrier oil
    4 drops basil oil
    3 drops rosemary oil
    3 drops thyme oil
    2 drops coriander oil
    1 drop ginger oil
    1 drop peppermint oil

Place the carrier oil in a clean container and add the essential oils. Gently turn the container upside down several times or roll it between your hands for a few minutes to blend the ingredients together. Rub the mixture over your entire abdominal area twice daily or as needed.

Insect Bites

Most encounters with insects are nothing more than a nuisance. However, the bites and stings of many insects can cause pain, itching, redness, swelling, and soreness within a localized area. Allergic reactions can involve the entire body and may cause headache and fever. Certain insect bites bring with them the possibility of infection.

HELPFUL TREATMENTS

Always cleanse insect bites thoroughly to prevent infection and apply Insect Repellent and Bite Oil immediately. Repeat as necessary. For stings, remove the stinger by gently scraping rather than by pulling it out. Apply a cold compress or ice to the area to reduce itching and swelling, followed by Insect Repellent and Bite Oil. This oil is all-purpose and both repels insects and relieves the itching and swelling of insect bites. Apply the oil several times daily until the discomfort subsides. Aloe vera gel also can soothe bites. To prevent scarring, resist the urge to stratch insect bites.

Using an insect repellent can help you avoid the discomfort of insect bites and stings and avert allergic reactions. Aromatherapy is a safe, natural way to ward off the attack of insects. Many essential oils, such as basil, bergamot, eucalyptus, fennel, lavender, patchouli, peppermint, pine, tea tree, thyme, and ylang ylang are useful in treating insect bites. They all possess repellent properties. Apply Insect Repellent and Bite Oil before you go outside to prevent insect bites.

AROMATHERAPY BLENDS

The aromatherapy blend below is an essential oil formula you can prepare at home. For a quick review of general guidelines for using essential oils, see page 91.

❧ Insect Repellent and Bite Oil

    1 ounce carrier oil
    4 drops bergamot oil
    4 drops pine oil
    4 drops tea tree oil
    3 drops eucalyptus oil
    2 drops patchouli oil
    1 drop peppermint oil

In a clean container, add the essential oils to the carrier oil and blend. Apply the oil to insect bites to help them heal. To repel insects, apply the oil to your skin before going outdoors.

Note: Bergamot oil increases sensitivity to the sun, increasing the possibility of sunburn and uneven darkening of the skin. Omit it from the formula if your skin will be exposed to sunlight.

Insomnia

Insomnia is the chronic inability to sleep. It may take the form of having difficulty falling asleep or having difficulty remaining asleep throughout the night. Common causes of insomnia include emotional upset, excitement, stress, and worry. Dietary or eating habits are also often involved, especially eating late at night, eating sweets or spicy or stimulating foods, eating a poor or high-sugar diet, eating poor combinations of foods, and overeating. Other possible causes of insomnia include asthma, indigestion, hypoglycemia, muscular aches and pains, the consumption of caffeine or certain drugs, exercising too close to bedtime, and nutritional deficiencies, especially a copper or iron deficiency.

HELPFUL TREATMENTS

If you suffer from insomnia, it is a good idea to see your health care professional to rule out or obtain treatment for any underlying health problems. Avoid caffeine. If you feel you must consume foods and beverages that contain caffeine, do so before noon. Avoid sugar and spicy or stimulating foods. Do your exercising early in the day; exercising before bedtime can invigorate you, preventing you from falling asleep.

Meditating or reading before bedtime helps many people fall asleep. Bathing in Dead Sea salts or mineral bath salts before bedtime relaxes muscles and promote calmness. Enhance your relaxation by playing soft music and drinking a cup of sleep-inducing herbal tea thirty minutes before bedtime. Catnip, chamomile, hops, skullcap, spearmint, and valerian root teas are good choices for this.

Aromatherapy can calm your nerves and help you sleep more soundly. Many essential oils—including basil, chamomile, coriander, lavender, marjoram, neroli, orange, sandalwood, thyme, vetiver, and ylang ylang—reduce stress and promote relaxation, making it easier to fall asleep.

Before bedtime, enjoy a leisurely bath in Bedtime Bath Blend. Put Good Night Diffuser Blend in your diffuser. Following your bath, massage your skin with Nighttime Massage Oil. Apply Sweet Slumber Personal Blend before bedtime. Spray your pillow and sheets with Sweet Dreams Pillow Spray.

AROMATHERAPY BLENDS

The aromatherapy blends below are essential oil formulas you can prepare at home. For a more detailed explanation of how to put together and use these blends, see AIR FRESHENERS; BATHS; DIFFUSERS AND LAMPS; MASSAGE; and/or PERSONAL FRAGRANCES AND PERFUMES in Part Four. For a quick review of general guidelines for using essential oils, see page 91.

🐦 Bedtime Bath Blend

½ to 1 cup Dead Sea or mineral bath salts
4 drops chamomile oil
2 drops marjoram oil
2 drops ylang ylang oil
1 drop basil oil

Add all the ingredients to a bathtub filled with warm water and disperse well. Soak in the bath for twenty minutes.

🐦 Good Night Diffuser Blend

25 drops lavender oil
10 drops orange oil
8 drops German chamomile oil
8 drops marjoram oil
6 drops ylang ylang oil

Add the oils to a clean glass bottle and gently turn the container upside down several times or roll it between your hands for a few minutes to combine. Add some of the blend to your diffuser or lamp bowl as necessary.

🐦 Nighttime Massage Oil

4 ounces carrier oil
10 drops lavender oil
8 drops sandalwood oil
7 drops ylang ylang oil
6 drops marjoram oil
5 drops chamomile oil
3 drops thyme oil
2 drops coriander oil
2 drops vetiver oil

Place the carrier oil in a clean container, add the essential oils, and blend. Massage the oil into your skin before bedtime as needed.

🐦 Sweet Slumber Personal Blend

⅛ ounce jojoba oil
6 drops sandalwood oil
2 drops neroli oil
2 drops ylang ylang oil
1 drop coriander oil
1 drop vetiver oil

Blend the oils together well in a clean container. Apply a few drops to your pulse points before bedtime.

❧ Sweet Dreams Pillow Spray

1 ounce distilled water
4 drops lavender oil
2 drops chamomile oil
2 drops orange oil
2 drops ylang ylang oil

Pour the water into a spray bottle, add the essential oils, and shake to blend. Spray the mixture on your pillow and sheets or in your room before bedtime. Shake before each use.

Jock Itch

Jock itch (known to doctors as *tinea cruris*) is the common name for a ringworm infection that appears on the groin, particularly in men. The fungal organism that causes it belongs to the same family as the fungus that causes athlete's foot. Like other fungi, it thrives in moist, dark, warm places.

Inflamed bumps appear on the upper inner thigh. As these bumps dry out, they turn into a scaly rash that causes painful and embarrassing itching. Friction between the legs further irritates the skin. Wearing tight pants or undershorts, particularly ones made from synthetic fabrics, can contribute to jock itch. The infection can be spread by contact with an infected towel, article of clothing, or athletic supporter, especially if these items are shared.

HELPFUL TREATMENTS

If you are suffering from a case of jock itch, be sure to keep the groin area clean and dry. Wash all clothing that comes into contact with the affected area after each wearing. Never share clothing or athletic supporters.

Essential oils such as cypress, lavender, myrrh, patchouli, and tea tree fight fungi and can help control jock itch. Take a Jock Itch Bath at the first signs of jock itch; repeat once or twice daily until the symptoms subside. Apply Jock Itch Oil to the affected area twice daily.

AROMATHERAPY BLENDS

The aromatherapy blends below are essential oil formulas you can prepare at home. For a more detailed explanation of how to put together and use these blends, see BATHS and/or MASSAGE in Part Four. For a quick review of general guidelines for using essential oils, see page 91.

❧ Jock Itch Bath

4 drops lavender oil
3 drops tea tree oil
2 drops cypress oil
1 drop myrrh oil

Add the essential oils to a bathtub filled with warm water. Soak in the bath for fifteen to twenty minutes. Repeat daily, as needed.

❧ Jock Itch Oil

1 ounce carrier oil
5 drops tea tree oil
3 drops lavender oil
2 drops patchouli oil
1 drop myrrh oil

Place the carrier oil in a clean container and add the essential oils. Gently turn the container upside down several times or roll it between your hands for a few minutes to blend. Apply the mixture to the affected area several times daily, as needed.

Low Blood Pressure

Low blood pressure, or *hypotension,* is a condition in which the blood does not pump through the blood vessels with as much force as normal. It is less common than high blood pressure and, unless severe, usually poses no threat to health. It can be an inconvenience, however. When the brain does not receive a steady, sufficient supply of blood, dizziness may result, especially upon rising. Sometimes fainting occurs. People with low blood pressure often feel cold and may tire easily. Low blood pressure can indicate inadequate function of the adrenal glands.

HELPFUL TREATMENTS

If you have low blood pressure, always move from a lying position to a sitting position, and from sitting to standing, slowly, to prevent dizziness. Pace yourself. Dress warmly to prevent chills. Regular exercise, massage, and skin brushing will also help by improving circulation.

Aromatherapy can help by raising blood pressure, stimulating circulation, preventing or minimizing dizziness, and helping to overcome fatigue. Black pepper, peppermint, rosemary, and thyme oils can elevate low blood pressure and stimulate circulation. Black pepper and peppermint oils also reduce the possibility of fainting. Coriander oil counteracts dizziness.

Before bathing, dry brush your skin to stimulate circulation (see SKIN BRUSHING in Part Four). Follow this with a Low Blood Pressure Bath daily. Afterwards, massage Low Blood Pressure Massage Oil onto your skin.

AROMATHERAPY BLENDS

The aromatherapy blends below are essential oil formulas you can prepare at home. For a more detailed explanation of how to put together and use these blends, see BATHS and/or MASSAGE in Part Four. For a quick review of general guidelines for using essential oils, see page 91.

❧ Low Blood Pressure Bath

4 drops rosemary oil
3 drops thyme oil
2 drops peppermint oil

Add the essential oils to a bathtub filled with warm water. Soak in the bath for fifteen to twenty minutes. Repeat daily.

❧ Low Blood Pressure Massage Oil

1 ounce carrier oil
6 drops rosemary oil
3 drops coriander oil
2 drops peppermint oil
1 drop black pepper oil

Place the carrier oil in a clean container and add the essential oils. Gently turn the container upside down several times or roll it between your hands for a few minutes to blend. Massage the oil over your skin daily.

CAUTIONS

Certain essential oils can depress blood pressure. These include clary sage, lavender, and ylang

ylang. If your blood pressure is already low, you should avoid using these oils.

Menopause-Related Problems

Menopause marks the "change of life" for women, with the gradual cessation of their menstrual cycles. Some women start this change in their middle to late thirties, but the majority of women usually begin during their forties or fifties. Although this transition should be gradual and smooth, many women experience much difficulty. Such symptoms as depression, heavy periods, hot flashes, insomnia, and irregular cycles can continue for several years. Other common complaints include bloating, circulatory problems, constipation, vaginal dryness, and varicose veins. The onset of menopause is also often related to the development of osteoporosis.

Many women say that hot flashes are the most troublesome side effect of menopause. Hot flashes happen when blood vessels erratically dilate and constrict. Blood flow increases, body temperature rises, and the heart pumps faster. Sweating usually accompanies hot flashes.

Along with the physical symptoms of menopause, many women experience a fear of growing old, feeling less feminine, or losing their looks. While it is natural to have these concerns, maintaining a bright, optimistic attitude can ease your apprehensions. To a large degree, menopause is what you make it; your expectations of what you will encounter will influence your experience. You can improve with age and enter this new phase of your life with joy and enthusiasm. Besides, there are benefits: You no longer have to worry about unplanned pregnancy; if you've had PMS or painful periods, or had to interrupt your normal activities because of menstrual difficulties, you no longer need to worry about these things, either. Most women welcome these changes.

HELPFUL TREATMENTS

A healthy diet, an active lifestyle, and time out for relaxation and stress reduction can make the transition smoother. Evening primrose oil and other essential fatty acid supplements provide additional relief for some women.

Aromatherapy can diminish many of the discomforts you may experience. Rose, a feminine and nurturing oil, restores confidence, comforts the emotions, and regulates the menstrual cycle. Chamomile oil calms both the body and mind. Clary sage, fennel, geranium, and lavender oils restore hormonal balance. Other essential oils that can help you through menopause are coriander, cypress, jasmine, lavender, orange, patchouli, and ylang ylang.

Pamper yourself with Menopause Balancing Bath as you relax and restore balance to your life. Keep cool with Cool Flash Spray or Cool Down Compresses. Massage Menopause Balancing Body Oil onto your skin every day to fight fluid retention, restore balance, and ease your transition. Dab on Femininity Personal Fragrance throughout the day and celebrate your femininity.

AROMATHERAPY BLENDS

The aromatherapy blends below are essential oil formulas you can prepare at home. For a more detailed explanation of how to put together and use these blends, see BATHS; COMPRESSES; MASSAGE; and/or PERSONAL FRAGRANCES AND PERFUMES in Part Four. For a quick review of general guidelines for using essential oils, see page 91.

❧ Menopause Balancing Bath

2 drops chamomile oil
2 drops clary sage oil
2 drops lavender oil
1 drop cypress oil
1 drop fennel oil
1 drop geranium oil

Disperse the essential oils in a bathtub filled with warm water. Soak in the bath for twenty to thirty minutes.

❧ Cool Flash Spray

8 ounces distilled water
4 drops clary sage oil
3 drops chamomile oil
3 drops geranium oil
2 drops cypress oil
1 drop peppermint oil

Pour the water into a spray bottle, add the essential oils, and shake to blend. Spritz yourself whenever you feel a hot flash coming. Refrigerate the spray for even greater effect. Shake well before each use.

❧ Cool-Down Compress Blend

9 drops clary sage oil
9 drops lavender oil
6 drops chamomile oil
6 drops geranium oil
4 drops cypress oil
4 drops patchouli oil
2 drops peppermint oil
1 quart cool water

Add the essential oils to a small glass bottle and blend. Add three drops of the essential oil blend to the water. Soak a clean cloth in the water and apply it to your face, forehead, chest, or other areas of your body to prevent or cool down hot flashes. If you wish, you can apply an ice pack over the compress to keep it cool. Do not let the compress come in contact with your eyes.

❧ Menopause Balancing Body Oil

2 ounces carrier oil
8 drops orange oil
6 drops cypress oil
4 drops geranium oil
3 drops coriander oil
2 drops fennel oil
2 drops patchouli oil

Place the carrier oil in a clean container and add the essential oils. Gently turn the container upside down several times or roll it between your hands for a few minutes to blend. Apply the mixture over your entire body, especially on bloated areas.

❧ Femininity Personal Fragrance

⅛ ounce jojoba oil
3 drops clary sage oil
3 drops lavender oil
2 drops German chamomile oil
2 drops geranium oil
2 drops ylang ylang oil
1 drop coriander oil
1 drop jasmine absolute or enfleurage
1 drop rose oil

In a clean container, add the essential oils to the jojoba oil and combine well. Wear on pulse points as a fragrance.

Menstrual Problems

For most young women, menstruation begins sometime between the ages of eleven and fifteen. Every twenty-one to thirty-five days during her reproductive years, a healthy woman's ovaries will release an egg. If the egg is not fertilized, the woman will shed the lining of her uterus about two weeks later. This shedding is known as menstruation. A woman's monthly menstrual flow normally lasts three to seven days; the entire menstrual cycle continues until menopause, which usually occurs during the forties or fifties.

Although menstruation itself should not necessarily be painful, as many as two thirds of menstruating women say that they experience some sort of difficulty or pain each month with their menstrual cycle, such as menstrual cramps or heavy or prolonged bleeding. Other common menstrual problems include scant, late, or irregular periods.

MENSTRUAL CRAMPS

Painful periods, or *dysmenorrhea*, commonly involve abdominal and back pain; sometimes diarrhea, headaches, nausea, nervousness, and vomiting accompany cramps as well. Medical researchers are not certain about the cause of cramping, but many believe that high levels of prostaglandins, which are hormones secreted by the uterine lining, may be involved. These hormones affect the smooth muscle of the uterus, causing an increase in uterine contractions. In addition, when the uterus swells and constricts in spasms, it restricts blood flow into the pelvic region and diminishes the supply of oxygen to those tissues. This can contribute to cramping.

If your periods are extremely painful, consult your physician about the possibility of an underlying health problem. Pay attention to diet, especially to adequate levels of dietary fiber and fluids, which promote regularity (constipation often exaggerates the pain of menstrual cramps). Avoid sugar, fats (especially cooked fats), and any other foods that cause gas or make the lower abdomen uncomfortable; avoid alcohol and caffeine. This is especially important the week before menstruation. A regular exercise program is also beneficial. However, during the time you are experiencing cramps, take it easy and avoid strenuous exercise. Instead, do yoga or light stretching or take a walk.

Aromatherapy can help minimize menstrual pain by easing cramps, regulating menstrual cycles, and soothing the emotions. It can also help relieve the symptoms of PMS (see PREMENSTRUAL SYNDROME). Basil, chamomile, clary sage, cypress, fennel, ginger, helichrysum, juniper, marjoram, peppermint, rose, and ylang ylang oils help relieve pain, reduce swelling, and soothe the muscle spasms of cramps.

Several days before the anticipated onset of your period, begin bathing daily in Cramp Relief Bath. Repeat as often as necessary to reduce cramps. Apply Menstrual Cramp Massage Oil to your abdomen and back starting several days prior to your period, before pain and cramping begin, if possible. To relieve cramping, apply a Cramp-Soothing Compress to your abdomen as needed.

The aromatherapy blends that follow are essential oil formulas you can prepare at home. For a more detailed explanation of how to put together and use these blends, see BATHS; COMPRESSES; and/or MASSAGE in Part Four. For a quick review of general guidelines for using essential oils, see page 91.

❧ Cramp Relief Bath

5 drops marjoram oil
2 drops ylang ylang oil
1 drop fennel oil
1 drop rose oil

Disperse the oils in a bathtub filled with warm water. Soak in the bath for twenty to thirty minutes. Repeat as necessary.

❧ Menstrual Cramp Massage Oil

2 ounces carrier oil
6 drops chamomile oil
6 drops marjoram oil
4 drops ylang ylang oil
3 drops cypress oil
3 drops helichrysum oil

Place the carrier oil in a clean container, add the essential oils, and blend by gently turning the container upside down several times or rolling it between your hands. Massage the oil over your abdomen and back as necessary.

❧ Cramp-Soothing Compress

1 quart cool water
2 drops marjoram oil
1 drop chamomile oil
1 drop helichrysum oil
1 drop juniper oil

Pour the water into a two-quart glass bowl and add the essential oils. Soak a clean cloth in the water and apply it to your abdomen. Repeat as necessary.

❧ Rose Cramp Relief Oil

½ ounce carrier oil
6 drops rose oil

Place the carrier oil in a clean container. Add the rose oil and blend. Beginning several days before the anticipated onset of your period, massage the oil over your abdomen and back. Repeat as necessary.

HEAVY MENSTRUAL FLOW

Some women experience heavy menstrual flow or unusually long menstrual periods (also known as *hypermenorrhea* or *menorrhagia*) and clotting each month with their menstrual cycles. If this occurs for prolonged periods of time, doctors consider it *dysfunctional uterine bleeding*. Hormonal imbalances and thyroid disorders are two health problems that can cause heavy menstrual flow. It may also be a sign of endometriosis, fibroid tumors, pelvic infection, or other female reproductive problems. Over time, heavy periods can lead to iron-deficiency anemia and other nutritional deficiencies.

If you have unusually heavy periods, it is wise to consult your health care professional to rule out the possibility of an underlying health problem and to check for nutritional deficiencies, especially anemia. Regular exercise may be helpful, but avoid strenuous exercise while you are having your period.

Aromatherapy can help regulate menstrual cycles and reduce menstrual flow. Essential oils that minimize heavy flow are cypress, frankincense, geranium, and rose. Bathe in Flow-Minimizing Bath twice a day, as necessary. Massage Flow-Minimizing Oil over your abdomen frequently. Apply a Cool Cypress Compress over your abdominal area as needed to reduce heavy flow. If your flow is heavy, you should avoid using basil, clary sage, coriander, jasmine, juniper, myrrh, and thyme oils during your period. These essential oils encourage menstrual flow.

The aromatherapy blends that follow are essential oil formulas you can prepare at home. For a more detailed explanation of how to put together and use these blends, see BATHS; COMPRESSES; and/or MAS-SAGE in Part Four. For a quick review of general guidelines for using essential oils, see page 91.

🐦 Flow-Minimizing Bath

4 drops cypress oil
2 drops frankincense oil
2 drops geranium oil
1 drop rose oil

Add the oils to a bathtub filled with warm water. Soak in the bath for twenty to thirty minutes.

🐦 Flow-Minimizing Oil

2 ounces carrier oil
10 drops cypress oil
10 drops geranium oil
4 drops frankincense oil

Place the carrier oil in a clean container, add the essential oils, and blend. Massage the oil frequently over your abdomen and back, beginning before the onset of your period if possible.

🐦 Cool Cypress Compress

Add 4 drops of cypress oil to a two-quart glass bowl containing one quart of cold water and mix well. Soak a clean cloth in the water and apply it to the abdominal area. Repeat as needed.

SCANT OR IRREGULAR MENSTRUAL PERIODS

Amenorrhea, or lack of menstruation not due to pregnancy or menopause, is usually caused by stress. It can also result from anorexia, depression, extreme physical exertion, hypoglycemia, low protein intake, nutritional deficiencies, poor diet, shock, travel and jet lag, sudden or extreme weight loss, and a very low ratio of body fat to muscle.

Aromatherapy can help encourage menstrual flow and regulate menstrual cycles. If your period is scant or late and you know you are not pregnant, basil, clary sage, coriander, jasmine, juniper, myrrh, and thyme oils can help start or increase your flow. Aromatherapy can also help by reducing stress and helping your cycle return to normal (see STRESS). Bathe daily in Period-Promoting Bath. Massage Flow-Inducing Oil into your abdomen and back.

To help normalize your menstrual cycles, use chamomile, clary sage, coriander, fennel, geranium, jasmine, juniper, rose, and/or vetiver oil. Massage Cycle-Regulating Oil onto your skin, particularly on your abdomen and back, daily. Once or twice a week, take a Cycle-Regulating Bath. Wear Harmonious Hormone Personal Perfume daily.

The aromatherapy blends that follow are essential oil formulas you can prepare at home. For a more detailed explanation of how to put together and use these blends, see BATHS; COMPRESSES; MASSAGE; and/or PERSONAL FRAGRANCES AND PERFUMES in Part Four. For a quick review of general guidelines for using essential oils, see page 91.

🐦 Period-Promoting Bath

3 drops clary sage oil
2 drops basil oil
2 drops coriander oil
2 drops thyme oil

Disperse the oils in a bathtub filled with warm water. Soak in the bath for twenty to thirty minutes.

🐦 Flow-Inducing Oil

2 ounces carrier oil
8 drops clary sage oil
6 drops myrrh oil

4 drops juniper oil
2 drops coriander oil
2 drops jasmine absolute or enfleurage

In a clean container, add the essential oils to the carrier oil and blend. Massage the oil over your abdomen and lower back several times daily.

❧ Cycle-Regulating Oil

2 ounces carrier oil
8 drops chamomile oil
6 drops clary sage oil
4 drops geranium oil
3 drops coriander oil
2 drops fennel oil
2 drops jasmine absolute or enfleurage
2 drops vetiver oil

Place the carrier oil in a clean container and add the essential oils. Gently turn the container upside down several times or roll it between your hands for a few minutes to blend. Massage the oil into your skin daily.

❧ Cycle-Regulating Bath

4 drops clary sage oil
4 drops geranium oil
2 drops fennel oil
2 drops vetiver oil

Add the essential oils to a bathtub filled with warm water. Soak in the bath for fifteen to twenty minutes.

❧ Harmonious Hormone Personal Perfume

⅛ ounce jojoba oil
4 drops clary sage oil
3 drops geranium oil

2 drops jasmine absolute or enfleurage
2 drops rose oil
2 drops vetiver oil
1 drop fennel oil

In a small bottle, add the essential oils to the jojoba oil and blend. Apply the mixture as a fragrance every day.

Migraine

See HEADACHE.

Morning Sickness

An estimated half of all pregnant women experience morning sickness in the beginning of pregnancy. Although women with morning sickness often experience nausea and vomiting after rising in the morning, the condition unfortunately is not limited to the morning hours and can come and go throughout the day.

Bouts of morning sickness can continue for two weeks to three months or longer. Changes in hormone levels and metabolism, along with the liver's inability to process increased amounts of hormones, account for most cases of morning sickness. Emotional factors can intensify episodes of nausea or vomiting.

HELPFUL TREATMENTS

Eat dry toast or crackers first thing in the morning—before arising, if possible—to prevent nausea and vomiting. During the day, eat smaller meals at more frequent intervals so that there is some food in your stomach at all times. Ginger can be effective in discouraging morning sickness. Drink ginger tea or take ginger capsules.

Aromatherapy can help alleviate the discomfort of morning sickness. Inhale ginger oil directly from the bottle or use Morning Sickness Inhalant Blend. Sandalwood oil can soothe the digestive tract as well as the nerves.

AROMATHERAPY BLENDS

The aromatherapy blend below is an essential oil formula you can prepare at home. For a more detailed explanation of how to put together and use this blend, see INHALANTS in Part Four. For a quick review of general guidelines for using essential oils, see page 91.

❧ Morning Sickness Inhalant Blend

    10 drops ginger oil
    8 drops sandalwood oil

Add the ginger and sandalwood oil to a small glass bottle with an airtight cover and blend. Inhale directly from the bottle as necessary to fight nausea and prevent vomiting.

CAUTIONS

Essential oils are highly concentrated and can have powerful effects. Some essential oils stimulate menstrual flow and/or uterine contractions, and are therefore *not* recommended for use during pregnancy. These include basil, cedarwood, clary sage, coriander, jasmine, juniper, marjoram, myrrh, peppermint, and thyme. You should consult with your health care practitioner before using any essential oils during pregnancy.

Motion Sickness

Motion sickness causes tremendous discomfort for some travellers. They may exhibit such symptoms as headaches, nausea, queasiness, and vomiting while driving, flying, sailing, or riding as a passenger. Other complaints include cold sweats, dizziness, loss of appetite, sleepiness, and even lack of coordination in extreme cases. Symptoms can persist for several hours after travel ends.

Motion sickness commonly occurs as a result of certain postures or movements that rotate a mechanism in the inner ear, called the vestibular apparatus, in different directions at the same time. The vestibular apparatus is responsible for maintaining equilibrium. These rotations disturb normal balance and also send messages to the brain that conflict with the nerve impulses sent by the other sensory organs.

HELPFUL TREATMENTS

If you tend to suffer from motion sickness, it is best to remain as still as possible when travelling, and in a position that minimizes movement. Avoid reading or observing passing scenery. Some people find that focusing their eyes on a point on the horizon is helpful; fresh air may also offer relief.

Motion sickness is easier to prevent than it is to cure. Take ginger capsules before embarking on a trip. There are a number of over-the-counter and prescription motion sickness remedies available, but they can cause side effects (especially drowsiness) and in many cases, ginger capsules are just as effective, if not more so.

Use aromatherapy to minimize your discomfort and prevent nausea. Chamomile, ginger, and peppermint are the best essential oils for treating motion sickness. Peppermint and ginger oils help prevent nausea and vomiting, while chamomile oil calms the nerves and soothes the stomach. Breathe in Motion Sickness Inhalant Blend, beginning at least one hour before travel. Continue inhaling it every fifteen to thirty minutes throughout your trip.

AROMATHERAPY BLENDS

The aromatherapy blend below is an essential oil formula you can prepare at home. For a more detailed explanation of how to put together and use this blend, see INHALANTS in Part Four. For a quick review of general guidelines for using essential oils, see page 91.

❧ Motion Sickness Inhalant Blend

10 drops chamomile oil
10 drops ginger oil
10 drops peppermint oil

Add the oils to a small glass bottle with an airtight cover and blend. Inhale directly from the bottle, beginning an hour before travel. Repeat frequently.

Muscular Aches, Pains, and Injuries

Muscular aches and pain may result from a strenuous workout, overexertion of muscles, illness, or simply using your muscles without warming them up. Muscular aches and pains function as a warning signal sent by your body; it attempts to prevent serious injury by keeping you from using or overusing stressed muscles. When this signal is ignored, injury often occurs. Types of muscle injuries include a tear in the muscle tissue, fluid retention in or around the muscle, muscle spasms, or overstretching of the connective tissue surrounding the muscle.

Aches and pains can be localized in particular muscle groups, such as the neck or shoulders, as a result of injury, overuse, strain, trauma, or even emotional tension. They can cause burning, hot or cold sensations, numbness, tingling, and weakness in the muscles. Chronic muscular aches and pains may be a sign of a type of soft tissue rheumatism that affects the muscles, ligaments, tendons, or joints. Symptoms may include muscle aches, fatigue, pain, and stiffness, as well as the development of painful points on certain muscles. In addition to muscular problems, this condition—like any kind of chronic pain—can lead to anxiety, depression, headaches, and sleep disturbances.

HELPFUL TREATMENTS

To help prevent aches, pains, and injuries, warm up your muscles before engaging in strenuous physical activity, whether work, exercise, or sports. Try not to exceed your body's capabilities. Set reasonable fitness goals and work up to them gradually.

Massage Preventive Sports Rub into your muscles before working out to reduce or eliminate injuries, sore muscles, and strain. After exercise or physical work, take an After-Sports Bath. Then apply either Deep Heat Tingling Rub or Post-Workout Rub to your muscles to ease or prevent soreness, as needed.

Treat any suspected injury to the muscles by

applying ice or a cold compress. Use a cold Muscle Strain Compress for bruises, inflammation, sprains, swelling, and tennis elbow. After an injury that results in bruising, apply Bruise Blend several times a day to promote healing. Seek medical attention immediately for any serious injury.

For chronic muscular pain, use warm or hot compresses. Apply a hot Chronic Pain Compress to minimize the discomfort of chronic muscle aches or old injuries. Acupressure, acupuncture, hypnosis, massage, and relaxation techniques offer relief for many people with chronic muscular pain. If you have a tendency to injure the same spots again and again, physical therapy may help you to retrain your muscles.

Aromatherapy can comfort both acute and chronic muscular aches and pains. Many essential oils, including basil, bergamot, black pepper, chamomile, clary sage, coriander, cypress, eucalyptus, juniper, lavender, marjoram, rosemary, thyme, and vetiver can be used to relieve pain, reduce swelling, and ease muscle spasms. If you suffer from chronic muscular aches and pains, take a Chronic Pain Relief Bath daily or several times a week. In the morning, apply Daytime Muscle Ache Oil for an invigorating treatment; in the evening, rub on Nighttime Muscle Relief Oil for a relaxing effect.

AROMATHERAPY BLENDS

The aromatherapy blends below are essential oil formulas you can prepare at home. For a more detailed explanation of how to put together and use these blends, see BATHS; COMPRESSES; and/or MASSAGE in Part Four. For a quick review of general guidelines for using essential oils, see page 91.

❧ Preventive Sports Rub

1 ounce carrier oil
4 drops basil oil

4 drops rosemary oil
2 drops peppermint oil
1 drop ginger oil

Place the carrier oil in a clean container and add the essential oils. Gently turn the container upside down several times or roll it between your hands for a few minutes to blend. Massage the mixture onto your muscles before physical activity.

❧ After-Sports Bath

4 drops lavender oil
3 drops chamomile oil
2 drops marjoram oil
1 drop peppermint oil
1 cup Dead Sea salts (optional)
¼ cup seaweed or algae powder (optional)

Disperse the essential oils, and the Dead Sea salts and seaweed or algae powder, if desired, in a bathtub filled with warm water. Soak in the bath for twenty minutes after physical exertion.

❧ Deep Heat Tingling Rub

1 ounce carrier oil
4 drops peppermint oil
3 drops ginger oil
2 drops black pepper oil

In a clean container, add the essential oils to the carrier oil and blend. Use this rub to massage your muscles if they are sore following physical activity.

❧ Post-Workout Rub

1 ounce carrier oil
4 drops chamomile oil
4 drops marjoram oil
2 drops thyme oil
2 drops vetiver oil

Place the carrier oil in a clean container, add the essential oils, and blend. Massage the mixture into your muscles after physical exertion to prevent stiffness and pain.

ཝ Muscle Strain Compress

1 quart cold water
2 drops chamomile oil
2 drops marjoram oil
1 drop rosemary oil

Pour the water into a two-quart glass bowl, add the essential oils, and blend. Saturate a clean cloth in the water and apply it to the affected area, as needed. If you wish, you can apply an ice pack over the compress to keep it from getting warm.

ཝ Bruise Blend

1 ounce carrier oil
4 drops geranium oil
2 drops helichrysum oil
2 drops juniper oil
2 drops lavender oil
1 drop ginger oil

In a clean container, add the essential oils to the carrier oil. Blend well by gently turning the container upside down several times or rolling it between your hands. After an injury, massage the blend over the bruised area several times daily.

ཝ Chronic Pain Compress

1 quart hot water
2 drops helichrysum oil
2 drops marjoram oil
1 drop peppermint oil

Pour the water into a two-quart bowl and disperse the oils in the water. Saturate a clean cloth in the water and apply it to the affected areas, as needed.

ཝ Chronic Pain Relief Bath

3 drops clary sage oil
2 drops juniper oil
2 drops marjoram oil
1 drop coriander oil
1 drop vetiver oil

Add the essential oils to a bathtub filled with warm water. Soak in the bath for twenty to thirty minutes.

ཝ Daytime Muscle Ache Oil

2 ounces carrier oil
10 drops rosemary oil
8 drops eucalyptus oil
6 drops cypress oil
6 drops marjoram oil
4 drops peppermint oil
3 drops thyme oil

Place the carrier oil in a clean container and add the essential oils. Gently turn the container upside down several times or roll it between your hands for a few minutes to blend. Massage the oil into sore muscles as needed.

ཝ Nighttime Muscle Relief Oil

2 ounces carrier oil
10 drops chamomile oil
10 drops marjoram oil
4 drops clary sage oil
4 drops coriander oil
4 drops cypress oil
4 drops ylang ylang oil

Thoroughly blend all the ingredients together in a clean container. At bedtime, apply the oil to sore muscles as needed.

Premenstrual Syndrome (PMS)

Many women experience emotional, mental, and physical discomfort and distress each month, usually starting one to two weeks before menstruation begins. They suffer from premenstrual syndrome, or PMS, with its 150 or more possible symptoms.

The most common physical symptoms of PMS include backaches, blemishes, bloating and fluid retention, cramps, faintness, fatigue or lethargy, headaches, swollen or tender breasts, insomnia, nausea, poor concentration, and a swollen abdomen. Mentally and emotionally, PMS may produce anger, anxiety, aggression, depression, irritability, mood swings, nervousness, personality changes, increased sensitivity, suicidal thoughts, and violent actions.

The precise cause or causes of PMS are not well understood, but the syndrome is thought to be related to hormonal imbalance, especially high levels of estrogen and low levels of progesterone, as well as rapid fluctuations in hormone levels. Hypoglycemia, nutritional deficiencies, poor absorption of nutrients, thyroid imbalances, food allergies, and candidiasis can all contribute to the discomforts of PMS as well.

HELPFUL TREATMENTS

Some women have had success using nutritional supplements—vitamin A, the B vitamins (especially vitamin B6 and folic acid), calcium, magnesium, essential fatty acids, and evening primrose oil—to control PMS. Following a healthy diet that is low in sodium and sugar and contains no alcohol, animal products or byproducts, caffeine, chocolate, or processed foods also reduces the severity of symptoms in many women. If you suffer from PMS, concentrate on eating whole grains and fresh vegetables and fruits, and drink eight to ten glasses of pure, clean water daily throughout the month.

Aromatherapy helps to minimize the discomforts of PMS in several ways. It can reduce bloating and puffiness, ease emotional upset, and relieve many of the physical and emotional symptoms associated with PMS. Chamomile, coriander, cypress, fennel, geranium, juniper, marjoram, patchouli, and thyme oils help reduce bloating and fluid retention. Other essential oils that decrease symptoms of PMS include benzoin, chamomile, clary sage, coriander, fennel, geranium, juniper, marjoram, neroli, rose, and ylang ylang.

Bathe in PMS Bath Blend daily for one to two weeks before your period begins. Apply PMS Body Oil to your skin every day. Use PMS Personal Blend as your perfume throughout the month or as desired. If you suffer from fluid retention or bloating, bathe in Fluid-Retention Bath at the first sign of puffiness and once or twice daily thereafter, as needed. Apply Fluid-Retention Massage Formula over your abdomen several times daily.

AROMATHERAPY BLENDS

The aromatherapy blends below are essential oil formulas you can prepare at home. For a more detailed explanation of how to put together and use these blends, see BATHS; MASSAGE; and/or PERSONAL FRAGRANCES AND PERFUMES in Part Four. For a quick review of general guidelines for using essential oils, see page 91.

🍃 PMS Bath Blend

    2 drops chamomile oil
    2 drops geranium oil
    2 drops juniper oil

2 drops marjoram oil
2 drops ylang ylang oil

Disperse the essential oils in a bathtub filled with warm water. Soak in the bath for twenty to thirty minutes. Repeat as necessary.

❧ PMS Body Oil

4 ounces carrier oil
10 drops chamomile oil
10 drops clary sage oil
4 drops coriander oil
4 drops fennel oil
3 drops geranium oil
3 drops ylang ylang oil

Place the carrier oil in a clean container, add the essential oils, and blend. Massage the oil over your body daily, as needed.

Note: Clary sage oil can cause drowsiness and can also exaggerate the effects of alcohol. Avoid alcohol when using it.

❧ PMS Personal Blend

⅛ ounce jojoba oil
4 drops clary sage oil
3 drops geranium oil
2 drops neroli oil
2 drops ylang ylang oil
1 drop benzoin resin
1 drop rose oil

In a clean container, add the essential oils to the jojoba oil and combine. Wear the blend as a fragrance.

❧ Fluid-Retention Bath

4 drops chamomile oil
3 drops cypress oil

2 drops coriander oil
2 drops patchouli oil

Disperse the oils in a bathtub filled with warm water. Soak in the bath for fifteen to twenty minutes. Repeat as needed.

❧ Fluid-Retention Massage Formula

2 ounces carrier oil
6 drops cypress oil
5 drops chamomile oil
3 drops coriander oil
3 drops patchouli oil
2 drops fennel oil

Place the carrier oil in a clean container, add the essential oils, and blend well. Massage the oil over swollen or bloated areas as necessary.

Prostate Problems

The prostate is a gland that is part of the male reproductive system. Situated beneath the bladder and encircling the urethra, it controls the release of urine. The prostate gland also secretes seminal fluid.

An estimated one third to one half of all men over the age of fifty have an enlarged prostate gland or other prostate problems. An enlarged prostate, or *benign prostatic hypertrophy,* is an overgrowth of the prostate. The precise cause is not known, but it is believed to be related to changes in hormone levels that accompany aging. Alcohol and stress may accelerate the development of the problem. If the prostate becomes sufficiently enlarged, it begins to press against the urethra and can interfere with urination, making it impossible to empty the bladder completely. As a result, the frequency of urination and feelings of urgency increase, particularly during the night; however, urination may take much effort and the flow of urine may become weaker. The retention of urine in the bladder also increases the possibility of bladder infections and, if allowed to continue for prolonged periods of time, it can lead to kidney damage.

Prostatitis is the inflammation or infection of the prostate gland. Like an enlarged prostate, a prostate that is inflamed as the result of infection can block the flow of urine from the bladder, and the infection may migrate, via the urethra and the bladder, into the kidneys. Chronic inflammation of the prostate can weaken the bladder and make it more susceptible to infection.

Some cases of prostatitis are caused by bacterial infection; an infection elsewhere in the body can spread to the urinary tract. In other cases, the cause is unknown. Some researchers suspect that men who have had vasectomies are more likely to develop prostate infections. Other possible complicating factors include hormonal imbalances, lack of exercise, zinc deficiency, failure to eliminate toxins properly, poor circulation, poor diet, and the consumption of alcohol, antihistamines, caffeine, high-acid foods, and too little dietary fiber. Symptoms can include difficulty urinating, a diminishing volume or flow of urine, a frequent need or desire to urinate, incontinence, the need to get up during the night to urinate, and pain or a burning sensation while urinating. Fatigue, fever, lethargy, and pain in the legs, lower abdomen, or lower back can also be symptoms of prostatitis.

Prostatitis is often associated with cystitis, and may be accompanied by diminished sex drive, impotence, and sometimes premature ejaculation. If untreated, the condition can lead to obstruction of the bladder and severe health consequences.

HELPFUL TREATMENTS

If you are suffering from the symptoms of an enlarged prostate or prostate infection, you should consult your health care provider. You may require medical treatment. Also, the symptoms of prostate enlargement can be similar to those present in the earlier stages of prostate cancer, so it is important to have a professional evaluation.

Dietary changes can bring about relief of many prostate problems and may even prevent them from developing into more serious conditions. Eat a diet consisting of fresh vegetables, whole grains, nuts, seeds, legumes, brown rice, and sources of polyunsaturated fatty acids, such as cold-pressed olive, sesame, and sunflower oils. Supplementing your diet with essential fatty acids, ginseng, pumpkin seeds, brewer's yeast, vitamin B6, and/or zinc may also help. Avoid all alcohol, caffeine, fried or greasy foods, and refined carbohydrates. Avoid contact with pesticides. Increase your intake of water to two or three quarts per day, and be sure to get regular exercise.

Essential oils that can help with prostate problems are benzoin, jasmine, juniper, pine, and sandalwood. In addition, bergamot, cedarwood, chamomile, cypress, eucalyptus, lemon, myrrh, tea tree, and thyme oils can increase urination and fight infection. A Prostate Sitz Bath can diminish some of the discomfort. Alternating hot and cold sitz baths improves circulation to the prostate. After a sitz bath, apply Prostate Massage Oil to your abdomen, lower back, and the groin area.

AROMATHERAPY BLENDS

The aromatherapy blends below are essential oil formulas you can prepare at home. For a more detailed explanation of how to put together and use these blends, see MASSAGE and/or SITZ BATHS in Part Four. For a quick review of general guidelines for using essential oils, see page 91.

🐚 Prostate Sitz Bath

2 drops cedarwood oil
2 drops juniper oil
2 drops pine oil
1 drop cypress oil
1 drop sandalwood oil

Add the oils to a shallow tub filled with water. Sit hip-deep in the water for five to fifteen minutes. Alternate between using hot and cold water.

🐚 Prostate Massage Oil

1 ounce carrier oil
4 drops cedarwood oil
3 drops lemon oil
2 drops juniper oil
2 drops pine oil
1 drop myrrh oil

Place the carrier oil in a clean container and add the essential oils. Gently turn the container upside down several times or roll it between your hands for a few minutes to blend. Massage the mixture over your abdomen, lower back, and groin area. Repeat once or twice daily, as necessary.

Psoriasis

Psoriasis shows up as bright-red inflamed skin with raised dry, silvery scales. The new skin cells of psoriasis sufferers grow about five times faster than the old cells are shed. Crusty patches of skin result, usually appearing on the elbows, knees, lower back, buttocks, nails, scalp, or chest. In severe cases, psoriasis can cover the entire body.

Heredity plays a major role in the development of psoriasis, while emotional factors and stress often determine the frequency and severity of outbreaks. Bacterial infections, drugs, illnesses, liver dysfunction, skin injuries, sunburn, surgery, and certain viruses can also trigger or aggravate outbreaks of psoriasis.

HELPFUL TREATMENTS

Sunshine often reduces the symptoms of psoriasis, as does a vacation away from sources of stress. Some sufferers have noticed an improvement within three months after they start taking either soy lecithin or vitamin E capsules. Many people bathe in Dead Sea salts to keep their psoriasis under control. Adding essential oils to the Dead Sea salts increases their effectiveness.

Aromatherapy can often control psoriasis by diminishing stress, reducing inflammation, and soothing and softening the skin. The essential oils of benzoin, chamomile, clary sage, helichrysum, lavender, myrrh, and sandalwood reduce inflammation and irritation and soothe skin. Bergamot, cedarwood, juniper, neroli, orange, pine, rose, rosemary, rosewood, tea tree, and ylang ylang oils also benefit psoriasis.

For rough areas, use Psoriasis Skin Scrub several times weekly to smooth and soften skin and to remove dead skin. Bathe in Soothing Psoriasis Bath daily or several times a week until symptoms improve, then once a week to maintain results. Apply Psoriasis Skin Oil to the affected areas several times daily.

AROMATHERAPY BLENDS

The aromatherapy blends below are essential oil formulas you can prepare at home. For a more detailed explanation of how to put together and use these blends, see BATHS and/or MASSAGE in Part Four. For a quick review of general guidelines for using essential oils, see page 91.

Psoriasis Skin Scrub

2 tablespoons blue cornmeal, almond meal, or hazelnut meal
1 tablespoon honey
2 drops bergamot oil
2 drops rosewood oil
1 drop helichrysum oil
1 drop myrrh oil

In a small bowl, blend all the ingredients together into a paste, adding a few drops of water if necessary for the proper consistency. Massage the paste over the affected areas. Rinse thoroughly and apply Psoriasis Skin Oil. If large areas of the body are affected, you may double or triple the formula to yield the desired amount of scrub.

Soothing Psoriasis Bath

2 cups Dead Sea salts
4 drops bergamot oil
2 drops chamomile oil
2 drops helichrysum oil
2 drops tea tree oil

Disperse all the ingredients in a bathtub filled with warm water. Soak in the water for thirty minutes. Repeat several times a week until symptoms improve, then once a week to maintain results.

Psoriasis Skin Oil

1 ounce jojoba oil
½ ounce hazelnut oil
10 drops borage oil
10 drops evening primrose oil
8 drops bergamot oil
4 drops chamomile oil
4 drops helichrysum oil
4 drops sandalwood oil
2 drops clary sage oil

2 drops neroli oil
2 drops ylang ylang oil

Mix the jojoba, hazelnut, borage, and evening primrose oils together in a clean container. Add the essential oils and gently turn the container upside down several times or roll it between your hands for a few minutes to blend. Apply the mixture to the affected areas as needed.

Note: Bergamot oil increases sensitivity to the sun. Omit it from the formula if your skin will be exposed to sunlight.

Scalp Problems

See HAIR AND SCALP PROBLEMS.

Seborrhea

Seborrhea, or seborrheic dermatitis, affects areas of skin with abundant oil glands, such as the chest, ears, eyebrows, face, nose, and scalp. When these glands secrete abnormal amounts of oil (or sebum) and the skin cells grow at a faster than normal rate, the ducts through which the sebum normally flows to the surface of the skin can become blocked. The glands then produce even more oil. The result is red eruptions on the skin, with thick crusting and scaliness. The oily pinkish-yellow scales resemble dandruff and may itch and flake.

A diet high in fats and sugar, food allergies, heredity, hormonal imbalances, infection, nutritional deficiencies, stress, and a yeast organism called *Pityrosporon orbiculare,* which is normally present in hair follicles, may all play a role in the development of seborrhea. In infants, seborrhea on the scalp is called cradle cap.

HELPFUL TREATMENTS

Use an elimination diet or consult a nutritionist to determine if you have food allergies or nutritional deficiencies. Eating a healthy diet that focuses on fresh vegetables and fruits and whole grains often helps to control seborrhea. Avoid chocolate, dairy products, fried or greasy foods, nuts, refined foods, sugar, and white flour. Supplements of vitamin A, the B vitamins (especially vitamin B6 and biotin), flaxseed oil, and zinc have been found to bring relief for some seborrhea sufferers.

Essential oils that help with seborrhea include cedarwood, clary sage, geranium, juniper, patchouli, pine, rosemary, and tea tree. For seborrhea on the scalp, massage Seborrhea Scalp Soother into your scalp daily and shampoo with Seborrhea Shampoo either daily or several times a week to bring seborrhea under control. For seborrhea on the face or other parts of the body, apply Seborrhea Skin Oil daily, as necessary.

Jojoba oil is the preferred oil to use as a carrier oil for blends to treat seborrhea, because jojoba oil is similar in chemical composition to human sebum and is known to help regulate sebum secretion.

AROMATHERAPY BLENDS

The aromatherapy blends below are essential oil formulas you can prepare at home. For a quick review of general guidelines for using essential oils, see page 91.

Seborrhea Scalp Soother

1 ounce jojoba oil
4 drops cedarwood oil
4 drops pine oil
3 drops rosemary oil
3 drops tea tree oil

Place the jojoba oil in a clean container and add the essential oils. Gently turn the container upside down several times or roll it between your hands for a few minutes to blend. Massage the mixture into your clean scalp and leave it on for fifteen to thirty minutes or overnight. Then shampoo with Seborrhea Shampoo.

Seborrhea Shampoo

4 ounces unscented shampoo
8 drops clary sage oil
8 drops tea tree oil
4 drops juniper oil
4 drops rosemary oil

Add the oils to the unscented shampoo and mix thoroughly. Shampoo with this formula daily to control seborrhea.

Seborrhea Skin Oil

1 ounce jojoba oil
4 drops clary sage oil
3 drops geranium oil
3 drops patchouli oil
2 drops tea tree oil

In a clean container, add the essential oils to the jojoba oil and blend. Massage the oil over the affected areas one or more times daily, as needed.

Sinusitis

Sinusitis is an inflammation or infection of the sinus cavities, which are open spaces in the skull that are located above the eyes, behind the bridge of the nose, beneath the cheekbones, and in the upper nose. Sinusitis often accompanies or follows an upper respiratory infection such as a cold. Because the sinus cavities are connected to the nose and nasal passages, infections can easily spread into the sinuses. The sinus cavities become inflamed and filled with mucus; normal drainage is blocked and breathing may be impaired. Pressure builds within the sinuses, causing a dull or throbbing ache behind the forehead, around the eyes, and in the cheeks. Other symptoms of sinusitis may include headache, fever, earache, loss of the sense of smell, bad breath, and even toothache.

Sinusitis can be allergic in origin. Hay fever and food allergies, especially an allergy to milk and dairy products, can cause allergic sinusitis. An injury to your nasal passages or chronic insult from exposure to cigarette smoke, environmental pollutants, fragrances, and other irritants can cause or contribute to sinusitis, as can the presence of tiny growths called polyps in the nasal passages. Exposure to dampness and the consumption of certain foods, such as wheat, dairy products, sugar, and refined carbohydrates, may make a person more susceptible to sinusitis.

HELPFUL TREATMENTS

If you are prone to sinusitis, investigate the cause of the problem. Experiment with an elimination diet to see if food allergies may be involved. Dairy and wheat products are two of the most common troublemakers, so it is probably best to start by eliminating them from your diet. Also, as much as possible, avoid contact with noxious chemicals, environmental pollutants, and synthetic fragrances.

During an attack of sinusitis, eliminate dairy products, sugar, and wheat from your diet. Make sure you drink plenty of fluids. If your sinusitis does not improve within several days, you should consult your health care practitioner. Medical treatment may be required to clear a stubborn infection.

Aromatherapy can help to clear sinusitis by combatting infection, opening up nasal passages, reducing congestion, and relieving pain and discomfort. Basil, benzoin, cedarwood, eucalyptus, ginger, helichrysum, lavender, marjoram, peppermint, pine, rosemary, sandalwood, tea tree, and thyme oils soothe sinus inflammation and ease discomfort.

For instant relief, breathe Sinus Inhalant directly from the bottle whenever necessary. Prepare a Sinus Steam Inhalation several times daily. A Sinus Foot Bath will also help to open sinuses and restore normal breathing.

AROMATHERAPY BLENDS

The aromatherapy blends below are essential oil formulas you can prepare at home. For a more detailed explanation of how to put together and use these blends, see FOOT BATHS; INHALANTS; and/or STEAM INHALATIONS in Part Four. For a quick review of general guidelines for using essential oils, see page 91.

🕊 Sinus Inhalant

> 10 drops eucalyptus oil
> 10 drops lavender oil
> 5 drops cedarwood oil
> 5 drops peppermint oil
> 3 drops helichrysum oil

Drop the oils into a small glass bottle with an airtight cover. Blend by gently turning the container upside down several times or rolling it between your hands for a few minutes. Breathe directly from the bottle as needed.

❧ Sinus Steam Inhalation

    1 quart steaming water
    2 drops eucalyptus oil
    2 drops tea tree oil
    1 drop ginger oil
    1 drop thyme oil

Pour the water into a two-quart glass bowl and disperse the essential oils in the water. Hold your head over the bowl. If possible, drape a towel over both your head and the bowl to capture the steam. Breathe in the vapors for five to ten minutes. Repeat as necessary.

❧ Sinus Foot Bath

    2 drops pine oil
    1 drop basil oil
    1 drop ginger oil
    1 drop rosemary oil

Add the oils to a shallow tub or foot bath filled with warm water. Soak your feet in the water for fifteen to thirty minutes. Repeat as needed.

Skin Problems

Healthy skin is clear and radiant, with a smooth and soft texture. The muscles that support the skin are firm, supple, and resilient; the skin surface looks moist and is neither too oily nor too dry. Its coloring is even and the pores are only slightly visible.

If your skin doesn't look or feel like this, you may have a skin problem. With the stresses of modern life, pollution, and poor nutrition, maintaining healthy, attractive skin is a challenge. Fortunately, aromatherapy and a good skin care routine can improve the condition of your skin and help you make the most of your natural assets.

Your skin serves as more than an attractive covering for your body. As an important part of your immune system, your skin offers the first line of defense from outside invaders. It protects you from environmental assaults such as cold, heat, pollution, sun, and wind, and prevents most foreign chemicals and water from entering your body. It regulates your body temperature and insulates your internal organs. Through perspiration, it releases heat when you become too warm. Your skin is also an organ of elimination. Excess wastes that your kidneys, lungs, and intestines cannot process may be expelled through the skin.

Skin health relies on good circulation and an adequate supply of water—two factors that become increasingly important with age. Poor circulation prevents the normal cellular exchange of nutrients and wastes. If circulation to the skin is sluggish, the cells fail to receive sufficient nourishment and wastes build up. The production of new skin cells slows down and premature aging may begin. Blemishes or acne can occur. Broken capillaries or varicose veins may appear. Boosting circulation to your skin cells can restore a healthy, radiant glow to your complexion while warding off signs of premature aging.

Water is critically important for healthy skin. Your body consists of about 70 percent water, and your skin cells need a constant supply of fresh water to function properly and to continue looking moist and youthful. Dehydrated skin cells show up as lines, wrinkles, and dry, dull skin.

Skin is usually classified as either normal, dry, or oily. To determine your skin type, perform the following test in the morning before cleansing your face: Blot your forehead, your nose, your chin, and your cheeks, each with a separate single-thickness piece of tissue. Then examine the tissues. Oily spots on the tissue reveal an oily area. No oil on a tissue indicates a dry area. Normal skin may leave a minimal amount of oil on the tissues.

Although they are the most common skin types, normal, dry, and oily skins are not the only classifications of skin type. Mature skin is skin that has begun to show signs of aging, such as lines and wrinkles. Combination skin has both dry and oily areas. Usually, the area known as the T-zone—the forehead, nose, and chin—is oily, while the cheeks and throat are dry. Combination skin may require a two-part approach to skin care in which you treat each area with products designed for that skin type.

Sensitive skin can be either dry or oily. It is usually very fragile and delicate and requires special treatment. Many cosmetics are too harsh for sensitive skin and will often irritate it, causing blemishes, broken capillaries, chapping or cracking, irritation, or rashes. If you have sensitive skin, you should be extremely careful about skin care and the products you use.

As you get older, your skin changes. As skin matures, it becomes thinner and more fragile, more susceptible to broken capillaries, bruising, and other injuries. Discolorations or variations in pigment may appear. However, much of what people accept as normal or inevitable signs of aging is actually premature aging. Lines and wrinkles and dry or sagging skin are the first signs of premature aging. All skin will develop lines and wrinkles eventually, but if your skin is well cared for and supported by a healthy lifestyle, it should look relatively line-free until you are in your late thirties or early forties, or even longer.

Lines and wrinkles may also result from years of repeating the same facial expressions, such as smiling, frowning, pouting, pursing your lips, raising your eyebrows, and squinting. These repeated expressions eventually etch their marks into your skin. Gravity also has an effect. The development of lines and wrinkles can be greatly accelerated by the consumption of alcohol; exposure to cigarette smoke (especially through smoking, but also from secondhand smoke) and other environmental pollutants; chronic constipation, dehydration, or illness; the use of certain drugs; harsh cosmetics; hormone imbalances; bad dental work; lack of good skin care; poor circulation; poor diet; nutritional deficiencies; poor posture; a sedentary lifestyle; stress; and overexposure to the sun. Heredity and coloring also are factors. Fair skin and dry complexions usually age sooner than dark skin and oily complexions.

Any kind of skin can be helped by a good skin care regimen (see Taking Care of Your Skin, page 184). Whether you are treating a problem skin or want to maintain healthy, normal skin, you should drink eight to twelve glasses of pure, clean water every day, and eat plenty of fresh fruits and vegetables to get the nutrients your skin needs. Avoid unprotected exposure to the sun—use a sunscreen daily and wear protective clothing, hats, and sunglasses. Choose skin care products that are suited to your skin type.

Use the formulas in this section to make your own simple aromatherapy skin care products easily and inexpensively. They will not be as elaborate or refined as commercial products, but they will be pure and they will contain no preservatives, artificial colorings, fragrances, or any other unnecessary ingredients. Best of all, they will work. It may seem like a little more trouble at first; some of the products have to be made just before each application. However, when you see the condition of your skin improve, you will probably decide that it is well worth any extra effort.

NORMAL SKIN

Normal skin is neither too dry nor too oily; it is the ideal skin type. It is moist and clear, with a smooth texture and even color. Normal skin appears soft and is firm to the touch. Pores may be perceptible but are not large.

Essential oils that are helpful for normal skin include cedarwood, clary sage, elemi, frankincense, geranium, jasmine, lavender, neroli, palmarosa, patchouli, rose, rosemary, rosewood, sandalwood, and vetiver. To maintain healthy normal skin, use the aromatherapy blends that follow in your skin care regimen. Or see SKIN CARE AND CUSTOMIZING SKIN CARE PRODUCTS in Part Four. For a quick review of general guidelines for using essential oils, see page 91.

❧ Honey and Clay Cleanser for Normal Skin

    1 teaspoon French green clay powder
    1 teaspoon honey
    1 drop lavender oil
    1 drop rosemary oil

Blend all the ingredients into a paste in your palm. Massage the paste into your skin until it feels clean. Rinse with warm water.

❧ Normal Skin Toner

    8 ounces distilled water
    2 drops lavender oil
    1 drop palmarosa oil
    1 drop rosewood oil

Pour the distilled water into a clean bottle and add the essential oils. Shake to blend. Apply the toner to your skin with a cotton ball after cleansing. Shake well before each use.

❧ Facial Oil for Normal or Sensitive Skin

    1 ounce jojoba oil
    3 drops neroli oil
    2 drops rose oil
    2 drops sandalwood oil

Place the jojoba oil in a clean container and add the essential oils. Gently turn the container upside down several times or roll it between your hands for a few minutes to blend. Apply several drops to your face twice daily, after cleansing and toning.

❧ Facial Mask for Normal or Oily Skin

    1 teaspoon French green clay powder
    1 teaspoon honey
    1 drop palmarosa oil
    1 drop rosewood oil
    1 teaspoon enzyme powder (optional)

In the palm of your hand, combine the essential oils with the green clay and honey (and the enzyme powder, if desired) and blend well. Apply the mixture to clean facial skin and relax for fifteen minutes. Rinse well. Use this mask once a week.

DRY, MATURE, AND PREMATURELY AGING SKIN

Dry skin lacks oil and moisture, and may appear scaly or flaky. It is usually thin, even transparent, with few, or no, visible pores. Dry skin usually feels "tight" after washing. It may lack suppleness and resiliency. Dry skin is usually relatively problem-free during youth, but may show signs of aging sooner than normal or oily skin. Essential oils that benefit dry skin include benzoin, bergamot, cedarwood, clary sage, elemi, fennel, frankincense, geranium, jasmine, lavender, myrrh, neroli, palmarosa, patchouli, rose, rosemary, rosewood, sandalwood, and vetiver. If your skin is dry, use the aromatherapy blends in this section as part of your regular skin care regimen. Or see SKIN CARE AND CUSTOMIZING SKIN CARE PRODUCTS in Part Four for ways to use essential oils together with the skin care products you already use.

Mature or prematurely aging skin is often thin and transparent, and is usually dry or dehydrated. The coloring may be uneven. The skin may also have lost some of its muscle tone and may sag. Mature skin or prematurely aging skin is characterized by lines, wrinkles, dryness, and loss of elasticity.

If you feel that your skin is aging prematurely, examine your lifestyle for possible contributing factors. The most common of these are sun exposure, poor diet, insufficient water intake, improper skin care, repeated facial expressions, and nutritional deficiencies. Many lines and wrinkles are preventable; even existing ones may be minimized by changing your habits and your lifestyle. Watch yourself in the mirror. Do your lines correspond to certain facial expressions you make regularly? You can gain control over those expressions—and the lines they cause—by becoming aware of them. If you can stop making them, you can often reduce the depth of the lines, and certainly prevent them from becoming deeper. You may also wish to consult a nutritionist about improving your diet and finding any nutritional deficiencies you may have.

Mature or prematurely aging skin can benefit from clary sage, elemi, fennel, frankincense, geranium, helichrysum, jasmine, lemon, myrrh, neroli, palmarosa, rose, rosemary, rosewood, sandalwood, and vetiver oils. Use the aromatherapy blends in this section to make skin care products that are appropriate for your skin type, and apply Rejuvenating Facial Oil to your skin twice a day to encourage the formation of new skin cells. Or see SKIN CARE AND CUSTOMIZING SKIN CARE PRODUCTS in Part Four for ways to add the benefits of essential oils to the skin care products you already use. For a quick review of general guidelines for using essential oils, see page 91.

🐦 Jojoba Oil Cleanser for Dry Skin

> 1 ounce jojoba oil
> 2 drops myrrh oil
> 2 drops sandalwood oil
> 1 drop benzoin resin
> 1 drop fennel oil
> 1 drop frankincense oil

Place the jojoba oil in a clean container and add the essential oils. Gently turn the container upside down several times or roll it between your hands for a few minutes to blend. Massage the cleanser into your skin, then gently wipe it off with a warm, wet washcloth.

🐦 Dry Skin Toner

> 8 ounces distilled water
> 1 drop frankincense oil
> 1 drop rosewood oil
> 1 drop sandalwood oil
> 1 drop vetiver oil

Pour the water into a clean bottle, add the essential oils, and shake to combine. Apply the toner to your skin with a cotton ball after cleansing. Shake well before each use.

🐦 Facial Oil for Dry or Mature Skin

> 1 ounce jojoba oil
> 3 drops palmarosa oil
> 2 drops frankincense oil
> 2 drops myrrh oil
> 1 drop patchouli oil

In a clean container, add the essential oils to the jojoba oil and combine. Apply several drops of oil to your face, twice daily, after cleansing and toning, and at other times, as needed.

Taking Care of Your Skin

Your face is usually the first part of you that the rest of the world sees. It makes a lasting impression on other people and often determines their perception of you. You want your face to look its very best, and attractive skin makes a major contribution toward looking good.

Taking good care of your skin is your best assurance for maintaining healthy, youthful skin. Skin care is simple when you know what to do and when you establish a regular routine. The immediate and long-range benefits of a consistent daily skin care program—a healthy, radiant complexion that looks good now and for years to come—are well worth the commitment.

Simple skin care involves seven basic steps. You need to do some procedures, such as cleansing, toning, and moisturizing, twice a day. Others—scrubbing, steaming, and applying masks—you can do about once a week. Misting can be done as often as you like. A skin care routine may seem like extra work initially, especially if you haven't been caring for your skin. But once you become adjusted to your new program, it will feel as normal as brushing your teeth or taking a shower.

The seven basic steps of a good skin care regimen are:

1. Cleansing. Cleansing removes dirt and impurities from the surface of the skin. Cleansing is increasingly important for maintaining good skin today, as the level of environmental pollutants rises. Cleanse your skin once in the morning, to remove wastes your skin generates during sleep, and again at night, to remove bacteria, oils, makeup, dirt, and any other residues that collect on your face during the day. Use a cleanser formulated for your skin type. Dry skin cleansers moisturize as they clean skin; oily skin cleansers remove excess oil as they cleanse.

2. Scrubbing. A facial scrub gently exfoliates (sloughs off) dead skin cells that can contribute to blackheads, blemishes, dryness, and wrinkles. It also boosts circulation to your face and gives your complexion a healthy glow. Scrubs can be made from almond meal, cornmeal, hazelnut meal, jojoba beads, jojoba meal, or any other grain that gently removes dead skin cells. Avoid abrasive scrubs that can scratch or irritate your skin. One to three times a week, *gently* massage the scrub into your skin after cleansing. Scrubs are appropriate for all skins except sensitive skin or skin with broken capillaries. If you have either of those conditions, you should avoid using scrubs.

3. Toning. A toner removes residues left on your skin by your cleanser, mask, scrub, or tap water. A toner leaves your face moist, allowing for better absorption of your moisturizer or facial oil. After cleansing, scrubbing, or removing a mask, moisten a cotton ball with toner and glide it over your face and neck. Repeat this procedure until no traces of dirt remain. Men can splash their faces with toner or after-shave after cleansing or shaving. Gentle toners are made with floral or herbal waters. Avoid toners or astringents that contain alcohol, which can dry and irritate your skin.

4. Moisturizing. Moisturizers or facial oils create a protective barrier between your skin and the atmosphere, bacteria, makeup, and smog. They plump up your surface skin cells, prevent moisture loss, and give your skin a smooth, soft appearance. Every skin, even oily skin, needs a moisturizer or facial oil to protect it. Select one formulated for your skin type. Apply a small amount of moisturizer or several drops of facial oil to your face after cleansing and toning. If your skin is dry, you may wish to apply moisturizer or facial oil at other times, too, especially after misting (see below).

5. Misting. A facial mist replenishes the moisture that your skin constantly loses to the atmosphere, especially with air conditioning and heating and in dry climates. Facial mists usually contain herbal or floral waters. Avoid products that contain synthetic ingredients and alcohol. Spray your face as often as you like.

6. Steaming. Facial steaming once a week will deep cleanse your pores, moisturize your skin, and improve circulation to your face. To steam your face, add three to five drops of an essential oil or oils appropriate for your skin type (see page 216) to a glass bowl containing one quart of steaming water. Capture the steam by draping a towel over your head to create a "tent" and hold your face over the bowl for five to ten minutes. Follow with a scrub or facial mask.

7. Masks. A facial mask can nourish your skin, replenish moisture, normalize oil secretions, and invigorate your complexion. Once a week, apply a mask for your skin type and relax for ten to fifteen minutes. Both the mask and the relaxation will improve the condition of your skin. Rinse off with warm water. Apply toner and facial oil.

🐚 Facial Mask for Dry or Mature Skin

2 teaspoons honey
2 drops sandalwood oil
1 drop frankincense oil
1 teaspoon enzyme powder (optional)

In the palm of your hand, add the sandalwood and frankincense oil (and the enzyme powder, if desired) to the honey and blend well. Apply the mask to clean skin. Relax for fifteen minutes, then rinse thoroughly. Use this mask once a week.

🐚 Rejuvenating Facial Oil

1½ ounces jojoba oil
10 drops borage oil
10 drops vitamin E oil
3 drops geranium oil
3 drops neroli oil
3 drops rosewood oil
2 drops fennel oil
2 drops frankincense oil
2 drops sandalwood oil
1 drop vetiver oil

Mix the jojoba, borage, and vitamin E oils together. Add the essential oils and blend. Massage several drops of oil into your face every morning and evening after cleansing and toning.

OILY SKIN

Oily skin usually has a shiny appearance because its overactive oil glands produce too much oil. The pores are often enlarged and clog easily, so the skin must be kept extremely clean to avoid blemishes. Although oily skin is acne-prone during the teen and early adult years, its natural oils help it to maintain youthfulness longer than dry skin.

Essential oils that can improve the condition of oily skin include cedarwood, clary sage, cypress, elemi, frankincense, geranium, jasmine, juniper, lemon, neroli, orange, palmarosa, patchouli, peppermint, rosemary, rosewood, sandalwood, tea tree, thyme, vetiver, and ylang ylang. To help regulate oily skin and keep it clear, use the aromatherapy blends in this section in your skin care regimen (see also page 182 for Facial Mask for Normal or Oily Skin). Or see SKIN CARE AND CUSTOMIZING SKIN CARE PRODUCTS in Part Four.

❧ Clay Cleanser for Oily Skin

1 teaspoon French green clay powder
1 teaspoon water
1 drop cedarwood oil
1 drop ylang ylang oil

Hold the green clay powder in the palm of your hand. Add the water and essential oils and blend well to make a paste. Massage the cleanser into your skin until it feels clean. Rinse with warm water.

❧ Oily Skin Toner

8 ounces distilled water
2 drops geranium oil
2 drops ylang ylang oil
1 drop lemon oil

Pour the water into a clean bottle, add the essential oils, and shake to blend. Apply the toner to your skin with a cotton ball after cleansing. Shake well before each use.

❧ Facial Oil for Oily Skin

1 ounce jojoba oil
3 drops ylang ylang oil
2 drops lemon oil
2 drops rosewood oil
1 drop clary sage oil
1 drop geranium oil

Place the jojoba oil in a clean container and add the essential oils. Gently turn the container upside down several times or roll it between your hands for a few minutes to blend. Apply one or two drops of oil to your face twice daily after cleansing and toning.

CHAPPED OR CRACKED SKIN

Skin that is chapped or cracked is extremely dry and dehydrated. It may lack both oil and moisture. Skin conditions such as dermatitis; exposure to cold, sun, wind, or harsh chemicals or cosmetics; and dietary factors such as an insufficient intake of oil, essential fatty acids, water, or certain nutrients (especially vitamin A) can all cause chapped or cracked skin.

If your skin has chapped or cracked areas, make sure you are getting enough water and that your diet contains a sufficient quantity of cold-pressed vegetable oil, about one tablespoon a day for most people. Consult a nutritionist if you suspect a nutritional deficiency. Protect yourself from the weather, the sun, harsh chemicals, and detergents.

Essential oils that can soothe and help heal chapped and cracked skin are benzoin, bergamot, frankincense, and myrrh. Apply Chapped Skin Oil to the affected areas at least twice daily.

❧ Chapped Skin Oil

1 ounce jojoba oil
4 drops benzoin resin
3 drops frankincense oil
3 drops myrrh oil
2 drops bergamot oil

In a clean container, add the essential oils to the jojoba oil and blend. Apply the oil to chapped areas as necessary.

Note: Bergamot oil increases sensitivity to the sun. Omit it from the formula if your skin will be exposed to sunlight.

ALL SKIN TYPES

Some skin care products can be beneficial regardless of whether your skin is normal, dry, or oily. The following aromatherapy blends are recommended for all skin types.

❧ All-Purpose Skin Scrub

1 teaspoon almond meal or blue cornmeal
1 teaspoon honey
1 drop geranium oil
1 drop lavender oil

Blend all the ingredients together into a paste in your palm. After cleansing and before toning, massage the scrub over your skin for one minute, then rinse thoroughly. Use one to three times a week, depending on your skin type (see Taking Care of Your Skin, page 184).

❧ Floral Facial Mist

4 ounces distilled water
3 drops lavender oil
2 drops rosewood oil
1 drop chamomile oil
1 drop neroli oil
1 drop rose oil

Pour the distilled water into a spray bottle, add the essential oils, and shake to blend. Spray your skin with the mist frequently during the day. Shake well before each use.

❧ All-Purpose After-Shave

8 ounces distilled water
2 drops cedarwood oil
2 drops lavender oil
2 drops rosewood oil
1 drop elemi oil
1 drop vetiver oil

Add the essential oils to the water and blend. Splash the mixture on your skin after shaving. Shake well before each use.

CAUTIONS

Some essential oils can irritate skin, especially sensitive skin. These include bitter fennel, black pepper, cajeput, camphor, cardamom, cedarwood, citronella, cinnamon, clove, eucalyptus, fir, ginger, lemon, lemongrass, lemon verbena, melissa, parsley, pennyroyal, peppermint, pimento, pine, oregano, rosemary, sassafras, savory, tea tree, thyme, thuja, and wintergreen. If your skin is sensitive, you may wish to use these oils at lower levels than generally recommended, or simply avoid using them.

Sore Throat

A sore throat usually starts as a scratchy, aching, or swollen feeling inside the throat. The throat may be red and inflamed; the lymph nodes in the neck may be tender. Swallowing or talking may be difficult or painful. A sore throat may be accompanied by fatigue, fever, headache, and/or nausea, especially if it signals the beginning of a cold or the flu.

Most sore throats are caused by viral or bacterial infection. Other possible causes include allergies, asthma, and local irritation from exposure to cigarette smoke, environmental pollutants, or other irritants. Nutritional deficiencies, fatigue, and a weakened immune system are among the factors that make a person more susceptible to illnesses that can cause a sore throat.

HELPFUL TREATMENTS

Most sore throats respond well to bed rest, nutritional supplementation, and an increased consumption of liquids, especially water. Taking supplements of vitamin A, vitamin C, bioflavonoids, and zinc can speed your recovery. The herbs echinacea, garlic, and goldenseal are also helpful. Avoid eating foods containing sugar when you have a sore throat, because sugar encourages the growth of bacteria.

Benzoin, bergamot, clary sage, eucalyptus, geranium, ginger, lavender, lemon, myrrh, pine, rose, sandalwood, tea tree, and thyme are essential oils that can soothe your sore throat and accelerate healing. Several times a day, massage Sore Throat Massage Oil or Geranium Throat Rub on your throat and neck area to soothe the pain and to prevent the spread of infection. Gargle frequently with Sore Throat Gargle. Apply a warm Throat-Soothing Compress several times during the day.

AROMATHERAPY BLENDS

The aromatherapy blends below are essential oil formulas you can prepare at home. For a more detailed explanation of how to put together and use these blends, see COMPRESSES; MASSAGE; and/or MOUTHWASHES, GARGLES, AND GUM TREATMENTS in Part Four. For a quick review of general guidelines for using essential oils, see page 91.

❧ Sore Throat Massage Oil

> 1 ounce jojoba oil
> 4 drops geranium oil
> 2 drops bergamot oil
> 2 drops eucalyptus oil
> 2 drops helichrysum oil
> 2 drops lavender oil

Place the jojoba oil in a clean container and add the essential oils. Turn the container upside down several times or roll it between your hands for a few minutes to blend. Gently massage the oil over your neck and throat to soothe a sore throat or swollen glands.

Note: Bergamot oil increases sensitivity to the sun. Omit it from the formula if your skin will be exposed to sunlight.

❧ Geranium Throat Rub

> ½ ounce jojoba oil
> 10 drops geranium oil

Blend the geranium oil into the jojoba oil. Massage the mixture over the throat area. Repeat as necessary.

❧ Sore Throat Gargle

Add 1 drop of ginger, lavender, lemon, or tea tree oil to a glass of warm water and mix thoroughly. Gargle. Repeat every two hours or as needed.

❧ Throat-Soothing Compress

> 1 quart hot water
> 2 drops clary sage oil
> 2 drops geranium oil
> 1 drop sandalwood oil

Pour the water into a two-quart glass bowl and disperse the essential oils in the water. Saturate a clean cloth in the water. Apply the compress to your throat and neck as needed.

Stress

Stress is general term for a disturbance of your physical or emotional balance. Virtually any type of change can cause stress. Changes in climate, deadlines, exposure to environmental pollutants or toxins, family conflicts, financial or job pressures, and physical or emotional trauma all cause stress. Stress has been linked with most diseases as either a causative or contributing factor. Some common conditions that are closely related to stress are asthma, headaches, digestive disorders, ulcers, high blood pressure, depression, premenstrual syndrome, menstrual difficulties, autoimmune diseases, cancer, diabetes, cardiovascular disease, and weakened immunity.

When you encounter stress, your body releases hormones that set in motion what is known as the "fight or flight" response—that is, a group of physiological changes that prepare you to deal with a threat. Digestion ceases, your heart rate increases, and your blood pressure rises. Breathing becomes more rapid; palms sweat. Fats and sugars are released into the bloodstream, making cholesterol and blood sugar levels rise. The muscles become more rigid; blood prepares to clot.

In the modern world, only rarely do people need to fight or flee in response to the things that cause stress reactions, yet these bodily reactions still take place, and they can continue for hours after the "fight or flight" phase is over. This extreme physical reaction takes a toll on the body. If the stress is constant or prolonged, the body has no chance to recover, and stress overloads your organs and immune system, weakening your body's immune response. Constant or repeated stress eventually may exhaust one or more organs.

Stress is often aggravated by the inability to relax, the attempt to maintain too many commitments, overwork, and poor nutrition, especially a high-sugar diet that contains too many refined foods and sweets. The consumption of alcohol, tobacco, caffeine, and other drugs also can make the problem worse. Whether stress results from a major disaster or a minor annoyance, its impact is the same: Stress, especially chronic stress, lowers immunity, elevates blood pressure, and raises cholesterol levels; it depletes your body's supplies of vitamins and minerals, including vitamin A, the B vitamins, vitamin C, vitamin D, vitamin E, calcium, iron, magnesium, molybdenum, potassium, sulphur, and zinc. Stress also depletes your physical, mental, and emotional energies. Stress-induced problems such as backache, diarrhea, diverticulosis, fatigue, hair loss, headaches, heartburn, high blood pressure, impotence, indigestion, insomnia, muscular aches, and ulcers can interfere with your life. Emotional signs of stress may include anger, anxiety, depression, emotional exhaustion, fear, hostility, lethargy, and mental fatigue.

HELPFUL TREATMENTS

Since stress is a fact of life, the best anti-stress strategies involve learning ways of managing, minimizing, or eliminating stress-provoking situations. Stress management includes anything that relaxes you and takes your mind off the sources of your stress. Biofeedback, deep breathing, exercise, meditation, relaxation and visualization techniques, and yoga can help control or counteract stress. When you are experiencing stress, try to take time out for yourself and avoid taking on too many responsibilities. Diet is important, too. Eat plenty of fresh vegetables, complex carbohydrates, and whole grains, as well as fruits, seeds, nuts, and protein. Avoid alcohol, caffeine, cigarettes, drugs, refined or processed foods, and sugar. If you suspect that nutritional deficiencies are contributing to your stress, you may wish to see a nutritionist for an evaluation.

Stress reduction is one of aromatherapy's specialties. Aromatherapy treatments can calm and relax you, giving you a chance to slow down and determine what is causing your stress so that you can decide what to do about it. Essential oils such as bergamot, chamomile, jasmine, lavender, rose, and ylang ylang will relax you, while basil, benzoin, geranium, and rosemary oils will recharge, revitalize, and stimulate you. Rosemary and geranium oils also strengthen the adrenal glands, which are affected by stress. Other essential oils with general stress-reducing properties include clary sage, coriander, cypress, elemi, fennel, frankincense, helichrysum, marjoram, neroli, orange, palmarosa, rosewood, sandalwood, and vetiver.

Aromatherapy can help boost immunity. In addition, it provides relief for some of the stress-related conditions mentioned above. Taking time out for yourself is a key factor in combatting stress, and aromatherapy offers you wonderful ways to do just that. Aromatherapy baths, diffuser blends, inhalants, fragrances, massage oils, and treatments for skin, hair, and body all let you pamper yourself and improve the condition of your body as you reduce stress.

Take a Stress-Reducing Bath whenever you feel stressed. Apply Stress-Soothing Massage Oil to your skin daily. Arrange to receive massages with it, if possible. Use Stress-Buster Diffuser Blend in your home or office to keep stress under control.

AROMATHERAPY BLENDS

The aromatherapy blends below are essential oil formulas you can prepare at home. For a more detailed explanation of how to put together and use these blends, see BATHS; DIFFUSERS AND LAMPS; and/or MASSAGE in Part Four. For a quick review of general guidelines for using essential oils, see page 91.

Stress-Reducing Bath

2 drops chamomile oil
2 drops lavender oil
1 drop cypress oil
1 drop fennel oil
1 drop geranium oil
1 drop vetiver oil

Disperse the essential oils well in a bathtub filled with warm water. Enjoy a leisurely soak for twenty to thirty minutes.

Stress-Soothing Massage Oil

2 ounces carrier oil
4 drops bergamot oil
4 drops chamomile oil
4 drops lavender oil
4 drops sandalwood oil
3 drops marjoram oil
2 drops elemi oil
2 drops frankincense oil

Place the carrier oil in a clean container, add the essential oils, and gently turn the container upside down several times or roll it between your hands for a few minutes to blend. Massage the oil onto your skin daily.

Note: Bergamot oil increases sensitivity to the sun. Omit it from the formula if your skin will be exposed to sunlight.

Stress-Buster Diffuser Blend

15 drops lavender oil
10 drops clary sage oil
10 drops elemi oil
10 drops geranium oil
8 drops bergamot oil
8 drops orange oil
8 drops rosewood oil
6 drops ylang ylang oil
5 drops coriander oil

Combine all the oils in a small glass bottle with an airtight cover. Add some of the mixture to your diffuser or lamp bowl as necessary.

Stretch Marks

Stretch marks are thin, narrow, wavy reddish-pink, purple, or silvery sunken streaks or lines that form when the skin stretches to accommodate an increase in body size. As the skin stretches, the collagen and elastic fibers in the deep layers of the skin weaken and lose their normal criss-cross structure, becoming thinner and straighter. Initially, stretch marks appear as parallel grooves that are slightly raised, and they give the surface skin a loosely wrinkled appearance. Over time, they may flatten out and fade to a white or silvery-white color.

Stretch marks—medically known as *striae atrophicae, striae gravidarum, striae distensae, lineae atrophicae,* or *linear atrophy*—are usually associated with pregnancy. However, they may also result from obesity; bodybuilding or weight training; rapid growth, especially during puberty and adolescence; an endocrine disorder known as Cushing's syndrome; the topical application of steroid creams; or prolonged treatment with corticisteroid drugs.

Most commonly, stretch marks occur during pregnancy on the hips, thighs, abdomen, breast, buttocks, and lower back, although they may appear on any area of skin that experiences rapid growth or expansion.

HELPFUL TREATMENTS

Preventing stretch marks is easier than eliminating them. If you expect a weight gain or an increase in size, such as with pregnancy or a bodybuilding program, plan ahead by keeping your skin well lubricated. Essential oils that help prevent stretch marks are lavender, neroli, and vetiver. In addition, cocoa butter, flaxseed oil, rose hip seed oil, wheat germ oil, and vitamin E oil are useful in preventing stretch marks.

Massage Stretch Mark Oil into your skin daily. If you already have stretch marks, long-term daily treatment with Stretch Mark Oil may help them fade (only surgery can remove them).

AROMATHERAPY BLENDS

The aromatherapy blend below is an essential oil formula you can prepare at home. For a more detailed explanation of how to put together and use this blend, see MASSAGE in Part Four. For a quick review of general guidelines for using essential oils, see page 91.

❧ Stretch Mark Oil

1 ounce cocoa butter, melted
½ ounce flaxseed oil
¼ ounce rose hip seed oil
¼ ounce wheat germ oil
10 drops lavender oil
8 drops neroli oil
4 drops vetiver oil

Blend the melted cocoa butter, flaxseed oil, rose hip seed oil, and wheat germ oil. Transfer the mixture to a clean jar. As it begins to cool and solidify, add the essential oils. Allow the mixture to cool to a comfortable temperature before using it. Massage the oil into your skin once or twice daily.

Sunburn

Sunburn is the skin's response to overexposure to the ultraviolet (UV) rays of the sun. The skin becomes pink or red and may feel tight and dry. It may become sore and swell with inflammation. In severe cases, the skin may blister and peel. Although sunburned skin often turns into a suntan, it is important to remember that anytime the skin burns or tans, it has suffered damage. Sunburns, particularly severe ones, can predispose a person to developing skin cancer later in life.

HELPFUL TREATMENTS

When it comes to sunburn, prevention and precaution are more important than treatment. Minimize exposure to the sun, especially during the midday hours between 10:00 A.M. and 3:00 P.M., when the sun is strongest. Apply a sunscreen to all exposed skin thirty minutes before going outdoors. When swimming or exercising, reapply sunscreen frequently. Cover as much of your body as possible with protective clothing. Wear a hat and sunglasses that filter out UV rays. After spending time in the sun, apply after-sun products to reduce the drying effects the sun has on your skin.

If you do develop sunburn, aromatherapy can help relieve some of the discomfort and minimize the damage to your skin. Chamomile, eucalyptus, helichrysum, lavender, patchouli, and peppermint oils are especially helpful for soothing sunburn pain and cooling burned skin. Bathe in a Sunburn-Soothing Bath as soon as possible to help draw out the heat from your sunburn. To relieve sunburn pain and the dry, tight feeling, and to discourage peeling of the skin, apply Lavender Sunburn Oil or Sunburn Relief Skin Oil to the affected areas several times daily.

AROMATHERAPY BLENDS

The aromatherapy blends below are essential oil formulas you can prepare at home. For a quick review of general guidelines for using essential oils, see page 91.

🐾 Sunburn-Soothing Bath

8 drops lavender oil
2 drops chamomile oil
2 drops helichrysum oil
1 drop peppermint oil

Disperse the essential oils in a bathtub filled with cool water. If you wish, you can add ice cubes to keep the water cool. Soak for fifteen to twenty minutes. Repeat every few hours until the pain subsides.

🐾 Lavender Sunburn Oil

2 ounces carrier oil
40 drops lavender oil

Place the carrier oil in a clean container and add the lavender oil. Blend well. Apply the oil frequently to sunburned skin.

🐾 Sunburn Relief Skin Oil

2 ounces carrier oil
15 drops lavender oil
8 drops helichrysum oil
5 drops chamomile oil
2 drops patchouli oil

In a clean container, add the essential oils to the carrier oil. Gently turn the container upside down several times or roll it between your hands for a few minutes to blend. Apply often to the affected areas.

Teething

See TOOTHACHE.

Toothache

A toothache usually results when the pulp, the innermost layer of the tooth and the part that contains the blood and nerve supply, becomes irritated and inflamed. The ache may be a persistent dull, throbbing pain or a sharp, stabbing one, or it may hurt only when you chew or bite down on the tooth. Your tooth may be sensitive to heat or cold.

Toothaches commonly occur when decay erodes the tooth enamel (the outer covering of the tooth) and the dentin (the body of the tooth), the two layers that surround the pulp. A toothache may also be caused by gum disease, poor dental work, infection or inflammation of the pulp, death of the tooth's nerve, injury to a tooth, a loose tooth, loss of a filling or crown, or receding gums. A sinus infection can sometimes cause pain that mimics a toothache as well.

HELPFUL TREATMENTS

If you develop a toothache, you should consult your dentist as soon as possible. Failure to the treat the underlying cause of a toothache could result in the loss of the tooth.

Aromatherapy can provide temporary relief until you visit your dentist. Essential oils that help ease toothache pain include chamomile, myrrh, peppermint, and tea tree. Apply one drop of any of these or a drop of Toothache Oil to the tooth and the surrounding area to ease the pain. For additional relief, apply a Toothache Compress on your face near the aching tooth.

To soothe teething pain in babies, chamomile oil is one of the safest and most effective remedies.

Massage Baby's Teething Blend onto the affected gum area.

AROMATHERAPY BLENDS

The aromatherapy blends below are essential oil formulas you can prepare at home. For a more detailed explanation of how to put together and use these blends, see COMPRESSES and/or MASSAGE in Part Four. For a quick review of general guidelines for using essential oils, see page 91.

❧ Toothache Oil

⅛ ounce carrier oil
6 drops tea tree oil
4 drops chamomile oil
2 drops myrrh oil
2 drops peppermint oil

Place the carrier oil in a clean container and add the essential oils. Gently turn the container upside down several times or roll it between your hands for a few minutes to blend. Apply one drop on the aching tooth and the surrounding gum, as needed.

❧ Toothache Compress

1 quart hot water
2 drops chamomile oil
1 drop peppermint oil

Pour the water into a two-quart glass bowl and disperse the oils in the water. Saturate a clean cloth in the water and apply the compress to your face near the aching tooth. Repeat as often as necessary.

❧ Baby's Teething Blend

⅛ ounce sunflower oil
1 drop chamomile oil

Add the chamomile oil to the sunflower oil and blend. Massage a drop into your baby's gums as needed.

Vaginitis

Vaginitis is a general term for an inflammation or infection of the vagina. There are a number of different microorganisms that commonly cause vaginitis, including bacteria (*Gardnerella*), protozoa (*Trichomona*), and *Candida albicans,* which causes the type of vaginitis known as a yeast infection.

Symptoms of vaginitis can include a burning sensation, discharge or dryness, itching, and an unpleasant odor. Poor hygiene, sexually transmitted diseases or infections, and the use of products such as artificially fragranced bath oils or bubble baths, commercial douches, birth control devices (especially the diaphragm), spermicides, tampons, and vaginal deodorant sprays are all factors that can lead to or promote the development of vaginitis. Hormonal imbalances, certain drugs (especially antibiotics), and poor nutrition are often contributing factors.

A yeast infection occurs when *Candida albicans,* a fungus commonly referred to as yeast, multiplies uncontrollably in the vagina. This often happens as a result of a change in the normal acidity of the vaginal environment. Symptoms of a yeast infection include leukorrhea (a thick, white, even cheesy-looking vaginal discharge), a burning sensation, irritation, severe itching, and sometimes pain or discomfort during intercourse.

Antibiotics, birth-control pills, diabetes, pregnancy, excessive douching, steroids, and a diet high in alcohol, dairy products, refined carbohydrates, sugar, and yeast products are all factors that can create or contribute to the development of the type of highly acid internal environment in which the yeast organism flourishes. Nutritional deficiencies, particularly deficiencies of the B vitamins, can also be a factor.

HELPFUL TREATMENTS

Many doctors treat vaginitis with antibiotics (for bacterial vaginitis) or fungicidal preparations (for yeast infections). Unfortunately, if you take an antibiotic for bacterial vaginitis, it can actually increase the likelihood that you will then develop a yeast infection, because antibiotics destroy the beneficial bacteria that keep candida under control.

There are a number of precautions you can take to prevent vaginitis. First, always wash yourself thoroughly with a mild, unscented body soap and gently pat yourself dry. Wear cotton underwear. Avoid using fragranced bubble baths and bath oils, commercial douches, fragranced detergents and fabric softeners, deodorant tampons or sanitary pads, scented toilet paper, and vaginal deodorant sprays. Reduce the amount of sugar, cheese, dairy products, and foods containing yeast from your diet (if you already have a yeast infection, or are prone to recurring yeast infections, eliminate these foods entirely). Wipe from front to back following bowel movements. Always urinate before and after intercourse and after bathing.

If you have recurring yeast infections, they may be a sign of a systemic candida infection, which may require more than a localized cure (see CANDIDIASIS). Also, because a yeast infection can be passed back and forth between sexual partners, it may be necessary for your partner to receive treatment to completely clear up a yeast infection. Avoid sexual intercourse until symptoms subside completely.

Aromatherapy can relieve some of the discomforts of vaginitis. Some essential oils that are useful for vaginitis are benzoin, chamomile, juniper, lavender, myrrh, and tea tree. If you begin treating vaginitis when the symptoms first appear, you may halt the infection, or at least minimize the severity, the discomfort, and the duration of the symptoms.

Take a Vaginitis Sitz Bath at the first sign of symptoms and repeat once or twice daily thereafter, as needed. You can use Vaginitis Douche either alone or in conjunction with the baths. Tea tree oil suppositories, inserted vaginally, can help fight a yeast infection. These are available in many health food stores. If you are unable to find tea tree oil suppositories, you can use one or two drops of lavender or tea tree oil dropped onto the tip of an unscented tampon instead. If the area surrounding the vagina is tender or raw, apply Vaginitis Soothing Oil. If symptoms persist for more than one or two weeks, consult your health care professional.

AROMATHERAPY BLENDS

The aromatherapy blends below are essential oil formulas you can prepare at home. For a quick review of general guidelines for using essential oils, see page 91.

❧ Vaginitis Sitz Bath

> 2 drops juniper oil
> 2 drops tea tree oil
> 1 drop chamomile oil
> 1 drop lavender oil

Add the oils to a shallow tub filled with warm water. Sit hip-deep in the water for fifteen minutes. Repeat once or twice daily, as needed.

❧ Vaginitis Douche

> 1 quart warm water

> 1 tablespoon apple cider vinegar
> 2 drop lavender oil
> 2 drops tea tree oil

Add the vinegar, lavender oil, and tea tree oil to the warm water and mix well. Fill a douche bag or syringe with the mixture and douche. Repeat one to three times weekly, as necessary.

❧ Vaginitis Soothing Oil

> 1 ounce jojoba or sunflower oil
> 3 drops tea tree oil
> 2 drops lavender oil
> 1 drop chamomile oil

In a clean container, add the essential oils to the jojoba or sunflower oil and blend. Apply the oil externally to irritated areas several times daily, as needed.

Varicose Veins

Varicose veins occur when veins lose their tone and elasticity. They can occur anywhere in the body, but they are most common in the ankles, calves, and thighs. Varicose veins develop when the little valves in the veins that normally work to keep blood pulsing through the circulatory system become unable to close properly and no longer push the blood upward toward the heart. Blood stagnates in the veins, and the legs become congested, swollen, and inflamed. This prevents the delivery of adequate nutrients and oxygen to the tissues of the legs and the removal of wastes from the legs. The veins turn purple, cranberry, or dark blue in color and begin to bulge. The legs may feel hot and heavy and become sensitive to pressure.

Heredity is usually a primary factor in the development of varicose veins. Hormones also play a role. Varicose veins rarely appear before puberty, and women are more prone to develop varicose veins than men are. Many women develop them during pregnancy as a result of the extra pressure on their blood vessels, particularly those in the legs. The increase in blood flow during pregnancy also places a bigger burden on a woman's veins.

Other factors that may be related to the development of varicose veins include age, muscular atrophy, chronic constipation, excess weight, extremes of temperature, insufficient exercise, poor circulation, prolonged bed rest, the consumption of alcohol or spicy foods, and the wearing of constricting clothing or hosiery, high heels, or other unsuitable shoes. Sitting or standing in the same position for long periods of time is a problem because it can restrict proper blood flow into and out of the legs. Strenuous physical exertion or injury can damage a valve in a vein or cause blood clots that permanently destroy valves in the veins and impair circulation. In some cases, varicose veins can signal other health problems.

HELPFUL TREATMENTS

Walking is probably the best preventive measure as well as the best treatment for varicose veins. Exercises that elevate the legs are also beneficial. Exercise improves lymphatic drainage, improves muscle tone, and increases muscle size. Larger, more developed muscles exert more pressure on the veins, encouraging the flow of blood back toward the heart. Compression, such as that provided by support hose or stockings, also helps the veins push the blood supply upward from the legs to the heart.

Regular massage of the feet and legs can improve or prevent varicose veins. Deep breathing exercises increase circulation, aiding the delivery of nutrients and oxygen to the affected areas. A person with varicose veins should avoid standing or sitting in one position for a prolonged period of time. When varicose veins are painful, elevating the legs often affords some relief; relax with your legs elevated whenever possible. In severe cases, medical treatment such as injection sclerotherapy, which permanently closes off the varicose veins, or surgery to remove all or some portion of the affected veins may be necessary.

Used by itself or in conjunction with medical treatments, aromatherapy can diminish the discomfort and improve the appearance of varicose veins. Essential oils such as cypress, geranium, ginger, juniper, lemon, neroli, peppermint, and rosemary are especially effective in restoring good circulation to the areas with varicose veins. Use alternating applications of a Warm Compress for Varicose Veins with Cool Stimulating Compress for Varicose Veins to stimulate circulation, relieve inflammation and swelling, and ease pain. Cold constricts blood vessels, while heat dilates them; alternating the temperatures of the compresses helps to "exercise" the veins. Apply Varicose Vein Massage Oil to the affected areas twice daily and gently massage the skin above the varicose veins upward toward the heart. Bathe in Bath for Varicose Veins once a day to promote circulation to the legs and ease discomfort.

AROMATHERAPY BLENDS

The aromatherapy blends below are essential oil formulas you can prepare at home. For a more detailed explanation of how to put together and use these blends, see BATHS; COMPRESSES; and/or MASSAGE in Part Four. For a quick review of general guidelines for using essential oils, see page 91.

❧ Warm Compress for Varicose Veins

    1 quart warm water
    2 drops geranium oil

2 drops lemon oil
1 drop rosemary oil

Pour the water into a two-quart glass bowl and add the essential oils. Blend well. Soak a clean cloth in the water and apply the compress to the affected areas. Elevate your legs for fifteen minutes. Follow with a Cool Stimulating Compress for Varicose Veins.

❧ Cool Stimulating Compress for Varicose Veins

1 quart cool water
2 drops cypress oil
1 drop ginger oil
1 drop neroli oil
1 drop peppermint oil

Pour the water into a two-quart glass bowl and disperse the essential oils in the water. Soak a clean cloth in the water and apply it to your legs. Elevate your legs for fifteen minutes. Follow with Varicose Vein Massage Oil.

❧ Varicose Vein Massage Oil

1 ounce carrier oil
4 drops lavender oil
3 drops cypress oil
3 drops lemon oil
3 drops rosemary oil
2 drops juniper oil

Place the carrier oil in a clean container and add the essential oils. Gently turn the container upside down several times or roll it between your hands for a few minutes to blend.

Beginning directly above the varicose veins, massage your legs with the oil, using strokes directed upward toward the heart. Apply the oil to your legs once or twice daily.

❧ Bath for Varicose Veins

4 drops lemon oil
2 drops cypress oil
2 drops geranium oil
2 drops juniper oil

Disperse the oils in a bathtub filled with warm water. Soak in the bath for fifteen to twenty minutes.

Weakened Immune System

Your immune system is a complex mechanism that works to protect and heal your body from infection and injury. It involves the blood, bone marrow, lymphatic system, skin, spleen, thymus, and special immune cells. These special cells patrol your body to locate, identify, and destroy any foreign substances that threaten your health. They differentiate between cells and molecules that are "self" and those that are "non-self." When anything is identified as "non-self," the immune cells take action to eliminate it. They do this by stimulating the production of antibodies to protect you against foreign substances, or antigens, that can attack healthy tissues and upset your body's balance, causing illness. A weakened immune system is unable to respond adequately to the presence of antigens, rendering you more susceptible to illness of every kind.

Poor nutrition and nutritional deficiencies are common contributors to low immunity. High cholesterol levels, stress, and sugar consumption also weaken immunity. Other factors that can contribute to weakened immunity include the consumption of alcohol; exposure to environmental pollutants, pesticides, radiation, and food additives, colorings, and preservatives; obesity; food allergies; heavy metal poisoning; hormonal imbalances; chemotherapy treatment for cancer; vaccines; and the prolonged use of antibiotics, cortisone, steroids, and over-the-counter, prescription, or recreational drugs.

Signs that you may be suffering from lowered immunity include allergies, candidiasis, chemical sensitivities, chronic fatigue, chronic infections, colds, recurring asthma or bronchitis, and slower than usual healing from illness or injury.

The immune system may also become severely depressed as a result of certain medical conditions, including acquired immune deficiency syndrome (AIDS), AIDS-related complex (ARC), and certain types of cancer. Although these serious illnesses are beyond the scope of this book, people who suffer from them can usually still derive benefit from using essential oils. Even in cases where it cannot address an underlying physical problem, aromatherapy can often successfully combat stress and address emotional issues (see STRESS and/or EMOTIONAL ISSUES). However, if you have an illness that seriously impairs your immunity, you should consult with your health care provider before using any essential oils.

HELPFUL TREATMENTS

There are a number of nutrients that can help restore and revitalize your immune system. These include the antioxidants, such as beta-carotene, selenium, zinc, and vitamins A, C, and E. Other important nutrients are iron and vitamin B6. The herbs echinacea, goldenseal, and licorice root have immune-stimulating properties as well. A digestive enzyme supplement may also be helpful. Digestive enzymes support the immune system by improving the digestion, absorption, and assimilation of all the food and nutritional supplements you consume.

Modify your diet, if necessary, to focus on fresh vegetables and fruits, whole grains, and legumes; avoid any foods that trigger allergies. You may wish to consult a nutritionist to determine if you have any food allergies or nutritional deficiencies and to set up an immune-boosting program. Stress management and regular exercise will also strengthen immunity.

Aromatherapy can boost immunity by prompting your body to heal itself. Essential oils that improve immunity are bergamot, clary sage, elemi, eucalyptus, geranium, ginger, lavender, lemon, myrrh, orange, rosemary, rosewood, sandalwood, tea tree, thyme, and vetiver. These oils promote the production of white blood cells, increase immune response, and fight bacteria, fungi, and viruses.

Aromatherapy can also reduce stress and help stabilize emotions. Long-term emotional upset and stress can compromise the immune system, preventing it from performing properly. Essential oils can help you to bring your body and mind back into balance.

Take either a Morning Immunity Bath or an Evening Immunity Bath each day. Apply Immune-Boosting Massage Oil over your body once or twice daily.

AROMATHERAPY BLENDS

The aromatherapy blends below are essential oil formulas you can prepare at home. For a more detailed explanation of how to put together and use these blends, see BATHS and/or MASSAGE in Part Four. For a quick review of general guidelines for using essential oils, see page 91.

🐦 Morning Immunity Bath

    4 drops tea tree oil
    3 drops rosemary oil
    2 drops lemon oil
    1 drop ginger oil

Disperse the essential oils well in a bathtub filled with warm water. Soak in the bath for fifteen to twenty minutes.

🐦 Evening Immunity Bath

    4 drops tea tree oil
    2 drops clary sage oil
    2 drops orange oil
    2 drops rosewood oil

Add the oils to a bathtub filled with warm water and blend. Soak in the bath for fifteen to twenty minutes.

🐦 Immune-Boosting Massage Oil

    4 ounces carrier oil
    10 drops geranium oil
    10 drops tea tree oil
    8 drops lemon oil
    8 drops thyme oil
    6 drops myrrh oil
    5 drops elemi oil

Place the carrier oil in a clean container, add the essential oils, and blend gently. Massage the mixture over your body once or twice daily.

Yeast Infection

See VAGINITIS.

PART FOUR

Ways of Using Aromatherapy

Introduction

You can introduce aromatherapy and its many benefits into your life in a variety of ways—in baths, massages, personal fragrances, and many other forms. Aromatherapy can help you deal with emotional and physical problems, enhance the appearance of your skin and body, and freshen your home and office.

This part of the book describes the many different ways in which you can use aromatherapy. It will help you determine what will work best for your particular condition and for your lifestyle. Be willing to experiment. You'll have fun, and you'll reap the many rewards that aromatherapy has to offer. The possibilities are limited only by your imagination and your willingness to explore the wide world of aromatherapy.

Air Fresheners

Aromatherapy air fresheners can quickly fragrance your environment or create certain moods in your home or office. They can purify or cleanse the air in your home and remove unpleasant odors. They can also provide fast, effective relief for respiratory ailments or sinus congestion. Some aromatherapy air fresheners can help control germs in sickrooms.

To make an aromatherapy air freshener, fill a spray bottle almost full with distilled water. Add four to ten drops of the essential oil or oils of your choice for each ounce of water. Shake the bottle well to blend and spray it around the room. Spray as often as you wish. Shake the bottle well before each use.

Atomizers

An atomizer is a glass bottle with a metal sprayer that is operated by an attached rubber bulb. When you squeeze the bulb, it sends a fine cloud of fragrance through the sprayer and into the atmosphere. An atomizer provides a simple, convenient, and inexpensive way to dispense room-freshening and mood-creating essential oils quickly into your atmosphere.

To use an atomizer, fill an atomizer bottle with the desired essential oil or mixture of oils. Mist your room, home, or office. You can use your atomizer as often as you wish. Any of the diffuser blends mentioned in Part Three will work fine in an atomizer.

Baths

Plunging your body into a pool of warm water scented with soothing or energizing essential oils practically guarantees that you will step out feeling calm, refreshed, and rejuvenated. Surrendering your emotionally or physically depleted body and soul to an aromatherapy bath can restore and revitalize you. Let your worldly worries wash down the drain with the bath water! You'll emerge feeling refreshed, ready to conquer your chores, dive into your deadlines, or just sink into your sheets and sleep peacefully like a baby. Bathing regularly with essential oils helps to control stress, alleviate anxiety and tension, and minimize muscular aches and pains.

To prepare an aromatherapy bath, add a total of six to ten drops of an essential oil or oils to a bathtub filled with warm water. The amount of oil required depends on the essential oil you choose. Some oils, such as black pepper, eucalyptus, ginger, lemon, orange, peppermint, and thyme, can give the desired results with only two to three drops to a tub of water. If you are using a blend of several different oils, use no more than ten drops total.

You can make your bathing experience even more enjoyable by running your diffuser, putting on some soothing music, and turning *off* the telephone before you sink into an aromatherapy bath.

If you are preparing a bath for an infant or child, first dilute the essential oil by blending one to three drops of essential oil in one ounce of carrier oil. Add two to six drops of the resulting diluted oil to the tub.

Compresses

Compresses are useful for relieving pain and reducing inflammation and swelling. They can also help cool fevers or eliminate chills. Both chronic and acute conditions respond to compresses.

Hot compresses relax muscles, reduce stiffness, ease aches and pains, and dilate blood vessels, increasing circulation to the treated area. Use hot compresses for chronic conditions and for abscesses, backaches, chills, earaches, or toothaches, as well as for flareups of arthritis or rheumatism.

Cold compresses reduce swelling and inflammation and cause blood vessels to contract, decreasing circulation to the treated area. Use cold compresses for acute conditions and fevers, headaches, inflamed and swollen conditions, and as first aid for sprains, tennis elbow, and other injuries.

To make a compress, pour one quart of either cold or hot water, depending on the condition you're treating, into a two-quart glass bowl. Add three to six drops of an essential oil or an essential oil blend to the water. If you will be using the compress on an infant or child, add only one drop of essential oil. Soak a clean cloth in the water. Wring it out and apply the cloth to the affected area. You can wrap a towel or piece of plastic around the cloth to keep in warmth or prevent the compress from dripping. If you are using a cold compress, you can apply an ice pack on top of the compress to make it more effective. Replace the compress with a fresh one every five to fifteen minutes, as needed.

Diffusers and Lamps

A diffuser is a device that disperses minute molecules of essential oils throughout your room, home, or office. Most diffusers operate on electricity. They provide an almost effortless way of using aromatherapy. Simply add essential oils to the diffuser, plug it in, and within minutes you'll be breathing the fragrant aroma that is permeating your room. Use a diffuser to freshen the air, create a mood, fight infection from a cold or the flu, treat asthma or bronchitis, help you overcome emotional upsets, or simply enhance your well-being. Your choice of oils will determine the outcome.

To use most diffusers, you attach a bottle of essential oil, plug the diffuser in, and turn it on. Follow the directions that come with your diffuser. All of the diffuser blends mentioned in Part Three will work in any kind of diffuser.

Aromatherapy lamps have the same purpose as diffusers; they release minute molecules of essential oils into the air. A small bowl atop the lamp holds water and essential oils. Beneath the bowl is a heat source, either a candle or an electric light bulb that gently heats the water and essential oils and sends the aroma into the atmosphere.

To use an aromatherapy lamp, fill the bowl with water. Add five to twenty drops of an essential oil or essential oil blend. Turn on the electricity or light the candle and enjoy the sweet smell that wafts through your environment. The diffuser blends described in Part Three will work in lamps as well as in diffusers.

Facial Steam Baths

Facial steam baths are a delightful addition to your regular skin care program. They are a wonderful way to deep-clean your pores and add moisture to your skin. They also increase the circulation to your face.

Facial steam baths are similar to steam inhalations, except that their purpose is to improve your complexion. Steaming your face once a week will help prevent blemishes and blackheads, keep your skin looking moist, and give your complexion a healthy glow.

To prepare a facial steam bath, pour about one quart of steaming water into a large (approximately two-quart) glass bowl. Add three to five drops of an essential oil or combination of oils suitable for your skin type (see page 216). Hold your clean face over the bowl for five to ten minutes. To capture the steam, drape a towel over your head to create a "tent." Afterwards, apply a cleanser, scrub, or mask to remove any impurities that the steaming released from your pores.

Foot Baths

A hot foot bath brings welcome relief to tired, aching feet. Foot baths are one of the best treatments for athlete's foot and foot odor. They improve circulation. They can also diminish the discomfort of a variety of non-foot-related ailments, such as colds and flu, cramps, insomnia, low blood pressure, poor circulation, respiratory problems, scant or late periods, and sinusitis. A cold foot bath can revive you on a sweltering summer day when you've begun to wilt. Aromatherapy foot baths also make a practical alternative for people who are ill or disabled, or who have difficulty getting into a full-sized bathtub.

To prepare an aromatherapy foot bath, add five to ten drops of an essential oil or essential oil blend to a foot bath filled with water. If you are preparing a foot bath for a child, add only one or two drops of essential oil. Use hot or cold water, depending on the condition you're treating. If you do not have a foot bath, use a bowl large enough to immerse the feet. Soak your feet for ten to fifteen minutes. Repeat the procedure as necessary.

Hair Care and Customizing Hair Care Products

A healthy head of hair begins with a healthy scalp, and essential oils can help improve the condition of your hair and scalp by stimulating circulation to your scalp. Aromatherapy hair care products can make your hair shiny and healthy-looking. Although there are aromatherapy shampoos and conditioners on the market, they usually contain very low levels of pure essential oils. The best way to assure that you're getting the essential oils you want at levels that are effective is to make your own products.

The aromatherapy blends suggested under HAIR AND SCALP PROBLEMS in Part Three are easy to make and are effective. You can also make customized aromatherapy hair care products by adding your choice of essential oils to any unscented shampoo or conditioner. You can create your own scalp treatments to nourish your scalp and improve the condition of your hair.

The following are general guidelines to use for making your own customized hair care products:

- **Shampoos.** Add 5 drops of an essential oil or blend of essential oils appropriate for your hair type or condition to one ounce of unscented shampoo. For example, if you are making two ounces of shampoo, you would add a total of 10 drops of one or more essential oils; for four ounces, you would add 20 drops.

- **Conditioners.** Add 5 drops of an essential oil or blend of essential oils appropriate for your hair type or condition for each ounce of unscented conditioner.

- **Scalp treatments.** Add 10 drops of an essential oil or blend of essential oils appropriate for your hair type or condition to one ounce of jojoba oil. To use, simply massage the mixture into your scalp and hair and leave it on for fifteen to thirty minutes or overnight; then shampoo.

To find out which oils are appropriate for your hair type or condition, consult Table 3.1.

Inhalants

Inhalants are essential oils that you breathe directly from the bottle. The aromatic molecules of the essential oils will waft up your nose, into your brain, and into your respiratory system. You'll feel a difference quickly. Inhalants work well for asthma, aller-

gies, colds and flu, emotional conditions, sinusitis, and stress. You can inhale any single oil or make an inhalant from any of the blends mentioned in Part Three. Diffuser blends will work as inhalants, too.

To make an inhalant, simply place your choice of essential oils in a small glass bottle that has an airtight cover. Blend the oils by gently turning the container upside down several times or rolling it between your hands for a few minutes, not by vigorous shaking.

Depending on the condition you wish to treat, you can prepare an aromatherapy inhalant blend recommended in the appropriate entry in Part Three. Or, if no inhalant blend is suggested, choose two or three oils from the list of essential oils suggested for that condition and mix them together in a small bottle. To use the inhalant, simply open the bottle and inhale the aroma. You can also place two or three drops of the blend on a tissue or handkerchief and inhale it that way. You can carry an inhalant with you almost anywhere for a refreshing aromatherapy break.

Massage

Incorporating essential oils into massage is a marvelous way to ease muscular aches and pains, subdue stress and tension, and treat a variety of conditions in a pleasant, relaxing way. Besides feeling great, massage can soothe the nervous system, reduce blood pressure, relax muscles, diminish swelling, and stimulate blood and lymphatic circulation. It also can release cellular wastes from your muscles, relax your breathing, and slow a racing pulse.

If you receive professional massages, take your aromatherapy massage oil blends for your thera-

Table 4.1 Essential Oils for Hair Care

This table lists essential oils that are known to be helpful for specific hair types or conditions. Use the recommendations here to help you choose which oil or oils you want to try in customized hair products. A detailed discussion of each of the individual essential oils here may be found in Part Two. Essential oils that are useful for more than one condition appear under each condition for which they are appropriate.

Normal Hair	Dry Hair	Oily Hair	Dandruff	Hair Loss
Chamomile	Cedarwood	Bergamot	Cedarwood	Cedarwood
Lavender	Chamomile	Cedarwood	Clary Sage	Clary Sage
Thyme	Clary Sage	Clary Sage	Cypress	Rosemary
Ylang Ylang	Lavender	Cypress	Lemon	Ylang Ylang
	Rosemary	Juniper	Patchouli	
		Lavender	Pine	
		Lemon	Rosemary	
		Patchouli	Tea Tree	
		Pine		
		Rosemary		
		Tea Tree		
		Thyme		
		Ylang Ylang		

pist to use on you. You can also gain tremendous advantage from self-massage. Whether you massage deep into your own muscles or lightly spread the oils onto your skin, you will derive most of the benefits mentioned above.

To make your own massage and skin oils, add ten drops of an essential oil or essential oil blend to one ounce of a carrier oil and blend well. Place several drops in your hand and apply the oil over your body as you massage. If you are preparing an oil for use on an infant or child, dilute one to three drops of essential oils in one ounce of carrier oil.

Use the massage movements described below whenever you give yourself a massage or apply skin oil over your body.

MASSAGING YOUR BODY

You can massage yourself every day when you apply your skin or massage oils. Massaging your body boosts your circulation, and the aromatherapy blends will help moisturize your skin and improve its appearance. Use either long, sweeping strokes or short overlapping strokes. You can also make circular movements in an upward direction. You can knead an area or you can tap it with your fingertips.

When you massage your body, the direction of the strokes should always be toward your heart (see Figure 4.1). Massage from your feet upward toward your head. Stroke from your fingers toward your heart. Make a clockwise circle over your abdomen.

In addition to giving yourself a whole-body massage, you can target specific areas of your body for aromatherapy massage treatment. If you are having a problem affecting one organ or system of the body, such as your lungs or respiratory system, you

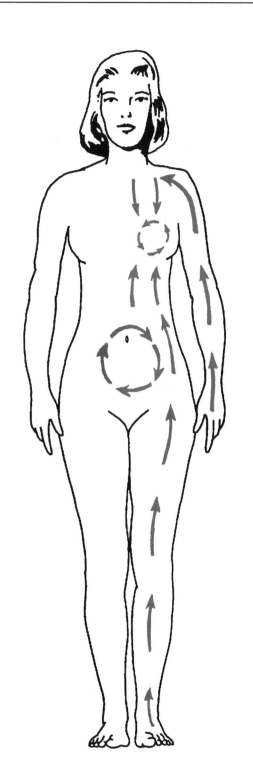

Figure 4.1   Massaging Your Body

body, such as your lungs or respiratory system, you can massage an aromatherapy blend over the specific organ or along the entire system. Figure 4.2 will help you to see where the major organs and systems of the body are located.

MASSAGING YOUR ABDOMEN

To give yourself an abdominal massage, move in a clockwise direction from your right side to your left. This follows the direction in which your large intestines eliminate wastes. Begin on your lower right abdomen just above your upper right thigh. Stroke upward and across your abdomen above your navel. Continue downward to the left side of your abdomen above your left leg. You can continue in a circle, spiralling inward over your small intestines. (See Figure 4.3.)

MASSAGING YOUR FACE

Massaging and touching your face properly can help counteract some of the effects of gravity and reduce facial tension. Facial massage also increases circulation to your skin and improves your complexion.

Always massage your skin gently, with upward motions, and use a facial oil to avoid stretching your skin. Figure 4.4 shows the basic direction of strokes for facial massage. Begin at the base of your neck and stroke upward toward your jawline. Make a circle around your mouth. Stroke your cheeks diagonally: along your jawline; from the corner of your mouth to your ears; from the corner of your nose to your temples. Beginning on your upper eyelids, make a circle from the inner corners, across your lids, under your eyes, and finish near your tear ducts. Stroke your forehead upward into your your hairline. Use these same movements anytime you touch your facial skin.

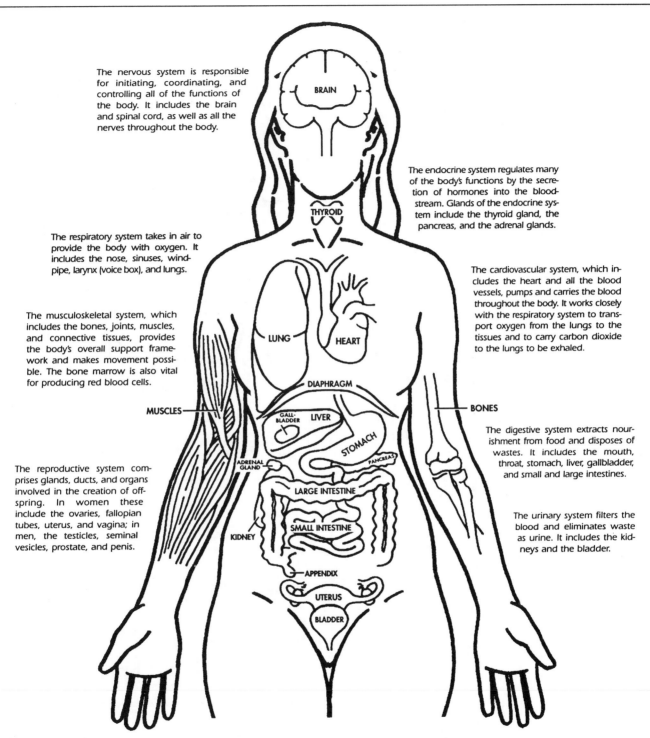

Figure 4.2 Anatomy of the Human Body

For certain conditions, it can be beneficial to massage an aromatherapy blend over the affected organ or system of the body. The diagram above indicates the relative locations of the major organs and systems of the body.

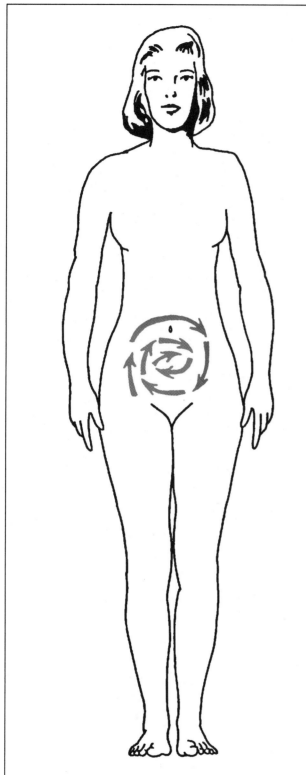

Figure 4.3   Massaging Your Abdomen

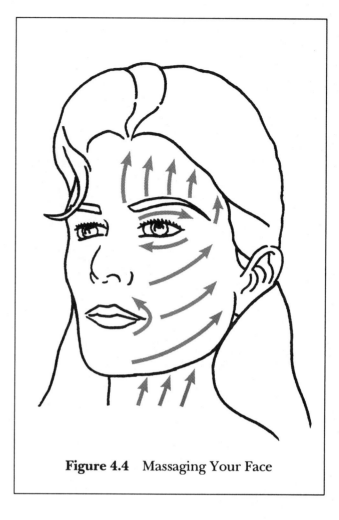

Figure 4.4   Massaging Your Face

Mouthwashes, Gargles, and Gum Treatments

Aromatherapy oral hygiene products can help you maintain or improve the condition of your mouth and teeth. They fight bacteria and infections, strengthen your gums, and help protect against gum disease.

The aromatherapy blends suggested under GUM DISEASE in Part Three are easy to make and are effective oral hygiene products. If you wish to make your own mouthwash or gargle fresh each day, add one or two drops of an essential oil to a four-ounce glass of water and mix well. Gargle or swish the mixture around in your mouth. To blend your own gum treatment oil, add ten to fifteen drops of essential oils to one-quarter ounce of a carrier oil and massage the mixture into your gums once or twice daily.

Personal Fragrances and Perfumes

You can easily create your own perfumes and fragrances with essential oils. Whatever your lifestyle, natural fragrances are a wonderful way of bringing aromatherapy into your daily life. Personal fragrances made with essential oils are not overpowering, as synthetic scents sometimes are. And unlike commercial fragrances, which are made almost exclusively of synthetic petrochemicals and can cause allergies and irritation, essential oils can be emotionally and physically therapeutic. These pleasing personal perfumes smell lovely and they can enhance your physical and emotional well-being.

You can make fragrances as intense or subtle as you desire, depending on your choice of essential oils and the amount of each oil you use. The easiest way to create your own fragrances is to follow the

formulas in this book, particularly the personal blends intended to influence the emotions that are listed in pages 127 through 140. You can also create your own blends by adding ten to twenty drops of essential oils to one-eighth ounce of jojoba oil. Jojoba oil is the best carrier oil for fragrances; it does not become rancid, so it cannot spoil your perfume.

Never apply pure essential oils as fragrances directly to your skin. Always dilute them in jojoba oil. Essential oils are highly concentrated and in their pure form can cause skin irritation.

Sitz Baths

Sitz baths can relieve congestion, pain, and spasms that occur in the pelvic area. They can help with ailments of the lower abdominal area, the intestinal tract, the reproductive organs, and the urinary tract. Conditions that respond well to sitz baths include constipation, cystitis, hemorrhoids, menstrual cramps, poor circulation, scant or late periods, and prostate problems.

To prepare a sitz bath, add five to ten drops of an essential oil or an essential oil blend to a sitz bath or a small tub filled with water. Sit hip-deep in the water for ten to thirty minutes. You may elevate your feet if you wish.

Skin Brushing

Skin brushing increases circulation, helps the body to eliminate cellular wastes, and improves the appearance of the skin. You can dry-brush your skin, or you can first apply a few drops of an aromatherapy skin oil, body oil, massage oil, or skin-brushing oil. It is best to brush before bathing everyday. Use a clean, firm natural-bristle brush.

Begin at your feet and stroke upwards toward your heart (see Figure 4.5). Apply enough pressure to stimulate circulation, but not so much that it hurts you. Make circles around your knees and at the top of your thighs, where lymphatic tissue is located. Brush your abdomen in a circle that follows the direction of your intestines: Start from your lower right abdomen and move upward and across your abdomen above your navel; then continue downward along your left side. Circle around your breast or chest. Brush upward from your hands to your shoulders. Make circles around your shoulder joint, another place where lymphatic tissue is located. From the base of your neck, stroke downward to your heart. On your back, stroke up and down along your spine.

Skin Care and Customizing Skin Care Products

Skin care is one of the most popular applications of aromatherapy. With the increasing awareness of the benefits of good skin care, along with competition to get ahead in the workplace, both men and women today want to look their absolute best. In addition, our desire to feel better about ourselves and stay physically fit is prompting many of us to take better care of our skin.

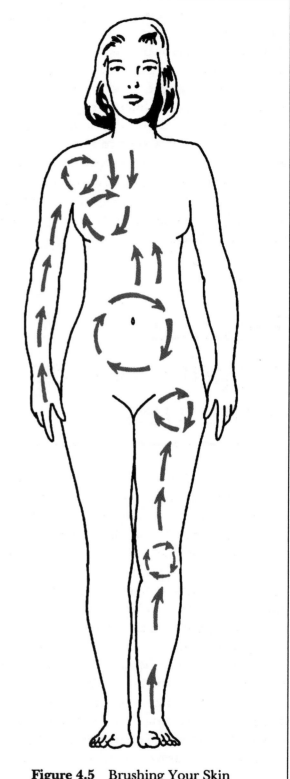

Figure 4.5   Brushing Your Skin

Many essential oils can improve the condition of your skin by increasing circulation to the surface. Good circulation will impart a healthy, youthful glow to your complexion. Some essential oils have cell-regenerating properties that can give your skin a more youthful appearance. They also have a positive impact on your emotions—and that will show up on your skin. Essential oils have minute molecules that can easily penetrate your pores and can affect the condition of your skin from the inside out.

You can buy commercial aromatherapy skin care products. However, I highly recommend that you make your own. Most ready-made aromatherapy products contain very low levels of essential oils, and some companies use synthetic oils instead of pure essential oils.

The aromatherapy blends suggested under SKIN PROBLEMS in Part Three are easy to make and are effective. However, if you would rather not make your own skin care products from scratch, the surest way to get pure aromatherapy products with effective levels of essential oils is to customize commercial cosmetics.

Customizing skin care products to suit your individual needs is simple. Whenever possible, start with unscented or fragrance-free products (see the list of recommended suppliers in the Aromatherapy Resource Guide in the Appendix for sources). Then choose a single essential oil or a combination of essential oils suited to your particular skin type or condition. A good general guide is to add a total of eight to ten drops of essential oil per ounce of product. For example, you might add sixteen to twenty drops of essential oil to two ounces of facial cleanser. For a single application of a product such as a facial mask, add only one or two drops of essential oil. Remember, *always* dilute essential oils before applying them to your skin.

The following are guidelines for customizing different types of skin care products with essential oils:

- **Cleansers.** To a single application of cleanser, add 1 drop of essential oil; to one ounce, add 8 to 10 drops of essential oil; to four ounces, add 30 to 40 drops of essential oil.

- **Facial Scrubs.** To a single application of a facial scrub, add 1 or 2 drops of essential oil; to one ounce, add 10 drops of essential oil; to four ounces, add 40 drops of essential oil.

- **Moisturizers.** To a single application of moisturizer, add 1 drop of essential oil; to one ounce, add 10 drops of essential oil; to four ounces, add 40 drops of essential oil. Or make a facial oil by adding 5 to 10 drops of any essential oil or essential oil blend you choose to one ounce of an unscented carrier oil, preferably jojoba oil.

- **Facial Masks.** To a single application of a facial mask, add 1 or 2 drops of essential oil; to one ounce, add 8 to 10 drops of essential oil; to four ounces, add 30 to 40 drops of essential oil.

To find out which essential oils are appropriate for your skin type or condition, consult Table 4.2.

Steam Inhalations

When you breathe in essential oils, they are immediately taken into your respiratory system. From there they can travel throughout your body. Aromatherapy inhalations can bring relief for respiratory ailments, anxiety, colds, the flu, headaches, sinusitis, sore throats, and stress. You can also use

Table 4.2 Essential Oils for Skin Care

This table lists essential oils that are known to be helpful for specific skin types or conditions. Use the recommendations here to help you choose which oil or oils you want to try in customized skin care products. A detailed discussion of each of the individual essential oils listed here may be found in Part Two. Essential oils that are useful for more than one condition appear under each condition for which they are appropriate.

Normal Skin	Dry Skin	Oily Skin	Mature Skin	Sensitive Skin
Cedarwood	Benzoin	Cedarwood	Elemi	Chamomile
Clary Sage	Bergamot	Clary Sage	Frankincense	Frankincense
Elemi	Cedarwood	Cypress	Geranium	Jasmine
Frankincense	Clary Sage	Elemi	Helichrysum	Neroli
Geranium	Elemi	Frankincense	Jasmine	Rose
Jasmine	Fennel	Geranium	Lemon	Rosewood
Lavender	Frankincense	Jasmine	Myrrh	Sandalwood
Neroli	Geranium	Juniper	Neroli	
Palmarosa	Jasmine	Lemon	Palmarosa	
Patchouli	Lavender	Neroli	Rose	
Rose	Myrrh	Orange	Rosemary	
Rosemary	Neroli	Palmarosa	Sandalwood	
Rosewood	Palmarosa	Patchouli	Vetiver	
Sandalwood	Patchouli	Peppermint		
Vetiver	Rose	Rosemary		
	Rosemary	Rosewood		
	Rosewood	Sandalwood		
	Sandalwood	Tea tree		
	Vetiver	Thyme		
		Vetiver		
		Ylang ylang		

an aromatherapy inhalation simply for relaxation or pleasure.

To prepare a steam inhalation, place a large (aproximately two-quart) ovenproof glass or ceramic bowl on a trivet or a thick potholder on a tabletop. Pour about one quart of steaming water into the bowl. Add three to six drops of an essential oil or essential oil blend. If you are preparing an inhalation for an infant or child, add only one drop of essential oil. Sit in a comfortable position and hold your head over the bowl and breathe in the vapor for five to ten minutes. If possible, capture the steam by draping a towel over your head and the bowl, creating a "tent." Keep your face far enough from the bowl so that the steam does not irritate or burn your skin (if you are using the inhalation on a child, be particularly careful about this). If necessary, you can allow the water to cool for a few minutes to a more comfortable temperature. Repeat as necessary.

Appendix

Aromatherapy Resource Guide

The following list of organizations and suppliers is included to help you find and use the products discussed in this book. I recommend them because I have found their products and services to be of good quality. Please be aware that addresses and phone numbers may be subject to change.

RECOMMENDED SUPPLIERS

Ahava
2001 West Main Street
Stamford, CT 06902
(800) 252–4282
(203) 357–1914
Dead Sea salts and related products.

Alba Botanica
P.O. Box 12085
Santa Rosa, CA 95406
(800) 347–5211
(707) 575–3111
Unscented skin and body care products.

Aroma Vera
5901 Rodeo Road
Los Angeles, CA 90016–4312
(800) 669–9514
(310) 280–0407
Essential oils; carrier oils; diffusers and lamps; unscented skin and body care products.

Arrowhead Mills
P.O. Box 2059
Hereford, TX 79045
(800) 858–4308
(806) 364–0730
Unrefined organic carrier oils.

Aztec Secret Health & Beauty
P.O. Box 19735
Las Vegas, NV 89132
(702) 369–8080
Clays.

Body Gold
3232 San Mateo Boulevard NE, Suite 190
Albuquerque, NM 87110
(505) 281–9701
Unscented body lotion.

Dr. Grandel
626 West Sunset Road
San Antonio, TX 78216
(800) 543–5230
(512) 829–1763
Carrier oils; unscented enzyme mask.

Desert King Jojoba Corporation
1550 East Missouri Avenue
Suite 201
Phoenix, AZ 85014
(602) 264–2300
Jojoba oil (minimum purchase one gallon).

Earth Science
23705 Via del Rio Road
Yorba Linda, CA 92687
(800) 222–6720
(714) 692–7190
Carrier oils; unscented skin, body, and hair care products.

Hobe Labs
201 South McKemy Avenue
Chandler, AZ 85226
(800) 528–4482
(602) 257–1950
Carrier oils.

International Flora Technologies
2267 South Coconino Drive
Apache Junction, AZ 85220
(602) 983–7907
Jojoba oil and other carrier oils (minimum purchase one gallon).

Leydet Oils
4611 Awani Court
Fair Oaks, CA 95628
(916) 965–7546
Essential oils; diffusers and lamps.

Lifetree Aromatix
3949 Longridge Avenue
Sherman Oaks, CA 91423
(818) 986–0594
Essential oils.

Magick Botanicals
3412 West MacArthur, Suite J-L
Santa Ana, CA 92704
(714) 957–0674
Unscented skin, body, and hair care products.

Masada
P.O. Box 4871
North Hollywood, CA 91607
(800) 368–8811
(818) 503–4611
Dead Sea salts and related products.

Mode de Vie
2701 Sol y Luz Loop
Santa Fe, NM 87505
(505) 438–6298
French green clay, seaweed powder, shea butter.

Natural Oils International
12350 Montague Street
Pacoima, CA 91331
(818) 897–0536
Carrier oils.

Nature's Gate
9200 Mason Avenue
Chatsworth, CA 91311
(818) 882-2951
(800) 327-2012
Unscented skin, body, and hair care products.

Omega Nutrition
6505 Aldrich Road
Bellingham, WA 98226
(800) 661-3529
(604) 322-8862
Unrefined organic oils.

Original Swiss Aromatics
P.O. Box 6842
San Rafael, CA 94903
(415) 459-3998
Essential oils; calophyllum inophyllum oil; diffusers and lamps; clays.

Orjene Natural Cosmetics
5-43 48th Avenue
Long Island City, New York 11101
(800) 886-7536
(718) 937-2666
Unscented skin, body, and hair care products; unscented products for men.

Oshadhi
15 Monarch Bay Plaza, Suite 346
Monarch Beach, CA 92629
(800) 933-1008
In California, call (714) 240-1104.
Essential oils; diffusers and lamps.

The Preferred Source
3637 West Alabama, Suite 146
Houston, TX 77027
(800) 880-6457
(713) 622-2190
Diffusers and lamps.

Prima Fleur Botanicals
1201-R Andersen Drive
San Rafael, CA 94901
(415) 455-0957
Essential oils (minimum purchase one ounce) and calophyllum inophyllum oil.

Santa Fe Fragrance
P.O. Box 282
Santa Fe, NM 87504
(505) 473-1717
Essential oils (bulk and small quantities); exotic rare absolutes; electric and ceramic candle diffusers; fixative-grain alcohol diluent for perfumes and colognes; carrier oils; sea salts; clays; botanical cosmetic and toiletry ingredients.

ShiKai
P.O. Box 2866
Santa Rosa, CA 95405
(800) 448-0298
(707) 584-0298
Unscented body lotion.

Source Vital
3637 West Alabama, Suite 146
Houston, TX 77027
(800) 880-6457
(713) 622-2190
Essential oils; carrier oils; unscented skin and body care products; Dead Sea salts; seaweed and algae products.

Spa Health Consultants
30 Hillside Avenue
Springfield, NJ 07081
(800) 777-7546
(201) 379-1959
Unscented skin and body care products; seaweed and algae products.

Thursday Plantation
PO Box 5613
Montecito, CA 93150-5613
(800) 848-8966
(805) 684-2615
Tea tree oil; tea tree oil suppositories.

Time Labs
P.O. Box 3243
South Pasadena, CA 91031
(208) 232-5250
Essential oils; diffusers and lamps.

Windrose Aromatics
12629 North Tatum Boulevard, Suite 611
Phoenix, AZ 85032
(602) 861-3696
Essential oils; diffusers and lamps; unscented skin and body care products; clays.

PUBLICATIONS

Beyond Scents Newsletter
1830 South Robertson Boulevard, Suite 203
Los Angeles, CA 90035
(800) 677-2368
(310) 838-6122

Common Scents Newsletter
P.O. Box 3679
South Pasedena, CA 91031
(818) 457-1742

Inside Aromatherapy Newsletter
P.O. Box 6723
San Rafael, CA 94903
(415) 479-9121

International Journal of Aromatherapy
The Alliance News Quarterly
P.O. Box 750428
Petaluma, CA 94975-0428
(707) 778-6762

Scentsitivity Newsletter
P.O. Box 17622
Boulder, CO 80308
(303) 258-3791

EDUCATION

Aroma Research Institute of America (ARIA)
P.O. Box 282
Santa Fe, NM 87504
(505) 473-1717

Aromatherapy Institute and Research
P.O. Box 2354
Fair Oaks, CA 95628
(916) 965-7546

Aromatherapy Seminars
1830 South Robertson Boulevard, Suite 203
Los Angeles, CA 90035
(800) 677-2368
(310) 838-6122

Aromatic Concepts
12629 North Tatum Boulevard, Suite 611
Phoenix, AZ 85032
(602) 861-3696

Beauty Kliniek
3268 Governor Drive
San Diego, CA 92122
(619) 457-0191

Pacific Institute of Aromatherapy
P.O. Box 6723
San Rafael, CA 94903
(415) 479-9121

Quintessence Aromatherapy
P.O. Box 4996
Boulder, CO 80306
(303) 258-3791

The Preferred Source
3637 West Alabama, Suite 146
Houston, TX 77027
(800) 880-6457
(713) 622-2190

Time Labs
P.O. Box 3243
South Pasadena, CA 91031
(818) 300-8096

AROMATHERAPY ORGANIZATIONS

The American Alliance of Aromatherapy
P.O. Box 750428
Petaluma, CA 94975-0428
(707) 778-6762

The American Society for Phytotherapy
   and Aromatherapy
P.O. Box 3679
South Pasadena, CA 91031
(818) 457-1742

International Federation of Aromatherapists
Department of Continuing Education, Room 8
Royal Masonic Hospital
RavensCourt Park
London W6 OTN
England
081-864-8066

National Association for Holistic Aromatherapy
P.O. Box 17622
Boulder, CO 80308
(303) 258-3791

Recommended Reading

Blevi, Viktor, and Gretchen Sween. *Aromatherapy.* New York: Avon Books, 1993.

Davis, Patricia. *Aromatherapy, An A–Z.* Essex, England: C.W. Daniel, 1988.

Fischer-Rizzi, Suzanne. *Complete Aromatherapy Handbook.* New York: Sterling Publishing, 1990.

Harvey, John, Lilias Folan, Annemarie Colbin, Roberta Wilson, Don Campbell, Kay Gardner, Shakti Gawain, Ohashi, Dan Millman, Michael Hutchison, and Terry Patten. *The Big Book of Relaxation.* Edited by Larry Blumenfeld. Roslyn, NY: The Relaxation Company, 1994.

Lavabre, Marcel. *Aromatherapy Workbook.* Rochester, VT: Healing Arts Press, 1990.

Lawless, Julia. *The Encyclopaedia of Essential Oils.* Rockport, MA: Element, Inc., 1992.

Rose, Jeanne. *The Aromatherapy Book.* Berkeley, CA: North Atlantic Books, 1992.

Ryman, Danièle. *Aromatherapy: The Complete Guide to Plant and Flower Essences for Health and Beauty.* New York: Bantam Books, 1993.

Sellar, Wanda. *The Directory of Essential Oils.* Essex, England: C.W. Daniel, 1992.

Worwood, Valerie Ann. *The Complete Book of Essential Oils and Aromatherapy.* San Rafael, CA: New World Library, 1991.

Bibliography

Arctancer, Steffen. *Perfume and Flavor Materials of Natural Origin.* Elizabeth, NJ: By the author, 1960.

Atkinson, Holly. *Women and Fatigue.* New York: G.P. Putnam's Sons, 1985.

Baker, Don, and Emery Nester. *Depression.* Portland, OR: Multnomah Press, 1983.

Balch, James, and Phyllis Balch. *Prescription for Nutritional Healing.* Garden City Park, NY: Avery Publishing Group, 1990.

Bell, Robert. *Dictionary of Classical Mythology.* Santa Barbara: ABC Clio, CA, 1982.

Benjamin, Ben, with Gale Borden. *Listen to Your Pain.* New York: Viking Press, 1984.

Berger, Stuart. *Dr. Berger's Immune Power Diet.* New York: New American Library, 1985.

Blevi, Viktor, and Gretchen Sween. *Aromatherapy.* New York, Avon Books, 1993.

Bricklin, Mark. *Rodale's Encyclopedia of Natural Home Remedies.* Emmaus, PA: Rodale Press, 1982.

Brooke, Elisabeth. *Herbal Therapy for Women.* London, England: Thorsons Publishing, 1992.

Cooley, Donald G., ed. *Family Medical Guide,* 5th ed. New York: Better Homes and Gardens Books, 1976.

Cunningham, Scott. *Magical Aromatherapy.* St. Paul, MN: Llewellyn Publications, 1989.

Davidson, Paul. *Chronic Muscle Pain Syndrome.* New York: Villard Books, 1989.

Davis, Patricia. *Aromatherapy, An A–Z.* Essex, England: C.W. Daniel, 1988.

Davis, Patricia. *Subtle Aromatherapy.* Essex, England: C.W. Daniel Company, 1991.

Dobelis, Inge, ed. *Magic and Medicine of Plants.*

Pleasantville, NY: Reader's Digest Association, 1986

Dorland, W.A. Newman. *Dorland's Illustrated Medical Dictionary,* 27th ed. Ed. Elizabeth J. Taylor, Douglas M. Anderson, Joseph M. Patwell, Katharine Plaut, and Kathleen McCullough. Philadelphia: W.B. Saunders Co., 1988.

Drury, Susan. *Tea Tree Oil: Nature's Miracle Healer.* Lindfield, Australia: Unity Press, 1989.

Egide, Stacey, ed. *A Guide to the Art of Aromatherapy.* Petaluma, CA: Tisserand Aromatherapy USA, 1993.

Ehrmantraut, Harry. *Headaches: The Drugless Way to Lasting Relief.* Berkeley, CA: Celestial Arts, 1987.

Finnegan, John. *The Facts About Fats.* Berkeley, CA: Celestial Arts, 1993.

Fischer-Rizzi, Suzanne. *Complete Aromatherapy Handbook.* New York: Sterling Publishing, 1990.

Garrison, Robert, Jr., and Elizabeth Somer. *The Nutrition Desk Reference.* New Canaan, CT: Keats Publishing, 1990.

Gattefossé, René-Maurice. *Gattefossé's Aromatherapy.* Essex, England: C.W. Daniel Company, 1937; reprint, 1993.

Genders, Roy. *A History of Scent.* London, England: Hamish Hamilton, 1972.

Gerson, Joel. *Standard Textbook for Professional Estheticians.* Bronx, NY: Milady Publishing, 1986.

Grieve, M. *A Modern Herbal,* Vols. 1 and 2. New York: Dover Publications, 1971.

Groom, Nigel. *The Perfume Book.* New York: Chapman & Hall, 1992.

Guiness, Alma, ed. *Family Guide to Natural Medicine.* Pleasantville, NY: Reader's Digest Association, 1993.

Hogan, Elizabeth, ed. *Sunset Western Garden Book.* Menlo Park, CA: Lane Publishing, 1988.

Junemann, Monika. *Enchanting Scents.* Wilmot, WI: Lotus Light, 1988.

Kowalchik, Claire, and William Hylton, eds. *Rodale's Illustrated Encyclopedia of Herbs.* Emmaus, PA: Rodale Press, 1987

Lanctôt, Guylaine. *How to Have Great Legs at Any Age.* New York: New Chapter Press, 1988.

Lautié, Raymond, and André Passebecq. *Aromatherapy: The Use of Plant Essences in Healing.* Wellingborough, England: Thorsons Publishing Group, 1979.

Lavabre, Marcel. *Aromatherapy Workbook.* Rochester, VT: Healing Arts Press, 1990.

Lavabre, Marcel. "Essential Oil Distillation." *Beyond Scents Newsletter,* Volume 1, Issue 3, Summer 1993.

Lavabre, Marcel. "Essential Oil Production: Traditional Versus Modern Distillation." *Beyond Scents Newsletter,* Volume 1, Issue 2, Spring 1993.

Lavabre, Marcel, and Michael Scholes. *Aromatherapy Seminars Advanced Certification Course.* Los Angeles: Aromatherapy Seminars, 1992.

Lawless, Julia. *The Encyclopaedia of Essential Oils.* Rockport, MA: Element, Inc., 1992.

Lee, William, and Lynn Lee. *The Book of Practical Aromatherapy.* New Canaan, CT: Keats Publishing, 1992.

Livingston, Lida, and Constance Schrader. *Wrinkles.* Englewood Cliffs, NJ: Prentice-Hall, 1978.

Maple, Eric. *The Magic of Perfume.* New York, NY: Samuel Weiser, 1973.

McArdle, William, Frank Katch, and Victor Katch. *Exercise Physiology: Energy, Nutrition, and Human Performance.* Philadelphia: Lea & Febiger, 1986.

Mee, Charles L., Jr., ed. *Massage: Total Relaxation.* Alexandria, VA: Time-Life Books, 1987.

Morris, Edwin. *Fragrance.* Greenwich, CT: ET Morris & Co., 1984.

Murray, Michael, and Joseph Pizzorno. *Encyclopedia of Natural Medicine.* Rocklin, CA: Prima Publishing, 1991.

National Academy Press. *Jojoba.* Washington, D.C.: National Academy Press, 1985.

Novick, Nelson Lee. *Super Skin.* New York: Clarkson N. Potter, Inc., 1988.

Olsen, Cynthia. *Australian Tea Tree Oil Guide.* Pagosa Springs, CO: Kali Press, 1992.

Pearsall, Paul. *SuperImmunity.* New York: McGraw-Hill Book Company, 1987.

Pugliese, Peter. *Advanced Professional Skin Care.* Bernville, PA: APSC Publishing, 1991.

Quirin, K.W., and D. Gerard. "Supercritical CO_2 Extraction of Natural Products used in Cosmetics and Perfumery." *Zeitschrift für die Chemisch-Technische Industrie, die Technische Chemie und Spezialchemikalien,* 24 October 1991.

Rector-Page, Linda. *Healthy Healing,* rev. ed. Privately printed, 1990.

Reynolds, James E.F., ed. *Martindale: The Extra Pharmacopoeia,* 30th ed. London, England: Pharmaceutical Press, 1993.

Rimmel, Eugene. *The Book of Perfumes.* Philadelphia: J.B. Lippincott, 1866.

Ronsard, Nicole. *Beyond Cellulite.* New York: Villard Books, 1992.

Ronsard, Nicole. *Cellulite.* New York: Bantam Books, 1975.

Rose, Jeanne. *The Aromatherapy Book.* Berkeley, CA: North Atlantic Books, 1992.

Ryman, Danièle. *Aromatherapy: The Complete Guide to Plant and Flower Essences for Health and Beauty.* New York: Bantam Books, 1993.

Sagarin, Edward. *The Science and Art of Perfumery.* New York: McGraw-Hill Book Company, 1945.

Schnaubelt, Kurt. Aromatherapy Course. San Rafael, CA: Pacific Institute of Aromatherapy, 1985.

Scholes, Michael. Beyond Scents Home Study Course. Los Angeles: Aromatherapy Seminars, 1991.

Sellar, Wanda. *The Directory of Essential Oils.* Essex, England: C.W. Daniel Company, 1992.

Serrentino, Jo. *How Natural Remedies Work.* Point Robert, WA: Hartley & Marks, 1991.

Shayevitz, Myra, and Berton Shayevitz. *Living Well*

with Emphysema and Bronchitis. Garden City, NY: Doubleday & Company, 1985.

Soltanoff, Jack. *Natural Healing.* New York: Warner Books, 1988.

Thompson, C.J.S. *The Mystery and Lure of Perfume.* London, England: John Lane The Bodley Head Limited, 1927.

Tisserand, Maggie. *Aromatherapy for Women.* New York: Thorsons Publishers, 1985.

Tisserand, Robert. *The Art of Aromatherapy.* Rochester, VT: Inner Traditions, 1979.

Tisserand, Robert. *The Essential Oil Safety Data Manual.* E. Sussex, England: The Tisserand Aromatherapy Institute, 1988.

Todd, Pamela. *Forget-Me-Not: A Floral Treasury.* Boston: Bulfinch Press, 1993.

Turin, Alan C. *No More Headaches!* Boston: Houghton Mifflin Company, 1981.

Trueman, John. *The Romantic Story of Scent.* London, England: Aldus Books Limited, 1975.

Valnet, Jean. *The Practice of Aromatherapy.* New York: Destiny Books, 1980.

Verrill, A. Hyatt. *Perfumes and Spices.* Boston: L.C. Page & Company, 1940.

Weinstein, Alan. *Asthma.* New York: McGraw-Hill Book Company, 1987.

Wellness Encyclopedia, The. Boston: Houghton Mifflin Company, 1991.

Wilson, Roberta. *The Cellulite Control System.* Los Angeles, CA: By the author, 1988.

Wilson, Roberta. *The Cellulite Control Guide.* Albuquerque, NM: By the author, 1994.

Wilson, Roberta. *The Facial Rejuvenation Program.* Santa Monica, CA: By the author, 1984.

Worwood, Valerie Ann. *Aromantics.* London, England: Pan Books, 1987.

Worwood, Valerie Ann. *The Complete Book of Essential Oils and Aromatherapy.* San Rafael, CA: New World Library, 1991.

Zohary, Michael. *Plants of the Bible.* Cambridge, MA: Cambridge University Press, 1982.

Index